Osteoporosis in Older Persons

Gustavo Duque · Douglas P. Kiel
Editors

Osteoporosis in Older Persons

Pathophysiology and Therapeutic Approach

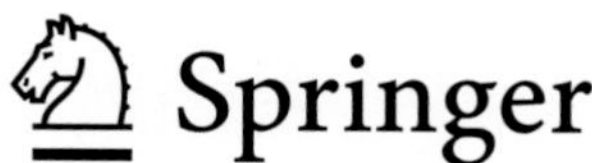

Gustavo Duque, MD, PhD
Assistant Professor
Division of Geriatric Medicine-Jewish
General Hospital
Lady Davis Institute for Medical Research
McGill University
Montreal, QC
Canada

Douglas P. Kiel, MD, MPH
Instiute for Aging Research
Hebrew SeniorLife
Harvard Medical School
Boston, MA
USA

British Library Cataloguing in Publication Data

Osteoporosis in older persons : pathophysiology and
therapeutic approach
1. Osteoporosis 2. Osteoporosis – Pathophysiology
3. Osteoporosis – Treatment 4. Older people – Diseases
I. Duque, Gustavo II. P. Kiel, Douglas
618.9′76716

ISBN-13: 9781846285158

Library of Congress Control Number: 2007930543

ISBN: 978-1-84628-515-8 e-ISBN: 978-1-84628-697-1

9 8 7 6 5 4 3 2 1

Springer Science+Business Media
springer.com

To my lovely and devoted parents, Maximo and Rubiela, who always inculcated in me the humility to respect the feeble, the curiosity to understand nature, and the respect for God who is the Great Architect of everything that is described in this book.

GD

Foreword

Although osteoporosis has been defined as "a metabolic bone disease characterized by low bone mass and microarchitectural deterioration of bone tissue leading to enhanced bone fragility and a consequent increase in fracture risk," it is not clear that osteoporosis represents a single disease as much as a similar response of bone to different pathophysiologies. In the 1940s Fuller Albright and colleagues recognized "osteoporosis of old age" and distinguished it from osteoporosis associated with the postmenopausal state, as well as from osteoporosis from disuse, osteoporosis from malnutrition, and other forms of osteoporosis. He nevertheless pointed out that it was unclear how much of osteoporosis is due to old age per se, in view of the fact that "in many cases osteoporosis of disuse, of malnutrition, of the postmenopausal state and of senility are inseparably superimposed." In this volume, Duque and Kiel have gathered an international panel of experts to highlight the unique features of senile osteoporosis and consideration of this disease spans the very basic through the clinical and the epidemiologic.

As an organ which harbors stem cells, bone may clearly influence not only its own regeneration but also the regeneration of other tissues, notably the hematopoietic system. Nevertheless even restricting consideration of bone to its own reparative capacity it is clear that specific changes occur during the aging process which influence the extent and direction of stem cell plasticity leading to increased cells of the adipose lineage relative to cells of the osteoblastic lineage. Using modern concepts of stem cell biology it should be possible in coming years to understand fully the regulation of this process and possible ways of reversing this.

Many animal models are available to study osteoporosis, however, perhaps among the most interesting, from a pathophysiologic perspective are rodent models of accelerated aging. Several are associated with single gene defects and may give considerable insight not only into the general process of aging but into the aging process in bone. Parallel studies on the genetic basis of osteoporosis in humans may be considerably more complex since multiple genes are likely to contribute, with each gene subject to unique gene-environment interactions. Nevertheless advances in genetic and genomic technology make this an active area of investigation and one which could lead to new approaches to diagnosis, prevention, and therapy.

Aging individuals can also be exposed to a unique hormonal milieu which in particular may result from changes in sex steroids and changes in calcium-regulating hormones, and much of this information has been gleaned from epidemiologic studies of large cohorts. In part sex steroid changes in elderly women do simulate the superimposition of postmenopausal osteoporosis on senile osteoporosis although even in elderly women (and certainly in men) the sex steroid hormonal milieu may evolve with age.

The realization that vitamin D as a steroidal hormone has actions beyond calcium homeostasis has increased our appreciation of the clinical significance of vitamin D deficiency which appears to be a more prevalent problem than previously thought. In part this high incidence of vitamin D deficiency does simulate the superimposition of osteoporosis of malnutrition on senile osteoporosis, however restricted exposure to ultraviolet light clearly plays a role in the pathophysiology of vitamin D deficiency. Vitamin D deficiency appears to be a reversible condition contributing to the evolution of osteoporosis once it is recognized.

The unique features of senile osteporosis can also clearly be seen in the clinic. Thus, although vertebral (and other) fractures continue to exact a high toll in aging individuals, the high incidence of hip fractures, a source of considerable costs to the health care system and a source of significant mortality, becomes a hallmark for osteoporosis of the aged. This relatively distinct clinical picture in the elderly is accompanied by distinct risk factors including muscle weakness, an increased risk of falls, and the high use of psychotropic agents.

Along with the unique clinical picture comes the unique challenges associated with therapy. Thus, specific considerations regarding non-medical therapy apply to the elderly as do specific considerations regarding pharmacologic and surgical therapy. All of these issues are expertly and comprehensively addressed in this book and make a clear and compelling case for the existence of a unique and increasingly important form of osteoporosis which has been termed senile osteoporosis.

D. Goltzman, MD
Professor of Medicine
Past-President American Society for Bone and Mineral Research
Director, Centre for Bone and Periodontal Research
McGill University
Montreal, Quebec
Canada

Preface

With the aging population increasing worldwide, there is a growing interest in age-related diseases and their functional and mental consequences. Osteoporosis is a common disease in older persons with significant impact on their functionality and quality of life. Additionally, osteoporotic fractures represent an important burden to health care budgets around the world.

Since the first description by Riggs and colleagues of a particular syndrome known as "senile osteoporosis," there has been a common agreement that there is a type of osteoporosis closely associated with the aging process. There is considerable controversy regarding the concept of "senile osteoporosis." Several experts in the field think that it is just "osteoporosis," a condition and disease that mostly affects post-menopausal women but also affects men after the age of 60. Unfortunately, because most of the resources and interventions have focused on post-menopausal women, a significant number of old men and women are not receiving appropriate treatment.

Fortunately, the concept of senile osteoporosis has been reconsidered as a real syndrome that affects a significant percentage of the elderly population. In fact, new findings on the pathophysiology, epidemiology, and treatment of senile osteoporosis have demonstrated that this entity is independent of the estrogen-related osteoporosis known as post-menopausal. This book focuses on these new findings in a bench to population model.

From the bench side, the fact that with aging there is a shift in the differentiation of mesenchymal stem cells within the bone marrow, from predominant osteoblastogenesis in the young bone to increasing adipogenesis in the old bone, has improved the understanding of the pathophysiology of senile osteoporosis. This process is independent of estrogen levels, as demonstrated by lack of increasing bone marrow adipogenesis in estrogen receptor knock-out mice. In fact, the increasing levels of bone marrow adipogenesis starts in humans even when normal serum levels of estrogens are present in the third and fourth decade of life, suggesting that this is an age-related process independent of sex hormones.

One additional feature in the pathophysiology of senile osteoporosis is the fact that it affects men and women after the sixth decade of life in a similar manner. Although estrogens seem to play a role in the pathophysiology of osteoporosis in men, it is well known that the predominant changes in bone cells in osteoporosis in men correspond mostly to those seen in age-related bone loss than in peri-menopausal women.

In this book, the chapters dedicated to bone biology illustrate the particular cellular and molecular features of senile osteoporosis from mice to human. Additionally, the authors look at the potential role that hormones, both calciotropic and sexual, may play in the pathophysiology of this syndrome.

Concerning the predominant fractures seen in older adults, the chapters on epidemiology make a complete appraisal of the particular incidence of osteoporotic fractures in the elderly. In fact, hip fractures are the predominant fracture after the seventh decade of life. This type of fracture correlates with the pathophysiology of osteoporosis, because the hip neck area is mostly dependant on osteoblast activity, which is severely affected by the aging process in bone. By contrast, the incidence of fractures owing to increasing osteoclastic activity, a typical feature of post-menopausal osteoporosis, decreases in the older population. These differences in the incidence and type of osteoporosis fractures in the elderly could correlate with genetic determinants of osteoporosis in older adults. The chapter on genetics of osteoporosis focuses on the identification of the genes that are directly associated with osteoporosis in older adults.

Concerning the treatment of osteoporosis, although there is increasing awareness about the importance of preventing fractures in older adults, the evidence shows that the number of patients at risk who are not receiving treatment is increasing. It is probably owing to a combination of factors that include ageism, lack of evidence of the effectiveness of the treatment in old patients, and treatments mostly directed to the regulation of osteoclastic activity that, although effective in geriatric populations, have not been shown to be effective in non-vertebral fractures, the most prevalent in the older population. One of the important messages throughout this book is that clinicians should be aware of the importance of treating of osteoporosis in older adults in order to prevent fractures, disability, and even death.

The chapter on pharmacological treatment of osteoporosis highlights very important points. First, osteoporosis, once diagnosed or suspected, should be treated independently of the patient's age. Second, there is poor evidence on most of the treatments available specifically in the older population, and furthermore in some cases treatment effectiveness in older persons is doubtful because most of the therapeutic agents regulate bone resorption without increasing bone formation. Third, the optimal therapeutic agent for osteoporosis in older individuals would be the one that decreases bone resorption while increasing bone formation. In their conclusion the authors state that the optimal therapeutic agent for senile osteoporosis does not exist yet, and that more research should be pursued in order to find the right approach to the particular features of senile osteoporosis.

A particularly unique aspect of this book is the inclusion of two chapters on falls. This important geriatric syndrome has been historically separated from the osteoporosis syndrome because of the fact that very few osteoporosis clinics considered the importance of fall prevention as a pivotal intervention to prevent fractures. As explained by the authors of the chapters, there could not be an effective preventive or therapeutic intervention for fractures in the elderly without an assessment of the risk of falls and the initiation of preventive measures. There are important links between the risk of falls and that of fractures. Probably the most relevant at this time is vitamin D, which has been proven essential for the prevention of both falls and fractures. Indeed, vitamin D is mentioned extensively in some of the chapters of this book as an essential intervention in the elderly population at risk. The evidence supporting this notion is reviewed in the chapters on calciotropic hormones as well as the one on the treatment of falls. Furthermore, because falls result from the interaction between multiple factors, non-pharmacological interventions are also considered in this book, where one chapter is dedicated to a review of the evidence on the effectiveness of non-pharmacological interventions for fall prevention.

Finally, we wanted to include a chapter on the surgical interventions for osteoporotic fractures. We know that this is an important element when caring for patients with fractures. Its understanding would help the clinician to interact with their surgical colleagues when treating old patients with acute fractures. Using outstanding illustrations, the author explains in detail the characteristics of fracture stabilization in the hip and the particular challenges the surgeon faces when treating fractures in very old patients. Additionally, a review on the potential alternatives for surgical treatment of vertebral fractures was included.

In summary, this textbook has brought together experts in the field of osteoporosis in older persons from four continents. We feel that we have reviewed the evidence supporting the notion that senile osteoporosis exists as a real geriatric syndrome with a particular pathophysiology and treatment. We expect that the information included in this book will be useful to all health professionals involved in the care of our aging population in order to understand the particular features of this syndrome and the importance of its prevention. This was our intention and we hope that after reading its chapters the reader will join us in this purpose.

Gustavo Duque, MD, PhD
Douglas P. Kiel, MD, MPH

Acknowledgments

The editors would like to thank Myra Miller for her assistance in the preparation of this work. We remain grateful to Melissa Morton from Springer for her outstanding support to this project and for her understanding that older adults suffer of a particular syndrome that must be identified and treated. To Eva Senior for her gentle guidance in the development of this project. Finally, we would like to thank all the authors of these book chapters who, like us, share the same interest on the subject of osteoporosis in older adults. Without their collaboration this project would have never been successful.

Gustavo Duque, MD, PhD
Douglas P. Kiel, MD, MPH

Contents

Contributors

Timothy Bhattacharyya, MD
Assistant Professor of Orthopaedic Surgery, Harvard Medical School, Orthopaedic Trauma Service, Departments of Orthopaedic Surgery, Brigham and Women's Hospital and Massachusetts General Hospital, Boston, MA, USA

Heike A. Bischoff-Ferrari, MD, MPH
Assistant Professor, Department of Rheumatology and Institute of Physical Medicine and Rehabilitation, University Hospital Zurich, Zurich, Switzerland

Christopher M. Bono, MD
Assistant Professor of Orthopaedic Surgery, Harvard Medical School, Chief, Spine Service, Department of Orthopaedic Surgery, Brigham and Women's Hospital, Boston, MA, USA

Steven Boonen, MD, PhD
Professor of Medicine, Leuven University Center for Metabolic Bone Diseases and Division of Geriatric Medicine, Katholieke Universiteit Leuven, Leuven, Belgium

Jane A. Cauley, DrPH
Department of Epidemiology, Graduate School of Public Health, University of Pittsburgh, Pittsburgh, PA, USA

E. Paul Cherniack, MD
Geriatric Research Education and Clinical Center, Research Service, Miami Veterans Affairs Medical Center, Geriatrics Institute and Division of Gerontology and Geriatrics, Miller School of Medicine, University of Miami, Miami, FL, USA

Jacqueline C.T. Close, MD
Prince of Wales Hospital and Prince of Wales Medical Research Institute, University of New South Wales, Randwick, Sydney, NSW, Australia

Gianluca D'Ippolito, PhD
Assistant Professor, University of Miami Miller School of Medicine and Geriatric Research, Educational and Clinical Center and Research Service, Veterans Affairs Medical Center, Miami, FL, USA

Gustavo Duque, MD, PhD
Assistant Professor, Division of Geriatric Medicine-Jewish General Hospital, Lady Davis Institute for Medical Research, McGill University, Montreal, Quebec, Canada

Z. Elizabeth Floyd
Stem Cell Laboratory, Pennington Biomedical Research Center, Louisiana State University System, Baton Rouge, LA, USA

Jeffrey M. Gimble, MD, PhD
Stem Cell Laboratory, Pennington Biomedical Research Center, Louisiana State University System, Baton Rouge, LA, USA

Guy A. Howard, PhD
Professor, University of Miami Miller School of Medicine and Geriatric Research, Educational and Clinical Center and Research Service, Veterans Affairs Medical Center, Miami, FL, USA

David Karasik, PhD
Institute for Aging Research, Hebrew SeniorLife, Harvard Medical School, Boston, MA, USA

Moustapha Kassem, MD, PhD, DSc
Department of Endocrinology and Metabolism, University Hospital of Odense, Denmark

Douglas P. Kiel, MD, MPH
Institute for Aging Research, Hebrew SeniorLife, Harvard Medical School, Boston, MA, USA

Stephen R. Lord, PhD
Prince of Wales Medical Research Institute, University of New South Wales, Randwick, Sydney, NSW, Australia

Kenneth W. Lyles, MD
Duke University Medical Center, Geriatrics Research Education and Clinical Center, Veterans Affairs Medical Center, Durham, NC, USA

Louise Mallet, BScPharm, PharmD, CGS
Professor of Clinical Pharmacy, Faculty of Pharmacy, University of Montreal; Clinical Pharmacist in Geriatrics, Department of Pharmacy, McGill University, Montreal, Quebec, Canada

Manuel Montero-Odasso, MD, PhD
Assistant Professor of Medicine, Department of Medicine and Division of Geriatric Medicine, Parkwood Hospital, University of Western Ontario; Associate Scientist, Lawson Research Institute, London, ON; Vice-Director, Geriatric Fellowship, Faculty of Medicine, University of Buenos Aires, Argentina

Mark E. Nuttall, PhD
Centocor, Horsham, PA, 19044, USA

Rujuta H. Patel, PhD
Duke University Medical Center, Geriatrics Research Education and Clinical Center, Veterans Affairs Medical Center, Durham, NC, USA

Paul C. Schiller, PhD
Associate Professor, University of Miami Miller School of Medicine and Geriatric Research, Educational and Clinical Center and Research Service, Veterans Affairs Medical Center, Miami, FL, USA

Catherine Sherrington, BAppSc(Phty), MPH, PhD
School of Physiotherapy, University of Sydney, Sydney, Australia

Bruce R. Troen, MD
Geriatric Research Education and Clinical Center, Research Service, Miami Veterans Affairs Medical Center, Geriatrics Institute and Division of Gerontology and Geriatrics, Miller School of Medicine, University of Miami, Miami, FL, USA

Ken Watanabe, PhD
Department of Bone and Joint Disease, National Institute for Longevity Science (NILS), National Center for Geriatrics and Gerontology (NCGG), Japan

1 Biology of Bone

Paul C. Schiller, Gianluca D'Ippolito, and Guy A. Howard

Overview

Bone is an exquisitely sophisticated organ/tissue in mammals. Bone is generally viewed as the main component of the skeleton, providing mechanical and structural support to the rest of the organs and systems. This function is indispensable for life, both during the growth and development period as well as during adult life. However, bone also provides the unique architecture and microenvironment that preserves the niches that maintain immature stem cells. This inadequately recognized function is also essential, because these stem cells are required for tissue repair and regeneration during adult life. In this respect, besides providing mechanical support, bone holds and supports the main reservoir of cells needed to sustain tissue integrity and function throughout our lives. Thus, understanding how bone is made and maintained during life is central to developing adequate strategies to preserve a healthy skeleton as we age; so that proper mechanical support, structural integrity, and tissue repair capacity is maintained.

In this chapter we will present a general overview of the process of bone formation during development, describe bone repair during adult life, review the differentiation program of bone cells, discuss the dynamic process of bone turnover, summarize the mechanisms by which hormones and growth factors regulate bone cell differentiation and function, and briefly describe the roles of bone cells and the skeleton in stem cell biology and the effect of aging on them.

Growth and Development of Bones

The cellular events underlying the processes of bone maintenance, remodeling, and repair during adult life have their basis in the embryonic development of bone. The vertebrate skeleton, composed of cartilage and bone, is derived from cells of three distinct embryonic lineages. The craniofacial skeleton is formed by cranial neural crest cells, the axial skeleton is the product of paraxial mesoderm (somites), and the limb skeleton is derived from lateral plate mesodermal cells *(1)*. During vertebrate embryogenesis, neural crest-derived mesenchymal cells directly differentiate into osteoblasts, which will form the bones of the skull, maxilla, and mandible, and the subperiosteal bone-forming layers of long bones. The bones of the skull are created as these regions of ossification merge. A single bone can therefore be made up of many smaller bones that fuse together during ossification. This process is called intramembranous ossification. In contrast, bones of the vertebral column, pelvis, and upper and lower limbs are formed on an initial hyaline cartilage model, generally called anlagen. Initially there is an aggregation and differentiation of mesenchymal cells, followed by the proliferation, hypertrophy, and death of chondrocytes. Bone formation initiates in the collar surrounding the hypertrophic cartilage core, which is eventually invaded by blood vessels and replaced by bone tissue and bone marrow. This process, called endo (within)—chondral (cartilage) ossification, is characterized by a defined series of events.

Early during limb development, a layer of four to six cells, which surrounds a prechondrogenic core of undifferentiated cells, appears to give rise to the lineage of osteogenic cells responsible for the formation of all structural bone *(2)*. This bone is fabricated outside of the cartilage core, and it appears that the core is not replaced by bone, but rather, is replaced by marrow and vascular elements. Bone formation is a vascular-driven phenomenon that is characterized by the directional nature of osteoid secretion. Analysis of the cellular and molecular events of embryonic osteogenesis suggests that osteogenesis and chondrogenesis are independent events that are programmed early in development. Many of the molecules involved in regulating this process during development continue to play central roles during adult life.

The transcription factor Sox9 is one of the master regulators of chondrogenesis *(3,4)*. Sox9 transcripts are detected in all prechondrogenic mesenchymal condensations as early as 8.5 to 9.5 days of mouse embryonic development, and the expression peaks in cartilage primordia at 11.5 to 14.5 days. This transcription factor is central for the regulated expression of the genes that defines the chondrocytic phenotype and for the expression of cartilage-specific matrix proteins such as collagen II, IX, and XI and the large proteoglycan aggrecan *(5)*. Soon after their formation, chondrocytes in the central region of the cartilage undergo further maturation to hypertrophic chondrocytes, which exit the cell cycle and synthesize an extracellular matrix that is different in composition from that of proliferating chondrocytes. Collagen X, a marker for hypertrophic chondrocytes, is a distinctive component of this matrix *(6)*. Angiogenic factors (e.g., vascular endothelial growth factor [VEGF]) secreted by hypertrophic chondrocytes induce sprouting angiogenesis from the perichondrium *(7)*. Following the vessels, bone-forming osteoblasts, bone-resorbing osteoclasts, and hematopoietic cells arrive, and form the primary ossification centers.

Within the primary ossification centers, hypertrophic chondrocytes undergo apoptosis, the hypertrophic cartilage matrix is degraded, incoming osteoblasts replace the degraded cartilage with trabecular bone, and bone marrow is formed. Simultaneously, osteoblasts in the perichondrium form a collar of compact bone surrounding the middle portion (diaphysis) of the cartilage. At both ends (epiphyses) of the cartilage, secondary ossification centers are created, leaving a plate of cartilage (growth plate) between epiphysis and diaphysis. In the growth plate, a coordinated sequence of chondrocyte proliferation, hypertrophy, and apoptosis results in longitudinal growth of long bones. In a coordinated fashion, the growth of the epiphysis and radial growth of the diaphysis take place concurrently.

In adults, bone repair takes place in a fashion similar to endochondral ossification. The natural healing process involves infiltration of fibroblasts, an inflammatory response, cartilage formation, vascularization, osteoblast formation, infiltration by osteoblasts and osteoclasts, and matrix remodeling. A more detailed description of the mechanisms that regulate bone cell differentiation and function will be discussed in the following section and in subsequent chapters.

Bone Cell Differentiation

Bone is a dynamic connective tissue composed of an elegant assembly of functionally distinct cell populations. Their roles are to maintain the structural, biochemical, and mechanical integrity of bone as well as its central role in ion homeostasis, as a calcium basin, and as a stem cell reservoir. Bone is continuously modified and reshaped throughout our lifetime by the work of osteoblasts (bone-forming cells) and osteoclasts (bone cells that break down previously formed bone). A fraction of the active osteoblasts become incorporated within the newly laid down matrix and develop into specialized osteocytes within defined spaces termed lacunae. Osteocytes form a complex and organized network of interconnected cells throughout the mineralized bone matrix that supports bone structure and maintenance. Quiescent osteoblasts become flat and form a single layer of cells, which protects the surface of bone and are called lining cells. Osteoblasts and osteoclasts originate from distinct cell lineages, stromal and hematopoietic (monocyte/macrophage), respectively. And the molecular processes that lead their differentiation programs and functional development are beginning to be understood.

Osteoprogenitors, Osteoblasts, and Osteocytes

Marrow stromal cells (MSCs) can give rise to a variety of cell types (osteoblasts, chondroblasts, myoblasts, adipocytes, fibroblasts, etc.). Under appropriate stimulation, MSCs engage in a differentiation program leading to the production of osteoprogenitors, which in turn give rise to osteoblasts (Figure 1.1). Upon functional maturation, these are the cells responsible for bone matrix deposition in both intramembranous and endochondral bone formation. Osteoblastic differentiation involves an exquisite interplay of developmental cues, signaling proteins, transcription factors, and their co-regulatory proteins that support differentiation (Figure 1.1). This refined differentiation program is reflected by the fact that within the osteoblastic lineage, subpopulations of cells can respond selectively to physiologic signals. Experimental evidence indicates that osteoblasts from appendicular and axial bone exhibit distinct responses to hormonal, mechanical, or developmental cues. It remains to be determined whether these differences reflect the inherent properties of the selected cells at different stages of osteoblastic differentiation or the local, cellular, and tissue environments.

Although it has been generally thought that committed precursors are directionally engaged in a specific differentiation program, accumulating data indicates a certain degree of plasticity. Phenotypically committed cells may de-differentiate during proliferation and post-mitotically assume a different phenotype, primarily owing to effects of the local cellular environment *(8,9)*. The local environment may activate specific mechanisms, such as those involving modulation of gap-junctional intercellular communication *(10)*, that may contribute to phenotypic determination.

The main function of the osteoblast is to synthesize bone matrix. A functionally mature osteoblast is characterized by unique morphological and ultrastructural characteristics typical of a cell engaged in the synthesis and secretion of a connective tissue matrix. These cells show a large nucleus, enlarged Golgi, and extensive endoplasmic reticulum. They express high levels of alkaline phosphatase (ALP) and secrete an unmineralized osteoid composed primarily of type I collagen and specific bone matrix proteins. A single layer of inactive flattened osteoblasts, or

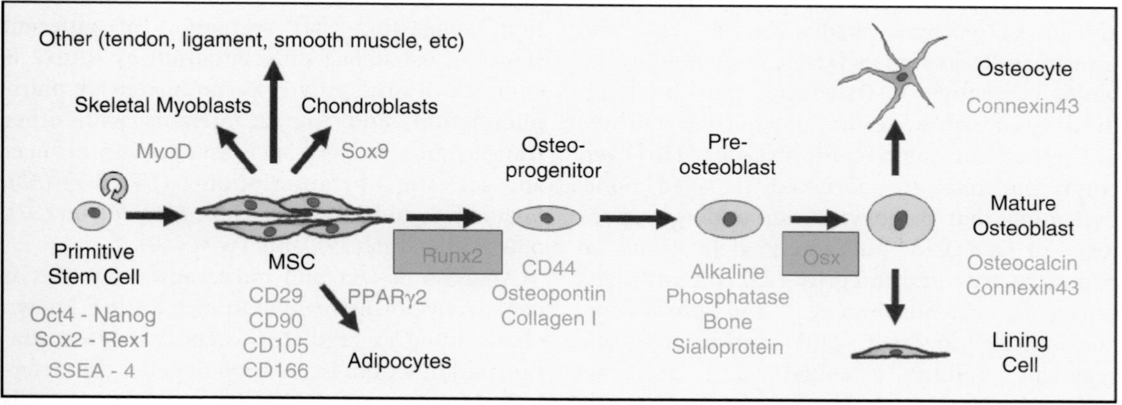

Figure 1.1. The osteoblastic differentiation pathway. The commitment of primitive stem cell to several lineages showing their differentiation potential, with an emphasis on the osteoblastic pathway is diagrammed. Some key transcription factors involved in establishing each phenotype are described (green), and the determinants of the osteoblastic phenotype Runx2 and Osx are boxed. Markers characteristic of each phenotypic stage are indicated (red).

bone lining cells, are observed on quiescent bone surfaces. These cells underlie the periosteum directly on the mineralized surface or form the endosteum separating bone from the marrow cavity.

The osteocyte is the terminal differentiation stage of cells in the osteoblastic lineage. It senses and mediates responses to support bone structure, biomechanical properties, and metabolic functions. Unique features distinguish these cells: they are strategically distributed throughout the mineralized bone matrix, each osteocyte resides within a lacuna, and osteocytes interconnect among themselves and with osteoblasts located on the bone surface via countless cellular extensions of filopodia processes that run through canaliculai. This extensive network of cytoplasmic interconnections contributes to ensure osteocyte viability and maintenance of functional properties. This network of cells is coupled molecularly and electrically mainly by intercellular communication mediated by gap junctions *(11–14)* comprised primarily of the gap-junction channel protein connexin 43 *(15–19)*. Connexin43-mediated gap-junctional communication is essential for osteoblast and osteocyte phenotypic maturation, activity, and survival *(18,20–22)*. Moreover, its inhibition may affect phenotypic determination of bone cells promoting the development of an adipocytic phenotype *(10)*.

The primary function of this osteoblast-lining cell-osteocyte functional syncytium is considered to be mechanosensory (i.e., to sense and transduce stress signals [stretching, bending] to biological activity). Osteocytes can be long-lived; in human bone that has not been turned over, they can survive for decades. However, empty lacunae are observed in aged bone, indicating that osteocytes can undergo apoptosis, a scenario potentially deleterious to bone structure and integrity *(23)*. Interestingly, estrogens, bisphosphonates, and physiologic mechanical loading, all anti-osteoporotic regimens, inhibit osteoblast and osteocyte apoptosis *(24–26)*.

The developmental expression pattern of transcription factors during osteoblastic maturation reflects their central roles as determinants of osteoblastic differentiation. Two transcription factors, Runx2 (Cbfa1/AML3) and Osterix (Osx; SP7), are absolutely required for osteoblast differentiation during both intramembranous and endochondral bone formation. Runx2 performs as a master regulator, because it mediates the temporal activation and/or repression of phenotypic genes as osteoblasts progress through stages of differentiation and cell growth *(27–29)*. Runx2 is a member of a small transcription factor family that shares DNA-binding domains of homology with Drosophila runt. In homozygous Runx2-deficient mice, bone tissue is not formed. Haploinsufficiency of Runx2 causes cleidocranial dysplasia (CCD) in both mice and humans *(30)*. This autosomal dominant disorder is characterized by a delay in closure of cranial sutures and fontanelles, hypoplastic or aplastic clavicles, dental anomalies that include delayed eruption of deciduous and permanent teeth, and supernumerary teeth of the permanent dentition *(30)*. In addition to the role of Runx2 in osteoblast differentiation, Runx2 activity is also required for bone matrix deposition by mature osteoblasts *(31)*, and some individuals with severe CCD have osteoporosis. Runx2 is targeted to the promoters and regulates the expression of several genes encoding bone-specific proteins, including osteocalcin (OC; an osteoblast-specific marker), bone sialoprotein, ALP, and type I collagen *(27)*. Interestingly, both overexpression of Runx2 and expression of a dominant-negative form of Runx2 in osteoblasts impair bone formation, suggesting that regulation of different stages of osteoblast differentiation by Runx2 is complex. Runx2 activity is modulated by phosphorylation, and Runx2 interacts with other transcription factors, such as signal transducer and activator of transcription-1 (STAT-1) *(32)*, Smads 1, 3, and 5 *(33–35)*, Hey1 *(36)*, Menin *(37)*, p300 *(38)*, Grg5 *(39)*, and Twist *(40)*.

Analysis of Osx-null mice shows that Osx is genetically downstream of Runx2. Little is known about how Osx regulates osteoblast differentiation and function. Expression of genes characteristic of mature osteoblasts is absent in cells surrounding chondrocytes in Osx-null mice, and instead these cells express genes characteristic of chondrocytes. Thus, Osx may be playing a role in directing precursor cells toward the osteoblast lineage and away from the chondrocyte lineage *(41,42)*.

The endochondral portion of the developing clavicle is particularly sensitive to a reduction in the level of Runx2, both in mice and humans *(43)*. In addition, no hypertrophy develops in cartilages of the axial skeleton and the proximal limbs in Runx2-null mice. In contrast, in the distal limbs, cartilage hypertrophy is reduced but does occur, and hypertrophy in hands and feet is initiated but is not maintained *(44,45)*. Because a low level of Runx2 expression can be detected in hypertrophic chondrocytes in wild-type growth plates, this has led to the hypothesis that Runx2, in addition to inducing osteoblast differentiation, is required or represents a limiting factor for chondrocyte hypertrophy. Furthermore, it may be required for VEGF expression and angiogenesis during endochondral ossification. Finally, Runx2 may control the expression of collagenase 3 (MMP-13) in hypertrophic chondrocytes *(46,47)*.

It has recently been determined that the Runx1 hematopoietic factor and the Runx3 gene (involved in neural and gut development) are also expressed in the skeleton, although their roles in bone formation are not known. Alterations in functions of various other non-bone-specific transcription factors have been also demonstrated to affect osteoblastic differentiation and function. These include activator protein-1 and its related molecules, Dlx5, Msx1, Msx2, Twist, Atf4, and nuclear steroid hormone receptors such as androgen receptors and estrogen receptors. As regulatory factors continue to be identified, the complexity of the molecular mechanisms that control gene expression in osteoblast lineage cells and drive the osteoblast maturation process are being further appreciated.

Regulators of Osteoblastic Cell Differentiation and Function

The osteoblastic differentiation program is subjected to a complex and intricate regulation by a number of growth factors, hormones, and cytokines, which mediate cues ranging from developmental signals to tissue homeostasis. As in other tissues, many signals simultaneously initiated by two or more of these factors have to be integrated for a unified phenotypic response. A detailed analysis of the mechanisms mediating all the osteogenic responses initiated by the action of extracellular regulators of osteoblast differentiation and bone development is beyond the scope of this section. We will present a brief overview of the main factors known to regulate osteoblastic cell differentiation and function.

Wnt Signaling Molecules

Engagement of MSCs toward osteoblastic differentiation, bone formation, and skeletal development appears to be initiated by activation of the Wnt/β-catenin signaling pathway *(48,49)*. β-Catenin is the downstream mediator of canonical Wnt signaling that forms transcription-regulating complexes with T-cell factor (TCF)/lymphoid enhancer factor (LEF) transcription factors. Key roles for this signaling pathway have been established in embryonic skeletal patterning, fetal skeletal development, and adult skeletal remodeling *(50–55)*. Recent work in which β-catenin was conditionally knocked out from cells at various stages of the osteoblast lineage suggests that β-catenin plays multiple critical roles in osteoblast differentiation *(56)*.

Parathyroid Hormone

Intermittent parathyroid hormone (PTH) therapy in animals and humans induces anabolic effects on bone formation. PTH mediates its effects in cells of the osteoblastic lineage via the type 1 PTH receptor (PTH1R), which is also activated by PTH-related peptide (PTHrP). Depending on the cellular context, binding to PTH1R causes the activation of at least the adenylate cyclase/protein kinase A (AC/PKA), protein kinase C (PKC), and mitogen-activated protein kinase (MAPK) signaling pathways *(57)*. Continuous administration of PTH produces bone loss caused by osteoclast activation as observed in hyperparathyroidism. Different signalling pathways are activated in osteoblast precursors by intermittent or chronic stimulation, respectively, which leads to important differences in downstream gene regulation patterns. Intermittent PTH and PTHrP treatment of MSC and preosteoblastic cell lines regulates their osteogenic differentiation capacity by modulating the expression of the transcription factors Runx2 and osterix and down-regulating components of the hedgehog signalling cascade *(58–60)*. The stimulatory effect on osteoblastic differentiation may depend on the cell differentiation stage, exposure time, and PTH dosage *(16,61)*.

PTH and PTHrP appear to also be involved in mechanotransduction by modulating intracellular Ca^{2+} via mechanosensitive channels *(62)*. Mechanical loading and PTH have synergistic effects on OC expression *in vitro* and on bone formation *in vivo* *(63)*. Moreover, mechanical stress induces PTHrP expression in osteoblast-like cells, which could be a potential mediator of the anabolic effects of mechanical force on bone *(64)*.

Vitamin D3

Vitamin D3 promotes osteogenic differentiation of MSCs by inhibiting proliferation and up-regulating osteogenic markers such as ALP and OC *(65,66)*. Surprisingly, vitamin D3 is not all together indispensable for normal bone development in embryogenesis as the skeleton of vitamin D receptor (VDR) mutant mice developed normally; however, they showed growth retardation, rickets, secondary hyperparathyroidism, and alopecia *(67)*. Vitamin D3-bound VDR interacts with Runx2 to up-regulate OC expression *(68)*. Overall, vitamin D3 stimulates the expression of many genes in bone cells like OC, ALP, osteopontin, CYR61, and thioredoxin reductase, and modifies osteogenic differentiation. But many of the programs induced may also be backed up by other systems.

Estrogen

Estrogens have a major impact both on bone formation during growth and development and bone metabolism in adults. Bone marrow stromal cells express estrogen receptor beta (ERβ) and two splice variants of ERα, suggesting they are targets of estrogen action. Furthermore, estrogens up-regulate ER expression in MSCs, and when overexpressed in the marrow stromal cells, ER induced osteogenic differentiation in response to estradiol.

The estrogenic compound genistein stimulates the proliferation and osteoblastic differentiation of bone marrow MSCs by activation of the NO/cGMP pathway *(69)*. The differentiation-inducing effects in MSCs might be mediated by downstream induction of BMP2 and BMP6 expression. Estrogens can up-regulate the expression of osteogenic marker genes like Runx2, ALP, collagen 1 (Col1), and transforming growth factor (TGF)β1 in MSCs. Estrogens inhibit osteoclast development and function via up-regulation of osteoprotegerin (OPG) expression in osteoblasts and inhibition of cytokine expression *(70)*. Estrogen deficiency leads to osteoporosis in women and men *(71)*. Although the influence of estrogens on osteoblast function might be important, the foremost function of estrogens in the maintenance of bone is still considered to be an anti-resorptive one.

Mechanical strain and estrogens activate ERα in bone cells *(72,73)*. ERα itself appears to be the mediator of such effects, as ERα knock out (KO) results in an impaired anabolic response to mechanical strain *in vivo* and *in vitro*.

Bone Morphogenetic Proteins (BMPs)

BMPs are members of the TGFβ superfamily of signal molecules, which mediate many diverse biological processes ranging from early embryonic tissue patterning to postnatal tissue homeostasis. Activation of BMP/TGFβ receptors initiates phosphorylation of the downstream effector proteins, known as receptor-regulated Smads, leading to signal transduction *(74)*. Although the same Smads are used by BMPs in all types of cells, association with different transcription factors account in part for the functional diversity of BMPs. These transcription factors are recruited by Smads to regulate the expression of specific subsets of target genes depending on the cell context. Runx2 is expressed in response to BMP/TGFβ, and acts as an integrator of BMP/TGFβ Smad signaling through the formation of Runx2–Smad complexes

(75,76). Although both BMP and TGFβ direct Runx2–Smad interactions, only the BMP-responsive Smads promote osteoblast differentiation together with Runx2. BMPs promote bone formation by stimulating the proliferation and differentiation of osteoblasts. It has been suggested that non-union of the bone, and delayed healing, may be the result of decreased levels of BMP activity. The BMP signalling cascade is closely regulated, with the inhibitory Smads blocking the intracellular signal cascade. Predominantly BMP-2 and BMP-7 have been shown to have potent stimulatory effects on osteoblastogenesis and, furthermore, proven clinical utility for bone regeneration *(77–79)*.

Growth Hormone(GH)/Insulin-Like Growth Factor (IGF)

GH is a peptide hormone secreted from the pituitary gland under the control of the hypothalamus. A large number, but not all, of its effects are mediated through IGF-I. Both GH and IGF-I play significant roles in the regulation of growth and bone metabolism and control bone mass. GH directly and through IGF-I stimulates osteoblast proliferation and activity, promoting bone formation. It also stimulates osteoclast differentiation and activity, promoting bone resorption. This results in an increase in the overall rate of bone remodeling, with a net effect of bone buildup. The absence of GH results in a reduced rate of bone remodeling and a gradual loss of bone mineral density. Bone growth primarily occurs at the epiphyseal growth plates and is the result of the proliferation and differentiation of chondrocytes. GH has direct effects on these chondrocytes, but primarily regulates this function through IGF-I, which stimulates the proliferation of and matrix production by these cells. GH-deficiency severely limits bone growth and hence the accumulation of bone mass. It is also known that GH effects on target tissue involve multiple components of the IGF system including the ligands, receptors, IGF binding proteins (IGFBP), IGFBP proteases and activators, and inhibitors of IGFBP proteases. Basic and clinical studies indicate there is a significant role for IGF-I in determining bone mineral density (BMD). Genomic studies resulting in IGF-I–deficient mice, and mice with targeted overexpression of IGF-I reinforce the essential role of IGF-I in bone development at both the embryonic and postnatal stages. Deficiency in the GH/IGF system that occurs with age has been proposed to play a major role in age-related osteoporosis. A thorough molecular dissection of the IGF regulatory system and its signaling pathway in bone may reveal novel therapeutic targets for the treatment of osteoporosis.

Leptin/β Adrenergic Receptors

Leptin was initially characterized as an adipocyte-secreted hormone that controls body weight *(80,81)*. KO animals for the leptin gene (ob/ob mouse) and the leptin receptor (db/db mouse), in addition to their body-mass phenotype, develop a high bone mass with an increase in trabecular bone volume *(83,84)*. This results from an increase in osteoblast function, not number, indicating that leptin in this context has no influence on osteoblast proliferation. There is strong evidence that leptin acts centrally via hypothalamic receptors to regulate bone mass. This is exerted via a neuroendocrine axis and the sympathetic nervous system by activating β2 adrenergic receptors on osteoblastic cells.

Leptin acts directly on human MSC by enhancing osteogenic differentiation and inhibiting the adipogenic pathway *(85)*. However, all together conflicting results are published with respect to the local effects of leptin on bone growth and regeneration. Thus it is still under debate if direct effects via leptin receptors on osteoblasts exert relevant effects.

Glucocorticoids

Glucocorticoid effects in bone metabolism are complex and vary significantly depending on the duration, concentration, and the time window of exposure *(86)*. Glucocorticoid receptor (GR) signalling is required during the earlier phase of osteoblastic differentiation but is dispensable in later phases. Physiologically, glucocorticoids *in vivo* are required for bone formation and stimulate osteogenic differentiation. Prolonged treatment at pharmacological doses induces osteoporosis *in vivo* and leads to an impairment of osteogenic differentiation *in vitro*, which is mediated via enhanced expression of dickkopf-1 (Dkk-1) and secreted-frizzled related protein 1, inhibitors of the canonical Wnt signalling pathway. This may favor alternative pathways of differentiation like adipogenesis *(87,88)*.

Thyroid Hormone

Thyroid hormone (T_3) is essential for the normal development of endochondral and intramembranous bone and plays an important role in the linear growth and maintenance of bone mass *(89)*. Thyroid hormone receptors (TR) are expressed in osteoblasts, chondrocytes of the growth plate, and MSC *(90,91)*. In MSCs three isoforms, TRα1, TRβ1, and TRβ2, are functionally expressed *(92)*. The effects of T_3 in osteoblastic cell lines and primary cultures are dependent upon species, cell type, anatomical origin, state of differentiation, confluence, and duration of treatment, but T_3 has been implicated in the increased synthesis of OC, type I collagen and ALP, and induction of MMP13, gelatinase B (MMP9), and the tissue inhibitor of MMP (TIMP) *(93,94)*. Mice expressing a nonfunctional TRα1 show delayed endochondral ossification and intramembranous bone formation during embryogenesis, and reduced postnatal linear growth. The results from KO and transgenic mice match those seen in hypo- and hyperthyroid animals, respectively, although overall the changes in growth plate and bone morphology are very complex and not yet completely unraveled.

Our increasing understanding of the downstream targets of osteogenic developmental signaling pathways, the molecular switches directing phenotypic commitment, and the network of transcription factors that regulate osteoblast differentiation are beginning to shed light on the complexity of control mechanisms for bone formation. The integration of the many osteogenic signaling pathways converges primarily through the Runx2 transcription factor, which identifies molecular mechanisms for coordinating activities from diverse developmental and physiological signals. Simultaneously, all this information is providing novel opportunities for therapeutic approaches for the intervention of metabolic and genetic disorders of the skeleton.

Monocyte/Macrophages and Osteoclastogenesis

The activity of osteoclasts, to degrade bone and cartilage, is required for skeletal modeling and remodeling. The osteoclast is a specialized multinucleated cell derived from cells in monocyte-macrophage lineage (Figure 1.2). The earliest identifiable precursor is the granulocyte-macrophage colony-forming unit (CFU-GM), which gives rise to granulocytes, monocytes, and osteoclasts. CFU-GM-derived cells differentiate to committed osteoclast precursors, which are post-mitotic cells that must fuse to form functional multi-nucleated osteoclasts. Osteoclasts are the principal, if not exclusive, bone-resorbing cells, and their activity has a profound impact on skeletal health. So, disorders of skeletal insufficiency, such as osteoporosis, typically represent increased osteoclastic bone resorption relative to bone formation. Prevention of pathological bone loss therefore depends on an understanding of the mechanisms by which osteoclasts

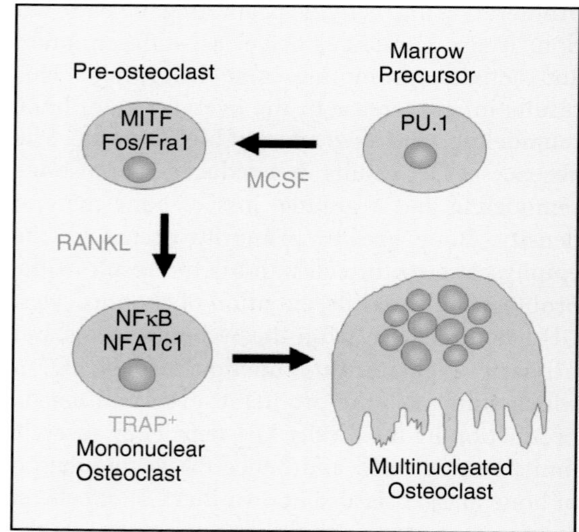

FIGURE 1.2. The osteoclastic differentiation pathway. The commitment of marrow precursors to the osteoclastic pathway is diagrammed. Some key transcription factors involved in establishing each phenotype are described (black), and the factors that induce osteoclastic determination, MCSF, and RANKL are included.

differentiate from their precursors and degrade the skeleton.

Osteoclast development follows vascular invasion of cartilage during embryogenesis and requires VEGF *(95)*. From this time forward, osteoclastogenesis and skeletal resorption continues through life. Osteoclast precursors in humans are characterized by the expression of CD14 and CD11b on their surface. In addition to several transcription factors required for B cell lineage development, two transcriptional factors are important in the regulation of osteoclastogenesis: PU.1 and microphthalmia transcription factor (MITF). The myeloid and B cell transcription factor PU.1 is the earliest characterized determinant of the macrophage/osteoclast lineage. Mice null for PU.1, in addition to having no B cells, lack osteoclasts and macrophages *(96)*. High levels of PU.1 are required for macrophage and osteoclast differentiation *(97)*. Downstream of PU.1, and interacting with it for osteoclast differentiation, is the MITF *(98)*.

Development of osteoclasts requires the concerted actions of a range of cytokines, steroids, and lipids, which act directly on precursors themselves and indirectly by targeting a combination of mesenchymal supportive cells and those in the lymphoid lineage. The capacity of mature osteoclasts to resorb bone is cytokine-driven and depends on their ability to recognize the matrix, polarize, and secrete acid and a collagenolytic enzyme.

So far, most genetic mutations that regulate bone mass, whether natural or generated by targeted deletions, are associated with the osteoclast. Mutations can be inherent to the osteoclast and precursor, or found in proteins that are produced by lymphoid or mesenchymal tissue, which regulate the survival, differentiation, and/or function of the mature bone-resorbing cell.

Modulators of Osteoclastic Cell Differentiation and Function

Osteoclastogenesis is regulated mainly by two cytokines: receptor activator of the NFκB ligand (RANKL) and macrophage colony-stimulating factor (M-CSF). RANKL is a glycoprotein produced by stromal cells that belongs to the TNF ligand super family. RANKL signal is mediated through the association to its receptor, RANK, a member of TNFR super family and a type I transmembrane protein. RANKL secreted by activated T cells is able to activate the monocytic cells to differentiate into osteoclasts through RANK receptor. RANK ligand can be inhibited by OPG, a soluble decoy receptor that also belongs to the TNFR super family *(99)*. Blocking RANKL causes osteoclast differentiation to be suppressed.

M-CSF is a secreted cytokine that promotes the proliferation and differentiation of precursors of the monocyte linage. M-CSF is able to recognize only one receptor, the tyrosine kinase c-Fms. Transgenic mice lacking c-Fms develop osteopetrosis *(100)* because of their inability to produce osteoclasts.

Most factors that induce osteoclast differentiation, such as PTHrP, interleukin (IL)-11, and prostaglandins, do so by inducing expression of RANKL on the surface of immature osteoblasts *(101)*. In addition, osteoclasts produce autocrine-paracrine factors that regulate osteoclast formation, such as IL-6. Several autocrine-paracrine factors that regulate osteoclast activity include annexin-II, macrophage inhibitory protein (MIP)-1α, eosinophil chemotactic factor, and osteoclast inhibitor factors 1 and 2. Most recently, the receptor for ADAM8 *(102)* and α9β1 integrin *(103)* have been shown to be involved in normal osteoclast activity. Osteoclast differentiation is controlled by exogenous hormones and cytokines as well as autocrine-paracrine factors that positively or negatively regulate osteoclast proliferation and differentiation.

In summary, bone cells from different origins, at different stages of differentiation, and with different and sometimes opposing functions, integrate into a network of cells that work together to orchestrate modeling, remodeling, and bone repair starting very early in development. Soluble signaling cytokines, hormones, and growth factors as well as cell-to-cell communication pathways (i.e., connexin43-gap junctional communication) play essential roles in maintaining tissue integrity and appropriate mechanical support (Figure 1.3).

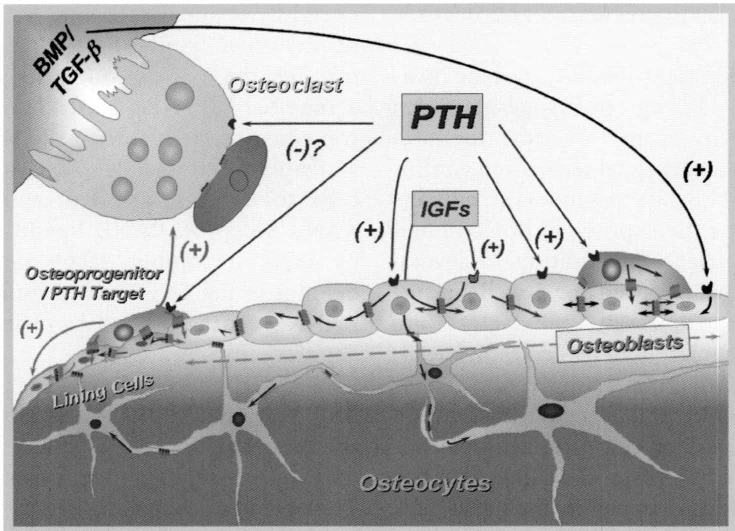

FIGURE 1.3. Bone cells working in concert. Bone cells with different and sometimes contrasting functions, integrate into a network to orchestrate modeling, remodeling, and repair of bone. Some soluble signaling hormones (PTH), morphogens (BMPs), and growth factors (IGF, TGF-β), as well as cell-to-cell communication pathways (i.e., connexin43-gap junctional communication [green channels between adjacent cells or cell processes]), are included in order to describe communication pathways utilized to coordinately maintain bone integrity. Systemic, paracrine, autocrine, and coupling factors make this environment unique for bone cell differentiation and function. Cytoplasmic signaling molecules can travel through mineralized matrix (red) thanks to the action of osteocytes and specialized cellular structures (i.e., gap junctions).

Bone Turnover

Bone mass is the result of a lifelong balance between the processes of bone formation and bone resorption, and in fact, most metabolic bone diseases, including osteoporosis, are a consequence of an unbalanced bone turnover. In normal conditions, bone resorption and bone formation in the adult bone represent not only the physiological response of the skeleton to injuries, such as fractures, but they also provide the mechanism for the renewal of aging bone tissue, as well as for the remodeling of the skeletal architecture to maximize its flexibility to stress and resistance to load.

Osteoporotic syndromes are characterized by a wide spectrum of bone turnover, ranging from accelerated to reduced remodeling rates. Although the status of bone remodeling is not a specific indication of any particular disorder, estimation of the processes of bone resorption and formation adds crucial information for the prognosis of the disease, as well as for the selection of the most appropriate therapeutic approach, thereby significantly affecting the clinical decision-making process. Higher rates of bone remodeling are in general associated with higher rates of bone loss, and in these conditions, an anti-resorptive treatment usually leads to better therapeutic responses than in disorders characterized by low remodeling rates.

During the process of bone resorption calcium salts are liberated from the bone, and if not reused by the osteoblasts for new bone formation, they enter the circulation and are cleared by the kidneys. Therefore, an increased bone turnover is usually associated with an increased urinary calcium output. Before current biochemical markers were introduced, urinary calcium excretion represented the only humoral index available to estimate the rate of bone turnover. Although a moderate hypercalcemia is still considered as a possible sign of increased bone remodeling rates, this parameter can obviously only provide a rough estimate of the real extent and nature of the remodeling process.

Measurement of Bone Turnover

Through the use of dual X-ray bone absorptiometry (DXA), it is possible to measure the BMD of individuals; thus providing information on the skeleton at that specific site and at that specific point in time. Although evaluation of BMD is critical in the clinical evaluation of the patient at risk for osteoporosis (and potentially for other metabolic bone diseases), BMD represents a static parameter that provides no insight into the rate of bone turnover in a given patient. The ability to complement the static measurement of BMD with an assessment of the dynamic process of bone turnover could, in principle, enhance the ability of BMD to predict risk of subsequent fractures. However, although it has been possible to measure BMD at various skeletal sites for almost 20 years, bone turnover *per se* could only be assessed in the past by a combination of calcium balance and isotope kinetic studies (both time-consuming and very expensive) or by tetracycline-based histomorphometry (both invasive and expensive as well). Thus, the more recent availability of biochemical markers for bone turnover represents a major methodological advance. These measurements are noninvasive, relatively inexpensive, generally available, can measure changes in bone turnover over short intervals of time, and can be assessed repetitively. As with any new technology, however, where they fit into a clinical approach to patients with known or suspected osteoporosis is an evolving area.

Bone Formation Markers

The major synthetic product of osteoblasts is type I collagen; however, osteoblasts also synthesize and secrete a variety of noncollagenous proteins, two of which are clinically useful markers of osteoblastic activity, and by inference, bone formation. Bone-specific isoform of ALP is an osteoblast product that is clearly essential for mineralization. Indeed, ALP deficiency, as in the disease hypophosphatasia, results in defective mineralization of bone and teeth *(104)*. Although bone-specific ALP has been used for years as a clinical indicator of bone turnover, the precise role of this enzyme in the mineralization process remains unclear. Studies suggest ALP may increase local concentrations of inorganic phosphate, destroy local inhibitors of mineral crystal growth, transport phosphate, act as a calcium-binding protein, or some combination of these events.

Circulating ALP activity is derived from several tissues, including intestine, spleen, kidney, placenta (in pregnancy), liver, bone, or from various tumors. Thus, measurement of total ALP activity does not provide specific information on bone formation. However, because the two most common sources of elevated ALP levels are liver and bone, a number of techniques, including heat denaturation, chemical inhibition of selective activity, gel electrophoresis, and precipitation by wheat germ lectin have been used to distinguish the liver versus bone isoforms of the enzyme. Most recently, assays have used tissue-specific monoclonal antibodies to measure the bone isoform, which has only 10–20% cross-reactivity with the liver isoform.

OC is another noncollagenous protein secreted by osteoblasts and is widely accepted as a marker for osteoblastic activity, and therefore, bone formation. However, it should be kept in mind that OC is incorporated into the matrix and is released into the circulation from the matrix during bone resorption, so the serum level at any one time has a component of both bone formation and resorption. Therefore, OC is more properly a marker of bone turnover rather than a specific marker of bone formation *per se*. To complicate matters, the function of OC has not been identified, although its deposition in bone matrix increases with hydroxyapatite deposition during skeletal growth. OC is measured in serum or plasma by radioimmunoassays, based on antibodies raised against bovine protein, which cross-react with the human molecule. Like ALP, OC levels vary with age. Thus, children in active stages of bone growth have higher circulating levels than adults, with a peak around the pubertal age for both sexes. Thereafter, serum OC stabilizes, until the fifth to sixth decade, when a significant rise occurs in females. This phenomenon is linked to the menopausal ovarian failure, is reproduced by oophorectomy, and represents a transient change. In fact, OC returns toward premenopausal levels 15–20 years after the menopause.

As noted previously, the major synthetic product of osteoblasts is type I collagen. Therefore, in principle, indices of type I collagen synthesis would appear to be ideal bone formation markers. Several such assays have been developed in recent years, directed against either the carboxy- or amino-extension peptides of the procollagen molecule. These extension peptides (carboxyterminal propeptide of type I collagen and aminoterminal propeptide of type I procollagen) guide assembly of the collagen triple helix, and are cleaved from the newly formed molecule in a stoichiometric relationship with collagen biosynthesis. However, because type I collagen is not unique to bone, these peptides are also produced by other tissues that synthesize type I collagen, including skin.

Bone Resorption Markers

In contrast to the bone formation markers, where the noncollagenous proteins produced by osteoblasts seem to be the most useful markers, it is the collagen degradation products, rather than specific osteoclast proteins, that are most useful as markers of bone resorption. As the skeleton is resorbed, the collagen breakdown products are released into the circulation and ultimately cleared by the kidney. The predominant amino acid of type I collagen is hydroxyproline, and assay of its level in the urine has been used for many years to assess bone resorption. However, hydroxyproline is not specific to bone collagen, and dietary protein sources can also contribute to urinary hydroxyproline excretion. Because of this, patients had to be on a collagen-free diet for 1–3 days before a 24-hour collection for hydroxyproline measurement. Moreover, a major drawback of urinary hydroxyproline measurements is that they require high-pressure liquid chromatographic (HPLC) methods, which are relatively time-consuming and expensive.

Nowadays, there are rapid and relatively inexpensive immunoassays for various collagen breakdown products, increasing the clinical use of bone resorption markers. These products are cross-linked N- and C-telopeptides of type I collagen from bone. Collagen is a triple helix, with the amino- and carboxy-terminals of the collagen chains connected to adjacent collagen chains by cross-links. During the process of collagen breakdown, these telopeptides are released into the circulation and cleared by the kidney. When osteoclasts resorb bone, they release a variety of collagen degradation products into the circulation that are metabolized further by the liver and the kidney. Thus urine contains these various telopeptides in specific forms that can be measured as both free and protein-bound moieties.

Finally, the only osteoclast-specific product that has been evaluated to any extend as a bone resorption marker is tartrate-resistant acid phosphatase (TRAP). Acid phosphatase is a lysosomal enzyme that is present in a number of tissues, including bone, prostate, platelets, erythrocytes, and the spleen. Osteoclasts contain a TRAP that is released into the circulation. However, plasma TRAP is not entirely specific for the osteoclasts, and the enzyme is relatively unstable in frozen samples. Because of these limitations, TRAP has not been used to any significant extent in the clinical assessment of patients, although the recent development of immunoassays using monoclonal antibodies specifically directed against the bone isoenzyme of TRAP may improve its clinical use.

Some of the issues regarding the use of various bone biochemical markers are as follows. First, urinary resorption markers are generally reported after normalization to creatinine excretion. This has certain limitations, including variability in the creatinine measurement that contributes to the overall variability in the measurement of the urinary markers. A second issue is that many of the bone turnover markers have circadian rhythms, so the timing of sampling is of some importance. Peaks levels usually occur between 4 and 8 AM *(105)*. Thus, for the urine markers, it is best to obtain either a 24-hour urine collection or, if that is inconvenient for the patient, a second morning void sample can be used.

Bone Turnover and Aging

In adults, a third consideration is that most of the bone turnover markers tend to be positively associated with age *(106)*, except for a significant decline from adolescence to approximately age 25 years, as the phase of skeletal consolidations is completed *(107)*. This issue must be kept in mind when normative data for each of the markers are established. A fourth issue is the potential for differential changes in the various bone formation or resorption markers in different disease states or in response to different therapies. Thus, for example, bone-specific ALP tends to show much larger increases in Paget's disease than OC; conversely, glucocorticoid therapy is associated with larger decrements in OC levels as opposed to bone-specific ALP levels *(108)*.

Finally, one has to be aware of the potential variability (technical and biological) of the various bone turnover markers. BMD can be measured by DXA with an accuracy of greater than 95% and a precision error for repeat measurements of between 0.5–2.5%. In contrast, the biochemical markers of bone remodeling are subject to intra- and inter-assay variability (technical variability) as well as individual patient biological variability.

Accordingly, bone biochemical markers assess balance between resorption and formation, and although bone turnover markers are generally inversely correlated with BMD, these correlations are not strong enough to have any value in terms of predicting bone mass for a given individual. Thus, these markers cannot and should not be used to diagnose osteoporosis or to predict bone mass; direct measurement of bone mineral density is extremely effective at accomplishing that.

Age-related fractures are the most common manifestation of osteoporosis and are responsible for the greatest proportion of the morbidity and mortality from this disease. Biochemical, biomechanical, and non-skeletal factors contribute to fragility fractures in the elderly. Over a lifespan, women lose approximately 42% of their spinal and 58% of their femoral bone mass *(109)*. Surprisingly, rates of bone loss in the eighth and ninth decades of life may be comparable with or even exceed those found in the immediate peri- and post-menopausal period of some women. This is because of the uncoupling in the bone remodeling cycle of older individuals, resulting in a marked increase in bone resorption but no change or a decrease in bone formation. This uncoupling has facilitated the efforts of the pharmaceutical industry in their search to produce effective therapeutic entities for the treatment of bone loss. Essentially, drugs that decrease bone resorption also tend to show decreased bone formation because of the coupling that exists between the two functions. And the opposite is true of drugs that tend to increase bone formation—they show an eventual increase in bone resorption. Thus, with the uncoupling that takes place in older individuals, pharmaceutical companies have been able to develop drugs that will decrease bone resorption without the concurrent or at least resultant decrease in bone formation.

Role of Bone and Bone Cells in Stem Cell Biology

As indicated earlier, although bone has been classically viewed as providing the structural support for the human body, and bone cells as being involved in maintaining bone and skeletal homeostasis; novel key roles for bone and bone cells in human physiology are being discovered in the area of stem cell biology. Cells of the stromal/osteoblastic lineage play central regulatory roles as part of the hematopoietic stem cell (HSC) niche *in vivo*. They are capable of directing stem cell self-renewal and proliferation, allowing a subsequent differentiation and repopulation of the hematopoietic system through Notch activation and BMP signaling *(110,111)*. Interestingly, this novel function of stromal/osteoblastic cells is stimulated by parathyroid hormone, a key regulator of bone and mineral homeostasis. Activation of PTH1R in a specific population of stromal/osteoblastic cells results in stimulation of Jagged 1 protein production and targeting to the cell surface. There it interacts with Notch on the surface of adjacent HSCs, triggering a biological response that results in increased HSC proliferation. Pharmacologic use of PTH increases the number of HSCs mobilized into the peripheral blood for stem cell harvests, protects stem cells from repeated exposure to cytotoxic chemotherapy, and expands stem cells in transplant recipients *(112)*.

All these cellular interactions take place within a specialized microenvironment in the bone marrow, the HSC niche. It is proposed that these niches localize at specific anatomical sites, requiring a unique micro-architecture that can only be structurally provided by bone tissue. Some of these structures are found in trabecular bone localized to the endosteal surface of bone *(113)*. Moreover, activated HSCs migrate out of the stromal/osteoblastic niche in trabecular bone and closer to specialized blood vessels, where they actually proliferate and begin to differentiate in close relationship to sinusoid endothelial cells *(114)*. This suggests that the stromal/osteoblast niche is a quiescent niche, where HSCs undergo self-renewal while proliferation and subsequent differentiation take place in the vascular niche some distance away from the stromal/osteoblast niche. This concept is consistent with an oxygen gradient and the effect of oxygen tension on stem cell physiology. The stromal/osteoblast niche is an environment of low oxygen tension anatomically at a distance from blood vessels, whereas the vascular niche provides a high oxygen tension environment. This agrees with the *in vitro* effects of oxygen observed on HSC differentiation, whereby low oxygen preserves a more developmentally primitive HSC and higher oxygen favors HSC differentiation *(115,116)*. This scenario may not only be true for the HSC compartment in bone marrow. MSCs represent a heterogeneous population of cells at different stages of differentiation. Developmentally primitive MSCs with a broad differentiation potential have been identified in human bone marrow *(117–119)*. Similarly, low oxygen tension favors a more primitive phenotype *(120)*, while inhibiting osteoblastic differentiation *(66)*. Thus, it is likely that the most primitive MSCs may also localize to a specific niche similar to that of the HSC niche, whereby the unique microenvironment is provide by specialized bone anatomical sites. Alternatively, both MSCs and HSCs may share the same niche, particularly because a population of human primitive MSCs *(119)* express PTH1R on their surface and respond to PTH stimulation.

References

1. Olsen BR, Reginato AM, Wang W. Bone development. Annu Rev Cell Dev Biol 2000;16:191–220.
2. Pechak DG, Kujawa MJ, Caplan AI. Morphological and histochemical events during first bone formation in embryonic chick limbs. Bone 1986;7:441–458.
3. Foster JW, Dominguez-Steglich MA, Guioli S, et al. Campomelic dysplasia and autosomal sex reversal caused by mutations in an SRY-related gene. Nature 1994;372:525–530.
4. Wagner T, Wirth J, Meyer J, et al. Autosomal sex reversal and campomelic dysplasia are caused by mutations in and around the SRY-related gene SOX9. Cell 1994;79:1111–1120.
5. Bi W, Deng JM, Zhang Z, et al. Sox9 is required for cartilage formation. Nat Genet 1999;22:85–89.
6. Iyama K, Ninomiya Y, Olsen BR, et al. Spatiotemporal pattern of type X collagen gene expression and collagen deposition in embryonic chick vertebrae undergoing endochondral ossification. Anat Rec 1991;229:462–472.
7. Gerber HP, Vu TH, Ryan AM, et al. VEGF couples hypertrophic cartilage remodeling, ossification and angiogenesis during endochondral bone formation. Nat Med 1999;5:623–628.
8. Park SR, Oreffo RO, Triffitt JT. Interconversion potential of cloned human marrow adipocytes in vitro. Bone 1999;24:549–554.
9. Doherty MJ, Ashton BA, Walsh S, et al. Vascular pericytes express osteogenic potential in vitro and in vivo. J Bone Miner Res 1998;13:828–838.
10. Schiller PC, D'Ippolito G, Brambilla R, et al. Inhibition of gap-junctional communication induces the trans-differentiation of osteoblasts to an adipocytic phenotype in vitro. J Biol Chem 2001;276:14133–14138.
11. Holtrop ME. The ultrastructure of bone. Ann Clin Lab Sci 1975;5:264–271.
12. Parfitt AM. The actions of parathyroid hormone on bone: relation to bone remodeling and turnover, calcium homeostasis, and metabolic bone disease. Part I of IV parts: mechanisms of calcium transfer between blood and bone and their cellular basis: morphological and kinetic approaches to bone turnover. Metabolism 1976;25:809–844.
13. Zhang D, Weinbaum S, Cowin SC. Electrical signal transmission in a bone cell network: the influence of a discrete gap junction. Ann Biomed Eng 1998;26:644–659.
14. Zhang D, Cowin SC, Weinbaum S. Electrical signal transmission and gap junction regulation in a bone cell network: a cable model for an osteon. Ann Biomed Eng 1997;25:357–374.
15. Schiller PC, Mehta PP, Roos BA, et al. Hormonal regulation of intercellular communication: parathyroid hormone increases connexin 43 gene

expression and gap-junctional communication in osteoblastic cells. Mol Endocrinol 1992;6:1433–1440.
16. Schiller PC, D'Ippolito G, Roos BA, et al. Anabolic or catabolic responses of MC3T3-E1 osteoblastic cells to parathyroid hormone depend on time and duration of treatment. J Bone Miner Res 1999;14:1504–1512.
17. Schiller PC, D'Ippolito G, Balkan W, et al. Gap-junctional communication mediates parathyroid hormone stimulation of mineralization in osteoblastic cultures. Bone 2001;28:38–44.
18. Schiller PC, D'Ippolito G, Balkan W, et al. Gap-junctional communication is required for the maturation process of osteoblastic cells in culture. Bone 2001;28:362–369.
19. Civitelli R, Beyer EC, Warlow PM, et al. Connexin43 mediates direct intercellular communication in human osteoblastic cell networks. J Clin Invest 1993;91:1888–1896.
20. Lecanda F, Warlow PM, Sheikh S, et al. Connexin43 deficiency causes delayed ossification, craniofacial abnormalities, and osteoblast dysfunction. J Cell Biol 2000;151:931–944.
21. Furlan F, Lecanda F, Screen J, et al. Proliferation, differentiation and apoptosis in connexin43-null osteoblasts. Cell Commun Adhes 2001;8:367–371.
22. Plotkin LI, Manolagas SC, Bellido T. Transduction of cell survival signals by connexin-43 hemichannels. J Biol Chem 2002;277:8648–8657.
23. Noble BS, Stevens H, Loveridge N, et al. Identification of apoptotic changes in osteocytes in normal and pathological human bone. Bone 1997;20:273–282.
24. Noble BS, Peet N, Stevens HY, et al. Mechanical loading: biphasic osteocyte survival and targeting of osteoclasts for bone destruction in rat cortical bone. Am J Physiol Cell Physiol 2003;284:C934–C943.
25. Plotkin LI, Aguirre JI, Kousteni S, et al. Bisphosphonates and estrogens inhibit osteocyte apoptosis via distinct molecular mechanisms downstream of extracellular signal-regulated kinase activation. J Biol Chem 2005;280:7317–7325.
26. Plotkin LI, Mathov I, Aguirre JI, et al. Mechanical stimulation prevents osteocyte apoptosis: requirement of integrins, Src kinases, and ERKs. Am J Physiol Cell Physiol 2005;289:C633–C643.
27. Ducy P, Zhang R, Geoffroy V, et al. Osf2/Cbfa1: a transcriptional activator of osteoblast differentiation. Cell 1997;89:747–754.
28. Otto F, Thornell AP, Crompton T, et al. Cbfa1, a candidate gene for cleidocranial dysplasia syndrome, is essential for osteoblast differentiation and bone development. Cell 1997;89:765–771.
29. Komori T, Yagi H, Nomura S, et al. Targeted disruption of Cbfa1 results in a complete lack of bone formation owing to maturational arrest of osteoblasts. Cell 1997;89:755–764.
30. Mundlos S, Otto F, Mundlos C, et al. Mutations involving the transcription factor CBFA1 cause cleidocranial dysplasia. Cell 1997;89:773–779.
31. Ducy P, Starbuck M, Priemel M, et al. A Cbfa1-dependent genetic pathway controls bone formation beyond embryonic development. Genes Dev 1999;13:1025–1036.
32. Kim S, Koga T, Isobe M, et al. Stat1 functions as a cytoplasmic attenuator of Runx2 in the transcriptional program of osteoblast differentiation. Genes Dev 2003;17:1979–1991.
33. Lee KS, Hong SH, Bae SC. Both the Smad and p38 MAPK pathways play a crucial role in Runx2 expression following induction by transforming growth factor-beta and bone morphogenetic protein. Oncogene 2002;21:7156–7163.
34. Zhang YW, Yasui N, Ito K, et al. A RUNX2/PEBP2alpha A/CBFA1 mutation displaying impaired transactivation and Smad interaction in cleidocranial dysplasia. Proc Natl Acad Sci U S A 2000;97:10549–10554.
35. Alliston T, Choy L, Ducy P, et al. TGF-beta-induced repression of CBFA1 by Smad3 decreases cbfa1 and osteocalcin expression and inhibits osteoblast differentiation. Embo J 2001;20:2254–2272.
36. Zamurovic N, Cappellen D, Rohner D, et al. Coordinated activation of notch, Wnt, and transforming growth factor-beta signaling pathways in bone morphogenic protein 2-induced osteogenesis. Notch target gene Hey1 inhibits mineralization and Runx2 transcriptional activity. J Biol Chem 2004;279:37704–37715.
37. Sowa H, Kaji H, Hendy GN, et al. Menin is required for bone morphogenetic protein 2- and transforming growth factor beta-regulated osteoblastic differentiation through interaction with Smads and Runx2. J Biol Chem 2004;279:40267–40275.
38. Sierra J, Villagra A, Paredes R, et al. Regulation of the bone-specific osteocalcin gene by p300 requires Runx2/Cbfa1 and the vitamin D3 receptor but not p300 intrinsic histone acetyltransferase activity. Mol Cell Biol 2003;23:3339–3351.
39. Wang W, Wang YG, Reginato AM, et al. Groucho homologue Grg5 interacts with the transcription factor Runx2-Cbfa1 and modulates its activity during postnatal growth in mice. Dev Biol 2004;270:364–381.

40. Bialek P, Kern B, Yang X, et al. A twist code determines the onset of osteoblast differentiation. Dev Cell 2004;6:423–435.
41. Nakashima K, Zhou X, Kunkel G, et al. The novel zinc finger-containing transcription factor osterix is required for osteoblast differentiation and bone formation. Cell 2002;108:17–29.
42. Akiyama H, Kim JE, Nakashima K, et al. Osteochondroprogenitor cells are derived from Sox9 expressing precursors. Proc Natl Acad Sci U S A 2005;102:14665–14670.
43. Huang LF, Fukai N, Selby PB, et al. Mouse clavicular development: analysis of wild-type and cleidocranial dysplasia mutant mice. Dev Dyn 1997; 210:33–40.
44. Inada M, Yasui T, Nomura S, et al. Maturational disturbance of chondrocytes in Cbfa1-deficient mice. Dev Dyn 1999;214:279–290.
45. Kim IS, Otto F, Zabel B, et al. Regulation of chondrocyte differentiation by Cbfa1. Mech Dev 1999;80:159–170.
46. Jimenez MJ, Balbin M, Lopez JM, et al. Collagenase 3 is a target of Cbfa1, a transcription factor of the runt gene family involved in bone formation. Mol Cell Biol 1999;19:4431–4442.
47. Porte D, Tuckermann J, Becker M, et al. Both AP-1 and Cbfa1-like factors are required for the induction of interstitial collagenase by parathyroid hormone. Oncogene 1999;18:667–678.
48. Logan CY, Nusse R. The Wnt signaling pathway in development and disease. Annu Rev Cell Dev Biol 2004;20:781–810.
49. Church VL, Francis-West P. Wnt signalling during limb development. Int J Dev Biol 2002;46:927–936.
50. Boyden LM, Mao J, Belsky J, et al. High bone density due to a mutation in LDL-receptor-related protein 5. N Engl J Med 2002;346:1513–1521.
51. Little RD, Recker RR, Johnson ML. High bone density due to a mutation in LDL-receptor-related protein 5. N Engl J Med 2002;347:943–944; author reply 944.
52. Kato M, Patel MS, Levasseur R, et al. Cbfa1-independent decrease in osteoblast proliferation, osteopenia, and persistent embryonic eye vascularization in mice deficient in Lrp5, a Wnt coreceptor. J Cell Biol 2002;157:303–314.
53. Holmen SL, Zylstra CR, Mukherjee A, et al. Essential role of beta-catenin in postnatal bone acquisition. J Biol Chem 2005;280:21162–21168.
54. Day TF, Guo X, Garrett-Beal L, et al. Wnt/beta-catenin signaling in mesenchymal progenitors controls osteoblast and chondrocyte differentiation during vertebrate skeletogenesis. Dev Cell 2005;8:739–750.
55. Hill TP, Spater D, Taketo MM, et al. Canonical Wnt/beta-catenin signaling prevents osteoblasts from differentiating into chondrocytes. Dev Cell 2005;8:727–738.
56. Hu H, Hilton MJ, Tu X, et al. Sequential roles of Hedgehog and Wnt signaling in osteoblast development. Development 2005;132:49–60.
57. Mannstadt M, Juppner H, Gardella TJ. Receptors for PTH and PTHrP: their biological importance and functional properties. Am J Physiol 1999;277: F665–F675.
58. Swarthout JT, D'Alonzo RC, Selvamurugan N, et al. Parathyroid hormone-dependent signaling pathways regulating genes in bone cells. Gene 2002;282:1–17.
59. Qin L, Qiu P, Wang L, et al. Gene expression profiles and transcription factors involved in parathyroid hormone signaling in osteoblasts revealed by microarray and bioinformatics. J Biol Chem 2003;278:19723–19731.
60. Wang BL, Dai CL, Quan JX, et al. Parathyroid hormone regulates osterix and Runx2 mRNA expression predominantly through protein kinase A signaling in osteoblast-like cells. J Endocrinol Invest 2006;29:101–108.
61. Locklin RM, Khosla S, Turner RT, et al. Mediators of the biphasic responses of bone to intermittent and continuously administered parathyroid hormone. J Cell Biochem 2003;89:180–190.
62. Mikuni-Takagaki Y, Naruse K, Azuma Y, et al. The role of calcium channels in osteocyte function. J Musculoskelet Neuronal Interact 2002;2: 252–255.
63. Sekiya H, Mikuni-Takagaki Y, Kondoh T, et al. Synergistic effect of PTH on the mechanical responses of human alveolar osteocytes. Biochem Biophys Res Commun 1999;264:719–723.
64. Chen X, Macica CM, Ng KW, et al. Stretch-induced PTH-related protein gene expression in osteoblasts. J Bone Miner Res 2005;20:1454–1461.
65. D'Ippolito G, Schiller PC, Perez-stable C, et al. Cooperative actions of hepatocyte growth factor and 1,25-dihydroxyvitamin D3 in osteoblastic differentiation of human vertebral bone marrow stromal cells. Bone 2002;31:269–275.
66. D'Ippolito G, Diabira S, Howard GA, et al. Low oxygen tension inhibits osteogenic differentiation and enhances stemness of human MIAMI cells. Bone 2006;39:513–522.
67. Erben RG, Soegiarto DW, Weber K, et al. Deletion of deoxyribonucleic acid binding domain of the vitamin D receptor abrogates genomic and non-

genomic functions of vitamin D. Mol Endocrinol 2002;16:1524–1537.
68. Paredes R, Arriagada G, Cruzat F, et al. Bone-specific transcription factor Runx2 interacts with the 1alpha,25-dihydroxyvitamin D3 receptor to up-regulate rat osteocalcin gene expression in osteoblastic cells. Mol Cell Biol 2004;24:8847–8861.
69. Pan W, Quarles LD, Song LH, et al. Genistein stimulates the osteoblastic differentiation via NO/cGMP in bone marrow culture. J Cell Biochem 2005;94:307–316.
70. Zallone A. Direct and indirect estrogen actions on osteoblasts and osteoclasts. Ann N Y Acad Sci 2006;1068:173–179.
71. Seeman E. Estrogen, androgen, and the pathogenesis of bone fragility in women and men. Curr Osteoporos Rep 2004;2:90–96.
72. Jessop HL, Sjoberg M, Cheng MZ, et al. Mechanical strain and estrogen activate estrogen receptor alpha in bone cells. J Bone Miner Res 2001;16:1045–1055.
73. Zaman G, Jessop HL, Muzylak M, et al. Osteocytes use estrogen receptor alpha to respond to strain but their ERalpha content is regulated by estrogen. J Bone Miner Res 2006;21:1297–1306.
74. Li X, Cao X. BMP signaling and skeletogenesis. Ann N Y Acad Sci 2006;1068:26–40.
75. Zaidi SK, Sullivan AJ, van Wijnen AJ, et al. Integration of Runx and Smad regulatory signals at transcriptionally active subnuclear sites. Proc Natl Acad Sci U S A 2002;99:8048–8053.
76. Afzal F, Pratap J, Ito K, et al. Smad function and intranuclear targeting share a Runx2 motif required for osteogenic lineage induction and BMP2 responsive transcription. J Cell Physiol 2005;204:63–72.
77. Lee MH, Kim YJ, Kim HJ, et al. BMP-2-induced Runx2 expression is mediated by Dlx5, and TGF-beta 1 opposes the BMP-2-induced osteoblast differentiation by suppression of Dlx5 expression. J Biol Chem 2003;278:34387–34394.
78. Ryoo HM, Lee MH, Kim YJ. Critical molecular switches involved in BMP-2-induced osteogenic differentiation of mesenchymal cells. Gene 2006;366:51–57.
79. Li T, Surendran K, Zawaideh MA, et al. Bone morphogenetic protein 7: a novel treatment for chronic renal and bone disease. Curr Opin Nephrol Hypertens 2004;13:417–422.
80. Green ED, Maffei M, Braden VV, et al. The human obese (OB) gene: RNA expression pattern and mapping on the physical, cytogenetic, and genetic maps of chromosome 7. Genome Res 1995;5:5–12.
81. Maffei M, Halaas J, Ravussin E, et al. Leptin levels in human and rodent: measurement of plasma leptin and ob RNA in obese and weight-reduced subjects. Nat Med 1995;1:1155–1161.
82. Wolf G. Leptin: the weight-reducing plasma protein encoded by the obese gene. Nutr Rev 1996;54:91–93.
83. Steppan CM, Crawford DT, Chidsey-Frink KL, et al. Leptin is a potent stimulator of bone growth in ob/ob mice. Regul Pept 2000;92:73–78.
84. Ducy P, Amling M, Takeda S, et al. Leptin inhibits bone formation through a hypothalamic relay: a central control of bone mass. Cell 2000;100:197–207.
85. Hess R, Pino AM, Rios S, et al. High affinity leptin receptors are present in human mesenchymal stem cells (MSCs) derived from control and osteoporotic donors. J Cell Biochem 2005;94:50–57.
86. Canalis E. Mechanisms of glucocorticoid action in bone. Curr Osteoporos Rep 2005;3:98–102.
87. Ohnaka K, Taniguchi H, Kawate H, et al. Glucocorticoid enhances the expression of dickkopf-1 in human osteoblasts: novel mechanism of glucocorticoid-induced osteoporosis. Biochem Biophys Res Commun 2004;318:259–264.
88. Ohnaka K, Tanabe M, Kawate H, et al. Glucocorticoid suppresses the canonical Wnt signal in cultured human osteoblasts. Biochem Biophys Res Commun 2005;329:177–181.
89. Bassett JH, Williams GR. The molecular actions of thyroid hormone in bone. Trends Endocrinol Metab 2003;14:356–364.
90. Stevens DA, Hasserjian RP, Robson H, et al. Thyroid hormones regulate hypertrophic chondrocyte differentiation and expression of parathyroid hormone-related peptide and its receptor during endochondral bone formation. J Bone Miner Res 2000;15:2431–2442.
91. Robson H, Siebler T, Stevens DA, et al. Thyroid hormone acts directly on growth plate chondrocytes to promote hypertrophic differentiation and inhibit clonal expansion and cell proliferation. Endocrinology 2000;141:3887–3897.
92. Gruber R, Czerwenka K, Wolf F, et al. Expression of the vitamin D receptor, of estrogen and thyroid hormone receptor alpha- and beta-isoforms, and of the androgen receptor in cultures of native mouse bone marrow and of stromal/osteoblastic cells. Bone 1999;24:465–473.
93. Salto C, Kindblom JM, Johansson C, et al. Ablation of TRalpha2 and a concomitant overexpression of alpha1 yields a mixed hypo- and hyperthyroid phenotype in mice. Mol Endocrinol 2001;15:2115–2128.

94. Pereira RC, Jorgetti V, Canalis E. Triiodothyronine induces collagenase-3 and gelatinase B expression in murine osteoblasts. Am J Physiol 1999;277:E496–E504.
95. Engsig MT, Chen QJ, Vu TH, et al. Matrix metalloproteinase 9 and vascular endothelial growth factor are essential for osteoclast recruitment into developing long bones. J Cell Biol 2000;151: 879–889.
96. Tondravi MM, McKercher SR, Anderson K, et al. Osteopetrosis in mice lacking haematopoietic transcription factor PU.1. Nature 1997;386:81–84.
97. DeKoter RP, Singh H. Regulation of B lymphocyte and macrophage development by graded expression of PU.1. Science 2000;288:1439–1441.
98. Luchin A, Suchting S, Merson T, et al. Genetic and physical interactions between Microphthalmia transcription factor and PU.1 are necessary for osteoclast gene expression and differentiation. J Biol Chem 2001;276:36703–36710.
99. Simonet WS, Lacey DL, Dunstan CR, et al. Osteoprotegerin: a novel secreted protein involved in the regulation of bone density. Cell 1997;89:309–319.
100. Dai XM, Ryan GR, Hapel AJ, et al. Targeted disruption of the mouse colony-stimulating factor 1 receptor gene results in osteopetrosis, mononuclear phagocyte deficiency, increased primitive progenitor cell frequencies, and reproductive defects. Blood 2002;99:111–120.
101. Blair HC, Zaidi M. Osteoclastic differentiation and function regulated by old and new pathways. Rev Endocr Metab Disord 2006;7:23–32.
102. Choi SJ, Han JH, Roodman GD. ADAM8: a novel osteoclast stimulating factor. J Bone Miner Res 2001;16:814–822.
103. Rao H, Lu G, Kajiya H, et al. Alpha9beta1: a novel osteoclast integrin that regulates osteoclast formation and function. J Bone Miner Res 2006;21: 1657–1665.
104. Whyte MP. Hypophosphatasia and the role of alkaline phosphatase in skeletal mineralization. Endocr Rev 1994;15:439–461.
105. McKane WR, Khosla S, Egan KS, et al. Role of calcium intake in modulating age-related increases in parathyroid function and bone resorption. J Clin Endocrinol Metab 1996;81:1699–1703.
106. Khosla S, Melton LJ, 3rd, Atkinson EJ, et al. Relationship of serum sex steroid levels and bone turnover markers with bone mineral density in men and women: a key role for bioavailable estrogen. J Clin Endocrinol Metab 1998;83:2266–2274.
107. Eastell R, Simmons PS, Colwell A, et al. Nyctohemeral changes in bone turnover assessed by serum bone Gla-protein concentration and urinary deoxypyridinoline excretion: effects of growth and ageing. Clin Sci (Lond) 1992;83:375–382.
108. Duda RJ, Jr., O'Brien JF, Katzmann JA, et al. Concurrent assays of circulating bone Gla-protein and bone alkaline phosphatase: effects of sex, age, and metabolic bone disease. J Clin Endocrinol Metab 1988;66:951–957.
109. Riggs BL, Wahner HW, Seeman E, et al. Changes in bone mineral density of the proximal femur and spine with aging. Differences between the postmenopausal and senile osteoporosis syndromes. J Clin Invest 1982;70:716–723.
110. Calvi LM, Adams GB, Weibrecht KW, et al. Osteoblastic cells regulate the haematopoietic stem cell niche. Nature 2003;425:841–846.
111. Zhang J, Niu C, Ye L, et al. Identification of the haematopoietic stem cell niche and control of the niche size. Nature 2003;425:836–841.
112. Adams GB, Martin RP, Alley IR, et al. Therapeutic targeting of a stem cell niche. Nat Biotechnol 2007. In Press.
113. Yin T, Li L. The stem cell niches in bone. J Clin Invest 2006;116:1195–1201.
114. Kiel MJ, Yilmaz OH, Iwashita T, et al. SLAM family receptors distinguish hematopoietic stem and progenitor cells and reveal endothelial niches for stem cells. Cell 2005;121:1109–1121.
115. Cipolleschi MG, Dello Sbarba P, Olivotto M. The role of hypoxia in the maintenance of hematopoietic stem cells. Blood 1993;82:2031–2037.
116. Cipolleschi MG, D'Ippolito G, Bernabei PA, et al. Severe hypoxia enhances the formation of erythroid bursts from human cord blood cells and the maintenance of BFU-E in vitro. Exp Hematol 1997;25:1187–1194.
117. Reyes M, Lund T, Lenvik T, et al. Purification and ex vivo expansion of postnatal human marrow mesodermal progenitor cells. Blood 2001;98:2615–2625.
118. D'Ippolito G, Howard GA, Roos BA, et al. Isolation and characterization of marrow-isolated adult multilineage inducible (MIAMI) cells. Exp Hematol 2006;34:1608–1610.
119. D'Ippolito G, Diabira S, Howard GA, et al. Marrow-isolated adult multilineage inducible (MIAMI) cells, a unique population of postnatal young and old human cells with extensive expansion and differentiation potential. J Cell Sci 2004;117:2971–2981.
120. Breyer A, Estharabadi N, Oki M, et al. Multipotent adult progenitor cell isolation and culture procedures. Exp Hematol 2006;34:1596–1601.

2
Aging and Bone

Jeffrey M. Gimble, Z. Elizabeth Floyd, Moustapha Kassem, and Mark E. Nuttall

Introduction

This chapter will provide a general overview of the aging process followed by the potential effect that aging may have in bone biology. Three important aspects will be considered: decreased number of osteoblasts, increasing adipogenesis, and significant osteoblast/osteocytes apoptosis during the aging process in bone.

Aging—A Definition

In clinical medicine, aging may be best defined by the words Supreme Court Justice Potter Stewart used to describe pornography: "I know it when I see it" (JACOBELLIS v. OHIO, 378 U.S. 184 (1964)). Every physician has witnessed the effects of aging, both in individual patients followed over a period of time and in their collective patient population base. Nevertheless, a number of definitions of aging have been offered, and these have been elegantly summarized in Carrington's review entitled: "Aging bone and cartilage: cross-cutting issues" *(1)*. In the clinical care setting, aging is generally associated with the loss of a wide range of physiological processes *(1)* (Table 2.1). These include decreased fertility *(2)*, decreased resilience in response to environmental stressors such as infections, surgery, or physical attack *(3)*, and decreased physical strength. Inevitably, aging is also associated with end of life and death *(2,4)*.

At the cellular level, several fundamental and interconnected processes accompany aging *in vitro* and *in vivo (1)* (Table 2.1). Hayflick first defined the process of cellular senescence, demonstrating that "normal" diploid cells can undergo a limited number of cell doublings *in vitro (5)*. These pioneering observations set the framework within which much of our understanding of aging is now predicated. Consequently, the Hayflick model for replicative senescence has been employed in biogerontology research to unravel mechanisms of age-related cellular defects *(6)*. Using this model, several investigators have reported an inverse relationship between the donor age and maximal proliferative potential of the cells *in vitro (7)*. The Kassem laboratory has characterised a Hayflick model for replicative senescence of human osteoblasts *(8,9)*. During continuous culture *in vitro*, human osteoblasts exhibited typical senescence-related phenotype including senescent-associated decrease in osteoblast marker production (alkaline phosphatase [AP], osteocalcin, collagen type I), decrease in mean telomere fragment length, and increase in the number of senescence-associated β-galactosidase (SA β-gal) positive cells *(10,11)*. With each progressive mitotic cycle, each telomere, located at the ends of individual chromosomes, decreases in length; and this has been associated with senescence *(12)*. It has been postulated that the telomere length acts as a "mitotic clock," and it is known that the overexpression of telomerase, the enzyme responsible for maintaining telomere length, leads to cell immortalization *(13)*. The Kassem laboratory has further examined the effect of donor age on the maximal proliferative potential of bone marrow stem cells (BMSC). An age-related decline in the maximal life span from

Table 2.1. Macro- and Micro-Manifestations of Aging (1)

Clinical	Cellular
Decreased fertility	Increased senescence
Decreased physical strength and/or mental acuity	Increased oxidative damage
Decreased resilience and stress response	Altered apoptosis or programmed cell death
Increased mortality	Increased AGEs

AGEs, advanced glycation end products.

41 ± 10 population doublings (PD) in young donors to 24 ± 11 PD in elderly donors was observed. These results thus suggest that human aging is associated with reduced maximal proliferation potential of BMSC. However, the proliferation potential of aged BMSC is still very high; thus, the contribution of the observed *in vitro* age-related decreased maximal proliferative potential of osteoblasts to age-related decreased bone formation *in vivo* is not clear.

It seems that the Hayflick model of replicative senescence is useful for studying some aspects of the aging process, and it has been employed extensively in biogerontology research to investigate changes at both the genetic and epigenetic levels. Somatic mutations increase *(1,4)* and DNA methylation and histone acetylation patterns alter *(14)*, leading to altered gene expression profiles and differentiation function. Other DNA changes accompany senescence in somatic cells. Reduced oxidative phosphorylation in the mitochondria of senescent cells leads to reduced energy availability and metabolic function *(15)*. In parallel, mitochondrial dysfunction results in elevated levels of free radicals in the form of reactive oxygen species (ROS), and this has long been postulated as a causative factor in cellular senescence and aging *(16,17)*. The generation of ROS has been associated with altered signal transduction responses to growth factors *(18)*. In addition, elevated levels of ROS cause increased expression of pro-apoptotic or programmed cell death regulators within differentiated cell types *(19)*. These changes may cause the cells to be more sensitive to exogenous stress to the endoplasmic reticulum and other subcellular organelles that lead to subsequent apoptosis *(20)*. An additional biochemical event associated with aging is the formation of advanced glycation end products (AGEs), formed through the non-enzymatic interaction of glucose with amino groups, known as the Maillard reaction *(21)*. Glycated forms of collagen and other proteins accumulate in tissues with low levels of cellular turnover, such as bone *(21)*. Whereas AGEs have been well established as the target for diagnostic and prognostic clinical testing in diabetes, they may have an equivalent potential as biomarkers for aging. Likewise, receptors for AGEs, also known as RAGEs, may be responsible for alterations associated with aging and chronic disease *(22,23)*. The gene for one of these receptors lies within the major histocompatibility locus and has been associated with the inflammatory response *(22)*; its activation induces the NFκB transcription factor responsible for regulating the expression of pro-inflammatory cytokines such as interleukin (IL)-6 and tumor necrosis factor (TNF)-α *(24)*. The accumulated impact of each of these biochemical events results in the cellular changes characterized as "aging."

Aging and Bone Physiology

Bone development is a dynamic process that begins in the embryo and extends throughout the lifetime of the individual (Figure 2.1). The osteogenic process in the embryo provides a paradigm for our understanding of the physiology of bone in the adult and the consequences of aging. The condensation of mesenchymal stem cells (MSCs) give rise to intramembranous and endochondral bone formation in the embryo *(25)*. In the former case, the progenitor/stem cells differentiate directly into osteoblasts, whereas in the latter, the cells form chondrocytes first, which subsequently mineralize their extracellular matrix and become osteoblasts *(25)*. These events are closely linked with angiogenesis and the secretion of angiogenic factors such as vascular endothelial growth factor (VEGF) in a coordinated and time dependent manner *(25)*. Bone accumulation reflects a lifelong balance or homeostasis between bone formation by osteoblasts and bone resorption by osteoclasts. As will be discussed further, multiple hormonal, cytokine, biomechanical, nutritional, and environmental factors influence these events. Shortly after birth, adipogenesis, or the formation

Events in the Progression of Bone Development

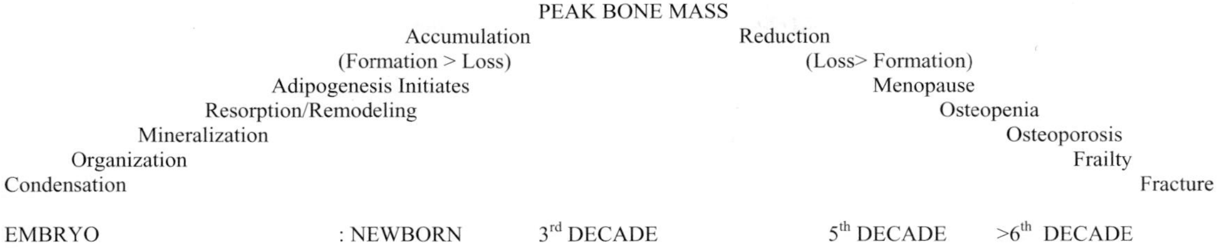

FIGURE 2.1. Events in the progression of bone development.

of fat cells, occurs within the marrow cavity of the distal phalanges and tarsal bones, and this advances proximally towards the skeleton of the thorax throughout life. These events are regulated, in part, by the body's hematopoietic demands. The human body reaches its peak bone mass during the third decade of life. After this point, bone mass decreases by as much as 1–2% per year. In women, the rate of loss is briefly accelerated during the years surrounding menopause. This puts women at greater risk of osteopenia and osteoporosis at a younger age than men. Extreme cases of osteoporosis are associated with frailty in the elderly and contribute to the high incidence of fracture in the aged population.

MSCs

The mesenchymal cells in the developing embryo give rise to the "anlagen," or condensation that ultimately forms bone. Alexander Friedenstein and his colleagues performed pioneering studies in the 1960s and 1970s identifying a subpopulation of bone marrow fibroblasts with the ability to differentiate along multiple lineage pathways, including adipocyte, chondrocyte, and osteoblast *(26)*. Over the years, these cells have been identified by many different names, including fibroblast stem cells *(27)*, mechanotyes *(26)*, nurse cells *(28)*, reticuloendothelial cells *(28,29)*, stromal cells *(30,31)*, stromal stem cells *(32,33)*, and Westin-Bainton cells *(29)*. Now recognized as mesenchymal stem cells or stromal cells *(34)*, it has been determined that MSCs continue to reside in the bone marrow microenvironment throughout life. Studies have documented that cloned MSCs retain their multipotent differentiation characteristics, consistent with the identification of a true "stem cell" *(35–37)*. These studies have led to a new appreciation of the existence of "adult" or "somatic" stem cells in multiple tissues of the body, terms that were formerly restricted to the progenitors of the hematopoietic lineages, (i.e., hematopoietic stem cells [HSCs]). A simple assay used to quantify the number of MSCs is based on their ability to form colonies when cultured *in vitro*, known as colony forming unit-fibroblast (CFU-F). Nucleated bone marrow cells are plated at limiting dilutions on a plastic surface and the number of cell "colonies" (defined as groups of more than 50 cells) with fibroblast morphology are determined after a 1- to 3-week expansion period. Based on this approach, studies have found that the number of murine bone marrow MSCs decreases with advancing age *(38)*. Likewise, in humans, the number of CFU-F decreases during the first decade of life *(39)*. In the later decades of life, between the ages of 20 to 70, the number of CFU-F remains relatively constant *(40,41)*. In conclusion, human studies show that with aging there is maintenance of CFU-F cell population size in the bone marrow, and that the observed decline in the number of CFU-F in early adulthood may represent changes in the skeletal dynamics from a modeling mode characteristic of skeletal growth and consolidation to a remodeling dynamic characteristic of the adult skeleton. This may also explain why experiments employing rodents showed a decline in the

CFU-F number as they continue to grow throughout their lifespan.

The Inverse Relationship Between Adipocytes and Osteoblasts

Clinical epidemiological observations have established that a relationship exists between adipocytes and osteoblast functions in the bone marrow microenvironment. Autopsy studies of large patient population bases of varying ages demonstrated that the percentage of the marrow cavity occupied by fat increased with advancing age *(42–46)*. Adipose accumulation was observed in the femur, iliac crest, and vertebral bodies. More recent, non-invasive studies using magnetic resonance imaging (MRI) have further documented the age-dependent increase in marrow fat *(47)*.

Work by Meunier et al. *(48)* in the early 1970s extended the initial pathological studies. Using bone marrow biopsies, they were able to draw a correlation between osteoporosis and the degree of adipogenesis in the iliac crest bone marrow cavity in a cohort of 84 subjects *(48)*. In the early 1990s, Beresford and colleagues performed pivotal studies regarding the differentiation of MSCs that provide a mechanistic understanding of these clinical observations *(49)*. They observed that cultures of bone marrow stromal cells could select the adipogenic or osteoblastic lineage pathways equally under controlled culture conditions. If, however, they delayed the addition of glucocorticoid or vitamin D3, they were able to promote osteoblast or adipoctye differentiation, respectively *(49)*. They concluded that the MSC response to nuclear hormone receptor ligands could regulate an inverse relationship between the number of adipocytes and osteoblasts in bone marrow *(49)*. Other laboratories later confirmed these important findings *(50)*. It is now recognized that a wide range of exogenous and endogenous factors can regulate MSC adipogenesis and osteogenesis in an inverse or reciprocal manner (Table 2.2). The levels of such factors may change with aging. Recent work by the Kassem laboratory has demonstrated that sera from elderly females are less able to support osteoblastic function in human MSCs as compared to that from younger females *(51)*. In contrast, both sera were equally effective in supporting adipocyte differentiation *(51)*. The specific serum components responsible for this remain to be determined.

Table 2.2. Pathways Regulating Bone Marrow MSC Adipogenic and/or Osteogenic Differentiation (52)

Nuclear hormone receptors	Transmembrane signal transduction pathways	Adipocyte-derived adipokines and factors
Vitamin D3	BMP	Adiponectin
Estrogen/Androgen	Insulin	Angiotensin
Glucocorticoids	Parathyroid hormone	Free fatty acids
LXR	TGF-β	Leptin
PPAR	Wnt Signaling	Oxidized LDLs

MSC, mesenchymal stem cell; BMP, bone morphogenetic protein; LXR, liver X recepter; TGF, transforming growth factor; PPAR, peroxisome proliferator-activated receptor; LDL, low-density lipoproteins.

Biochemical Signaling Pathways

Nuclear hormone receptors are a large family of transcription factors that control a broad range of physiological and metabolic responses. These proteins respond to small lipophilic ligands, which move easily across cell membranes as well as between cells and organs. These lipophilic activators range from fatty acids to steroids, making the nuclear hormone receptors important targets for therapeutic intervention in metabolic disorders *(53,54)*.

The peroxisome proliferator-activated receptor gamma (PPARγ) is activated by fatty acids derived from dietary and metabolic sources, and is the target of the anti-diabetic thiazolidinedione class of insulin-sensitizing drugs such as rosiglitazone and pioglitazone. PPARγ is essential for the development of adipose cells, including the adipose depots of the bone marrow *(55)*. *In vitro* studies using bone marrow-derived MSCs find that PPARγ-mediated induction of adipogenesis inhibits osteoblastic bone formation *(49,50)*. The reciprocal relationship between PPARγ activity and osteogenesis is particularly evident with increased age *(56,57)*. Recent evidence indicates that the use of thiazolidinediones in older diabetic adults may be associated with bone loss in women *(58)*. These studies indicate that therapeutic approaches to the treatment of diabetes that target PPARγ may lead to enhanced bone loss in women at risk for osteoporosis.

The glucocorticoid receptor is another nuclear hormone receptor whose activation has important therapeutic implications. Glucocorticoids are widely used because of their anti-inflammatory effects (reviewed in *59*). The side effects associated with long-term use of glucocorticoids includes increased fat accumulation and osteoporosis. *In vitro* studies show that dexamethasone treatment of bone marrow-derived mesenchymal cells leads to increased expression of genes required for adipogenesis *(60)*. These changes are associated with decreased expression of genes that regulate osteoblast formation, suggesting glucocorticoids stimulate production of bone marrow-derived adipocytes at the expense of bone formation. The effects of glucocorticoid receptor activation are particularly problematic in the aging population, which is associated with decreased osteoblast formation *(61)*.

Nuclear hormone receptors are closely linked with transmembrane signaling via the Wnt/β-catenin signaling pathway. Wnt pathways are important regulators of developmental and endocrine functions. Interaction between nuclear receptors and the Wnt pathway plays a prominent role in bone and adipocyte development. Activation of Wnt signaling blocks the formation of adipocytes by inhibiting the expression of PPARγ and C/EBPα *(62,63)*. Human studies of mutant forms of the Wnt co-receptor, the low-density lipoprotein (LDL)-related protein 5 (LRP5), demonstrate the importance of Wnt signaling in bone formation. Loss of LRP5 function is associated with decreased bone mass *(64)* whereas gain-of-function mutations in LRP5 lead to increased bone mass *(65)*. *In vitro* studies of MSCs attribute Wnt-dependent stimulation of osteogenesis to Wnt10b *(66)*, a Wnt signaling protein found in stromal vascular cells, but not adipocytes *(63)*.

The bone morphogenetic proteins (BMP) belong to the transforming growth factor beta (TGF-β) family and are important determinants of bone and fat formation. Recent studies of human bone marrow mesenchymal cells indicate BMP and Wnt signaling cooperate in regulating inhibition of adipocyte development *(67)*. In particular, BMP signaling regulates expression of Wnt10b and LRP5, both components of the Wnt pathway involved in inhibiting adipocyte formation.

Adipocytes secrete a number of proteins ("adipokines") that function as hormones through an endocrine pathway. Leptin is a 16-kDa peptide hormone that binds to the leptin receptor, a member of the cytokine receptor signaling pathway *(68)*. Originally identified as a satiety factor, leptin's role has expanded to include a range of effects, including the regulation of bone formation. Murine studies indicate that age-related loss of bone strength is accompanied by decreased serum leptin levels *(69)*. Studies of elderly men show that leptin exerts a modest effect on bone strength independent of fat mass *(70)*. Further studies demonstrate that MSCs exhibit high-affinity leptin binding when undergoing either adipogenesis or osteogenesis *(71)*. Leptin binding was decreased in mesenchymal cells derived from post-menopausal osteoporotic donors, supporting a role for leptin in determining bone strength in an elderly population.

Adiponectin is another adipocyte-secreted protein that links body weight with regulation of bone mass. Adiponectin is well-described as being secreted by white adipose tissue and having a positive effect on insulin sensitivity. Recent studies show that bone marrow-derived mesenchymal cells contain adiponectin receptors and also produce adiponectin *(72,73)*. The *in vitro* evidence suggests a complex role for adiponectin in regulating bone density. Adiponectin may act directly on bone via endocrine or autocrine pathways and indirectly via improvement of insulin sensitivity.

Resistin, a newly discovered adipokine associated with insulin resistance *(74)*, is also expressed in bone marrow-derived mesenchymal cells *(75)*. Resistin levels are inversely related to bone density *(76)* in aging men, suggesting a role for resistin in determining bone formation. Although the mechanism of action of these adipokines is not well understood, the relationship between bone and fat formation makes these proteins an important target for therapeutic intervention.

Why Fat?

The role of adipocytes in the bone marrow cavity remains an area of active investigation and speculation *(77)*. A number of teleological hypotheses have been posed:

a. That adipocytes fill up space in the marrow cavity that is not required for hematopoiesis. The marrow cavity occupies a greater volume of the adult organism relative to that of a newborn or child. Consequently, less than 100% of the volume may be required at any given time for blood cell production (passive role).
b. That adipocytes in the marrow contribute to the overall synthesis, processing, and storage of lipids and triglycerides (active role).
c. That adipocytes in the marrow serve as an energy reserve for local or systemic events requiring a rapid metabolic response (active role).
d. That adipocytes retain functions associated with other MSC lineages, such as HSC support, through the release of regulatory cytokines and the surface expression of HSC adhesion factors, and/or osteogenesis and mineralization (active role).
e. That adipocytes provide bone with mechanical advantages to withstand stresses associated with physical activity (active role).

Which Fat?

The bone marrow is just one of many adipose depots in the body (Table 2.3). Each serves a different function and has greatest importance at specific human developmental stages. Brown adipose tissue (BAT) acts as a non-shivering heat source, and is located around vital organs such as the heart, carotid arteries, kidneys, and gonads. During the critical period following birth, BAT provides neonatal humans with a survival advantage, allowing them to maintain their core body temperature with a minimum expenditure of energy. Later in life, human BAT stores disappear; however, this is not the case in small rodents or hibernating mammals. Changes in ambient temperature and daylight cycles signal the BAT stores in these animals to increase in size and activity. The BAT provides the necessary energy and heat to allow these animals to survive the winter without significant loss of body mass or function. Bone marrow adipose tissue displays some features in common with BAT. The Nobel Laureate, Charles Huggins, correlated the degree of bone marrow adiposity with the core temperature of the marrow cavity. He found that the femur and ulna (lower core temperatures) contained more marrow fat than the vertebra and ribs (higher core temperatures) *(78–80)*. Further independent studies have confirmed these initial findings *(81,82)*. In the armadillo, which has bony plates exposed close to the skin's surface, the marrow cavity transitions between a red (hematopoietic) and yellow (fatty) phenotype in accordance with the season and ambient temperature *(82)*. Comparable manipulation of the marrow fat can be achieved using hematopoietic stressors or stimuli. Under conditions of anemia, owing to exposure to phenylhydrazine, prolonged hypoxia, or in response to sickle cell disease, adiposity within the marrow cavity is reduced *(83–88)*. Under conditions of artificial polycythemia (hypertransfusion), in contrast, marrow adiposity is increased *(89)*.

Table 2.3. Adipose Tissue Depots in Man (93)

Type of adipose tissue depot	Function
Brown	Non-shivering thermogenesis
Bone marrow	Multiple—hematopoietic, energy and lipid metabolism, other?
Mammary	Lactation support
Mechanical	Weight-bearing stress protection
White	Energy reservoir

Bone marrow adipose tissue displays features in common with white adipose tissue (WAT) as well. In some species, such as rabbit, bone marrow fat plays an active role in clearing chylomicrons and triglycerides from the circulation *(90,91)*. Under conditions of extreme starvation or anorexia, bone marrow adipose depots are depleted to an extent equivalent to WAT *(92)*. It remains to be determined if bone marrow adipose tissue provides any weight-bearing advantage to bone from a biomechanical/bioengineering perspective.

What Makes It Bone Versus Fat?

Genetic factors exert considerable influence over the physiology and pathology of MSC differentiation and bone formation or loss. Specific genes have been identified that are associated with exceptionally strong or weak bone phenotypes. An example is LRP5, which functions as a receptor for the Wnt signal transduction pathway. In families with a dominant negative mutation in LRP5, inheritance of the gene leads to a condition known as osteoporosis-psuedoglioma, associated with defective bone formation *(64)*. Likewise, in families with a constitutively active mutation in LRP5, inheritance gives subjects a bone phenotype that appears to be impervious to fracture *(65,94)*. These clinical findings are consistent with *in vitro* and *in vivo* murine studies. Activation of Wnt signaling transduction inhibits the adipogenic pathway in cell models *(62,63)*. When transgenic mice over-express Wnt10b under the control of an adipocyte-specific promoter, their bone marrow lacks adipocytes and displays increased evidence of osteoblast activity *(66)*. At a broader level, genetic factors associated with ethnicity influence bone physiology. For example, the risk of osteoporosis is greater in Caucasian and Asian women as compared to those of African-American origins; however, the genetic basis for this remains an area of active investigation. Nevertheless, there is little evidence that this phenomenon is caused by bone instead of fat formation.

Epigenetic factors exert a level of influence comparable to genetic factors. Physical activity has a direct relationship to bone mass and bone health. In industrialized societies, even "healthy" individuals spend less time each day in physical activity as they enter the work force. An individual's level of high impact exercise correlates with increased bone formation and bone strength. Weight-bearing activities, such as gymnastics and high-impact exercise, enhance bone metabolism and remodeling. In contrast, enforced bed rest is associated with a reduction in bone mass and bone strength. Patients with chronic illness who are bed-ridden, a condition more frequently observed in aged populations, are therefore at increased risk of osteoporotic changes. With prolonged space flight, physicians and investigators have determined that weightlessness is detrimental to osteogenesis. The net bone loss may reflect both osteoblastic bone formation and/or enhanced osteoclastic bone resorption.

The physical environment also determines an individual's sun exposure and, consequently, the biosynthesis of vitamin D and its active metabolites. These nuclear hormone receptor ligands play a critical role in regulating calcium metabolism in the bone, intestine, and kidney, with subsequent consequences on parathyroid hormone action. Whether an individual works indoors or outdoors will have a direct bearing on vitamin D pathways. In many elderly, the hours spent outdoors decrease as fitness declines, resulting in low or inadequate levels of vitamin D receptor ligands.

Nutrition has been a target to offset the risk of vitamin D deficiency. We now fortify milk products with Vitamin D3 to insure that individuals receive a minimum daily level; however, because many elderly reduce their intake of dairy products for reasons of taste or lactose intolerance, this strategy is not always effective. Nutrition exerts other effects on bone and fat metabolism. Dietary components such as flavinoids and antioxidants have been linked to osteoblast differentiation and longevity (*see* apoptosis). Conjugated linoleic acid (CLA), a component of animal fats, has been found to reduce adipose tissue depots in animal models *(95)*. Independent studies indicate that CLA can increase bone mass *(96)*, and this appears to be mediated through effects inhibiting the formation and activation of osteoclasts via the receptor activator of the NFκB ligand (RANKL) signaling pathway *(97)*.

When dietary nutrition leads to a state where net energy consumption exceeds energy demands, it often results in obesity. Although obesity manifests as an abundance of extramedullary WAT, it correlates with enhanced bone mass *(98)*. Several factors may account for this. First, with increased weight, an individual's skeleton is forced to bear greater loads. Biomechanical stimuli may enhance bone formation relative to bone resorption. Second, obesity alters circulating hormone levels, directly or indirectly. Adipocytes express aromatase, allowing these cells to generate estrogenic-like compounds *(98)*. Adipocytes secrete insulin-like growth factors, and obesity is associated with hyperinsulinemia secondary to insulin resistance, both of which can lead to bone protection; clinical analyses support this hypothesis *(98)*. Obesity has also been associated with elevated levels of parathyroid hormone *(99)*. Third, adipokines such as leptin have been associated with positive effects on osteoblast differentiation and mineralization in murine *in vitro* and *in vivo* models while inhibiting adipogenesis *(100,101)*. These leptin effects seem to be mediated through peripheral mechanisms acting locally within the marrow microenvironment. Independent studies suggest that leptin administered by intra-ventricular injection causes bone loss through centrally mediated mechanisms involving the hypothalamus *(102,103)*. The development of leptin resistance and the activity of the blood brain barrier may account for the apparent discrepancy in these data. Another adipokine, adiponectin, has been associated with MSC differentiation and altered bone mineral density. Unlike other adipokines, adiponectin decreases with obesity *(104)*. When added to murine bone marrow stromal cells, adiponectin inhibited adipocyte differentiation through a COX2-mediated pathway *(105)*. Transgenic mice over-expressing adiponectin displayed increased bone mass owing to enhanced osteoblast activity and suppressed osteoclast function *(106)*. Both adiponectin and its receptors have been detected in human MSCs *(72)*, and adiponectin levels have been inversely correlated to bone mineral density in clinical studies *(104,107)*. As with leptin, the mechanism of adiponectin actions will require further investigation.

Menopause is associated with a rapid decline in circulating estrogen, and as a consequence there is trabecular bone loss, which results in a loss of bone strength. Paradoxically, there are increases in bone size (medullary bone and periosteal diameter) after menopause. The increase in size is caused by increased periosteal apposition, which partially preserves strength *(108)*. Loss of bone mass that follows the loss of ovarian function is associated with an increase in the rates of bone resorption and bone formation, with the former exceeding the latter, and an increase in the number of osteoclasts in trabecular bone. Post-menopausal bone loss is associated with excessive osteoclast activity. In addition to these marrow changes, menopause is associated with a gain in fat mass and a loss of lean body mass, but these changes in body composition are not prevented by hormone replacement therapy *(109)*. It is clear that the loss of ovarian function causes dramatic changes to bone marrow cell activity as well as extramedullary cell activity. In addition, menopause results in quite dramatic changes in susceptibility to certain diseases such as cardiovascular disease. It is complex to tease out what drives these changes because of the complexity of the cell systems involved and the interplay between different cell types. In terms of bone turnover, there appear to be effects on the development and activity of both osteoblasts and osteoclasts.

Data indicate that changes in estrogen status *in vivo* are associated with the secretion of mononuclear cell immune factors *in vitro* and suggest that alterations in the local production of bone-acting cytokines may underlie changes in bone turnover caused by surgically induced menopause and estrogen replacement *(110)*. There is now a large body of evidence suggesting that the decline in ovarian function with menopause is associated with spontaneous increases in pro-inflammatory cytokines. The cytokines that have obtained the most attention are interleukin (IL)-1, IL-6, granulocyte-macrophage colony-stimulating factor (GM-CSF), and TNF-α. The exact mechanisms by which estrogen interferes with cytokine activity are still incompletely known but may potentially include interactions of the estrogen receptor with other transcription factors, modulation of nitric oxide activity, antioxidative effects, plasma membrane actions, and changes in immune cell function. Experimental and clinical studies strongly support a link between the increased state of pro-inflammatory cytokine activity and post-menopausal bone loss *(111)*.

The production of IL-6 by stromal–osteoblastic cells, as well as the responsiveness of bone marrow cells to cytokines such as IL-6 and IL-11, is regulated by sex steroids. When gonadal function is lost, the formation of osteoclasts as well as osteoblasts increases in the marrow, both changes apparently mediated by an increase in the production of IL-6. These changes may also be due to an increase in the responsiveness of bone marrow progenitor cells not only to IL-6 but also to other cytokines with osteoclastogenic and osteoblastogenic properties. This is supported by both *in vitro* and *ex vivo* experimental data. Osteoclast formation in response to either IL-6 in combination with the soluble IL-6 receptor or IL-11 is significantly greater in cultures of bone marrow from ovariectomized mice than in cultures from mice that have undergone sham operations, even when the cultures have the same number of osteoblastic support cells and an IL-6 signal of the same magnitude. These findings indicate that not only the production of the osteoclast precursors but also their responsiveness to IL-6 (and to IL-11) are enhanced in a state of estrogen deficiency.

Studies of the effect of ovariectomy on the formation of osteoblast progenitors in cultures of bone marrow suggest that loss of ovarian function increased osteoblastic activity. The number of fibroblast CFUs is increased several-fold in ovariectomized mice. At this stage there is no mechanistic explanation for the observation that the formation of osteoclasts and the formation of osteoblast progenitors in the marrow increase simultaneously after the loss of ovarian function. It has been hypothesized that changes in levels of systemic hormones alters the sensitivity of osteoblast and osteoclast precursors to several cytokine signals by modulating glycoprotein 130 *(112)*. It is clear that there is still considerable work to be done before we fully understand the control of marrow cell development and activity under normal physiological condition and after menopause. It will be interesting to understand whether sex steroids themselves positively drive activity and/or development of osteoclast and osteoblast progenitors and menopause results in the removal of this activity or, paradoxically, whether gonadal steroids inhibit/control bone formation and resorption and menopause results in the relief of this repression.

Apoptosis and the Aging Bone

Apoptosis, or programmed cell death, has been postulated to act as a cellular mechanism accounting for the effects of aging on bone *(1)* (Table 2.4). Apoptosis is initiated by the activation of a proteolytic enzyme cascade, leading to cellular self-destruction. Unlike cell death caused by necrosis, apoptotic cell death is characterized by cell shrinkage and disintegration without damage to the neighboring cells. Pioneering studies by Jilka and colleagues demonstrated that cytokines such as TNF induced apoptosis in MSC-like cell lines *in vitro (113)*. To further address the mechanism, Weinstein, Jilka, and colleagues used an *in vivo* murine model to examine the potential apoptotic effects of glucocorticoids *(114)*. Chronic treatment with glucocorticoids activated apoptotic pathways in osteoblasts and osteocytes of the intact bone while reducing osteoblastogenesis *(114)*. Additional causes of osteoblast and osteocytes apoptosis have been identified. Thiazolidinedione compounds, known ligands for the peroxisome proliferator-activated receptor γ adipogenic transcription factor, stimulated osteoblast and osteocytes apoptotic events when administered to mice *(115)*. In rodents maintained under conditions simulating weightlessness, there was a rapid increase in the number of apoptotic osteoblasts within the bone; this was followed by increased numbers of osteoclasts and bone resorption *(116)*. The addition of AGEs to cultures of human MSCs led to increased numbers of apoptotic cells, and this correlated with a reduced capacity for differentiation *(117)*.

A number of agents antagonize apoptosis in osteoblasts and osteocytes. Endocrine factors such as parathyroid hormone and calcitonin increased bone formation by protecting osteoblasts from apoptosis in rodent models *(118,119)*. Similar actions are displayed by the active form of

Table 2.4. Cellular Apoptosis in the Marrow Microenvironment

Cell type	Agonists	Antagonists
Osteoblast/Osteocyte	Glucocorticoids and thiazolidinediones	Bisphosphonates, $1,25(OH)_2D_3$, calcitonin
	AGE	α-Linoleic acid
	TNF	CD40 ligand
	Weightlessness	TGF-β, IL-6, PTH
Osteoclasts	Bisphosphonates	
	β 3 integrin	
Adipocytes	CLA	Glucocorticoids
	TNF	
	Retinoic acid	

AGE, advanced glycated end product; TNF, tumor necrosis factor; TGF, transforming growth factor; IL, interleukin; PTH, parathyroid hormone; CLA, conjugated linoleic acid.

vitamin D ($1,25(OH)_2D_3$) *(120)* and cytokines including TGF-β and those acting through the gp130 receptor pathway, such as IL-6 and oncostatin M *(113)*. Pharmaceutical agents such as the bisphosphonates exert anti-apoptotic effects on osteoblasts through mechanisms involving the extracellular signal-regulated kinases (ERKs) and the connexin43 channel *(120)*. Likewise, lipids such as α-linoleic acid blocked apoptosis in human bone marrow-derived MSCs exposed to TNF-α or hydrogen peroxide *(121)*. It appeared that the α-linoleic acid prevented the generation of reactive oxygen species and subsequent activation of the NFκB and c-jun N-terminal kinase pathways *(121)*. Finally, because osteoblasts express the TNF receptor-related surface protein CD40, interaction with the CD40 ligand serves to protect them from apoptosis initiated by a variety of agents, including glucocorticoids, TNF-α, and proteasomal activators *(122)*.

Despite these findings, without apoptosis, bone formation may be impaired. Studies of mice deficient in the enzyme caspase-3, critical to the apoptotic cascade, found that they displayed reduced bone formation *in vivo* and reduced bone marrow-derived MSC differentiation *in vitro (123)*. These findings could be mimicked using a caspase-3 inhibitor in wild-type mice *(123)*. Biochemical studies implicated the TGF-β/Smad signal transduction pathway as the underlying mechanism *(123)*. Independent studies created a transgenic mouse over-expressing the bcl2 anti-apoptotic protein under an osteoblast-selective promoter *(124)*. Although the osteoblasts isolated from the transgenic bone were resistant to glucocorticoid-induced apoptosis, the cells displayed reduced mineralization. The transgenic mice were smaller than their wild-type littermates *(124)*. Thus, osteoblastic apoptosis is a complex phenomenon that may have both positive and negative effects on bone formation.

Apoptotic events influence the activity of other cell types within the bone marrow microenvironment. Osteoclasts undergo apoptosis in response to bisphosphonates or in the absence vitronectin, the natural ligand for α3β1 integrin *(125,126)*. Bisphosphonates are the accepted standard of care for the treatment of osteoporosis in the elderly. Whereas few, if any, studies have been performed on bone marrow-derived adipocytes, evidence from extramedullary adipocytes indicates that they are relatively resistant to apoptotic stimuli caused by induced levels of bcl2 *(127)*. Nevertheless, adipocytes undergo apoptosis in response to TNF-α *(128)*, although this occurs in a depot-specific pattern; adipocytes from omental fat were more susceptible than those from subcutaneous fat *(129)*. The relative apoptotic sensitivity of bone marrow adipocytes has not been reported. Additional agents exert apoptotic actions on adipocytes, including CLA, retinoic acid, botanical extracts, and cytokines acting through the gp130 receptor *(95,130,131)*. Some investigators postulate that pharmaceutical agents and/or functional foods targeting the adipocyte apoptotic pathway will have the combined benefit of reducing obesity while improving bone growth by reducing bone marrow adipogenesis and enhancing osteoblast function *(131)*.

References

1. Carrington JL. Aging bone and cartilage: cross-cutting issues. Biochem Biophys Res Commun 2005;328(3):700–708.
2. Kirkwood TB, Austad SN. Why do we age? Nature 2000;408(6809):233–238.
3. Miller RA. When will the biology of aging become useful? Future landmarks in biomedical gerontology. J Am Geriatr Soc 1997;45(10):1258–1267.
4. Busuttil RA, Dolle M, Campisi J, et al. Genomic instability, aging, and cellular senescence. Ann N Y Acad Sci 2004;1019:245–255.
5. Hayflick L. The limited in vitro lifetime of human diploid cell strains. Exp Cell Res 1965;37: 614–636.
6. Campisi J. From cells to organisms: can we learn about aging from cells in culture? Exp Gerontol 2001;36(4–6):607–618.
7. Cristofalo VJ, Allen RG, Pignolo RJ, et al. Relationship between donor age and the replicative lifespan of human cells in culture: a reevaluation. Proc Natl Acad Sci U S A 1998;95(18):10614–10619.
8. Kassem M, Ankersen L, Eriksen EF, et al. Demonstration of cellular aging and senescence in serially passaged long-term cultures of human trabecular osteoblasts. Osteoporos Int 1997;7(6): 514–524.
9. Kveiborg M, Rattan SI, Clark BF, et al. Treatment with 1,25-dihydroxyvitamin D3 reduces impairment of human osteoblast functions during

cellular aging in culture. J Cell Physiol 2001;186(2): 298–306.
10. Dimri GP, Lee X, Basile G, et al. A biomarker that identifies senescent human cells in culture and in aging skin in vivo. Proc Natl Acad Sci U S A 1995;92(20):9363–9367.
11. Allsopp RC, Chang E, Kashefi-Aazam M, et al. Telomere shortening is associated with cell division in vitro and in vivo. Exp Cell Res 1995; 220(1):194–200.
12. Harley CB, Futcher AB, Greider CW. Telomeres shorten during ageing of human fibroblasts. Nature 1990;345(6274):458–460.
13. Harley CB. Telomere loss: mitotic clock or genetic time bomb? Mutat Res 1991;256(2–6): 271–282.
14. Bandyopadhyay D, Medrano EE. The emerging role of epigenetics in cellular and organismal aging. Exp Gerontol 2003;38(11–12):1299–1307.
15. Lesnefsky EJ, Hoppel CL. Oxidative phosphorylation and aging. Ageing Res Rev 2006;5(4):402–433.
16. Harman D. Aging: a theory based on free radical and radiation chemistry. J Gerontol 1956;11(3): 298–300.
17. Finkel T, Holbrook NJ. Oxidants, oxidative stress and the biology of ageing. Nature 2000;408(6809): 239–247.
18. Li J, Holbrook NJ. Common mechanisms for declines in oxidative stress tolerance and proliferation with aging. Free Radic Biol Med 2003; 35(3):292–299.
19. Ikeyama S, Wang XT, Li J, et al. Expression of the pro-apoptotic gene gadd153/chop is elevated in liver with aging and sensitizes cells to oxidant injury. J Biol Chem 2003;278(19):16726–16731.
20. Li J, Holbrook NJ. Elevated gadd153/chop expression and enhanced c-Jun N-terminal protein kinase activation sensitizes aged cells to ER stress. Exp Gerontol 2004;39(5):735–744.
21. DeGroot J. The AGE of the matrix: chemistry, consequence and cure. Curr Opin Pharmacol 2004;4(3):301–305.
22. Schmidt AM, Stern DM. Receptor for age (RAGE) is a gene within the major histocompatibility class III region: implications for host response mechanisms in homeostasis and chronic disease. Front Biosci 2001;6:D1151–D1160.
23. Pricci F, Leto G, Amadio L, et al. Role of galectin-3 as a receptor for advanced glycosylation end products. Kidney Int Suppl 2000;77:S31–S39.
24. Yan SD, Schmidt AM, Anderson GM, et al. Enhanced cellular oxidant stress by the interaction of advanced glycation end products with their receptors/binding proteins. J Biol Chem 1994; 269(13):9889–9897.
25. Olsen BR. *Bone embryology, 6th edition*. Washington, DC: American Society for Bone and Mineral Research; 2006.
26. Friedenstein AJ. Precursor cells of mechanocytes. Int Rev Cytol 1976;47:327–359.
27. Friedenstein AJ, Chailakhjan RK, Lalykina KS. The development of fibroblast colonies in monolayer cultures of guinea-pig bone marrow and spleen cells. Cell Tissue Kinet 1970;3(4):393–403.
28. Foy H, Kondi A. Reticulo-endothelial cells as 'nurses' for plasma cells and erythroblasts in baboons. Nature 1964;204:293.
29. Westen H, Bainton DF. Association of alkaline-phosphatase-positive reticulum cells in bone marrow with granulocytic precursors. J Exp Med 1979;150(4):919–937.
30. Gimble JM, Pietrangeli C, Henley A, et al. Characterization of murine bone marrow and spleen-derived stromal cells: analysis of leukocyte marker and growth factor mRNA transcript levels. Blood 1989;74(1):303–311.
31. Weiss L, Sakai H. The hematopoietic stroma. Am J Anat 1984;170(3):447–463.
32. Owen M. Marrow stromal stem cells. J Cell Sci Suppl 1988;10:63–76.
33. Owen M, Friedenstein AJ. Stromal stem cells: marrow-derived osteogenic precursors. Ciba Found Symp 1988;136:42–60.
34. Caplan AI. Mesenchymal stem cells. J Orthop Res 1991;9(5):641–650.
35. Nuttall ME, Patton AJ, Olivera DL, et al. Human trabecular bone cells are able to express both osteoblastic and adipocytic phenotype: implications for osteopenic disorders. J Bone Miner Res 1998;13(3):371–382.
36. Pittenger MF, Mackay AM, Beck SC, et al. Multilineage potential of adult human mesenchymal stem cells. Science 1999;284(5411):143–147.
37. Grigoriadis AE, Heersche JN, Aubin JE. Differentiation of muscle, fat, cartilage, and bone from progenitor cells present in a bone-derived clonal cell population: effect of dexamethasone. J Cell Biol 1988;106(6):2139–2151.
38. Jiang D, Fei RG, Pendergrass WR, et al. An age-related reduction in the replicative capacity of two murine hematopoietic stroma cell types. Exp Hematol 1992;20(10):1216–1222.
39. D'Ippolito G, Schiller PC, Ricordi C, et al. Age-related osteogenic potential of mesenchymal stromal stem cells from human vertebral bone marrow. J Bone Miner Res 1999;14(7):1115–1122.

40. Stenderup K, Justesen J, Eriksen EF, et al. Number and proliferative capacity of osteogenic stem cells are maintained during aging and in patients with osteoporosis. J Bone Miner Res 2001;16(6): 1120–1129.
41. Justesen J, Stenderup K, Eriksen EF, et al. Maintenance of osteoblastic and adipocytic differentiation potential with age and osteoporosis in human marrow stromal cell cultures. Calcif Tissue Int 2002;71(1):36–44.
42. Custer RP AF. Studies on the structure and function of bone marrow. II. Variations in cellularity in various bones with advancing years of life and their relative response to stimuli. J Lab Clin Med 1932;17:960–962.
43. Hartsock RJ, Smith EB, Petty CS. Normal variations with aging of the amount of hematopoietic tissue in bone marrow from the anterior iliac crest. A study made from 177 cases of sudden death examined by necropsy. Am J Clin Pathol 1965;43:326–331.
44. Vost A. Osteoporosis: a necropsy study of vertebrae and iliac crests. Am J Pathol 1963;43: 143–151.
45. Hudson G. Bone-marrow volume in the human foetus and newborn. Br J Haematol 1965;11: 446–452.
46. Hudson G. Organ size of human foetal bone marrow. Nature 1965;205:96–97.
47. Babyn PS, Ranson M, McCarville ME. Normal bone marrow: signal characteristics and fatty conversion. Magn Reson Imaging Clin N Am 1998; 6(3):473–495.
48. Meunier P, Aaron J, Edouard C, et al. Osteoporosis and the replacement of cell populations of the marrow by adipose tissue. A quantitative study of 84 iliac bone biopsies. Clin Orthop Relat Res 1971;80:147–154.
49. Beresford JN, Bennett JH, Devlin C, et al. Evidence for an inverse relationship between the differentiation of adipocytic and osteogenic cells in rat marrow stromal cell cultures. J Cell Sci 1992;102 (Pt 2):341–351.
50. Dorheim MA, Sullivan M, Dandapani V, et al. Osteoblastic gene expression during adipogenesis in hematopoietic supporting murine bone marrow stromal cells. J Cell Physiol 1993;154(2):317–328.
51. Abdallah BM, Haack-Sorensen M, Fink T, et al. Inhibition of osteoblast differentiation but not adipocyte differentiation of mesenchymal stem cells by sera obtained from aged females. Bone 2006;39(1):181–188.
52. Gimble JM, Zvonic S, Floyd ZE, et al. Playing with bone and fat. J Cell Biochem 2006;98(2):251–266.
53. Takada I, Suzawa M, Kato S. Nuclear receptors as targets for drug development: crosstalk between peroxisome proliferator-activated receptor gamma and cytokines in bone marrow-derived mesenchymal stem cells. J Pharmacol Sci 2005; 97(2):184–189.
54. Nettles KW, Greene GL. Ligand control of coregulator recruitment to nuclear receptors. Annu Rev Physiol 2005;67:309–333.
55. Gimble JM, Robinson CE, Wu X, et al. Peroxisome proliferator-activated receptor-gamma activation by thiazolidinediones induces adipogenesis in bone marrow stromal cells. Mol Pharmacol 1996; 50(5):1087–1094.
56. Akune T, Ohba S, Kamekura S, et al. PPARgamma insufficiency enhances osteogenesis through osteoblast formation from bone marrow progenitors. J Clin Invest 2004;113(6):846–855.
57. Kawaguchi H, Akune T, Yamaguchi M, et al. Distinct effects of PPARgamma insufficiency on bone marrow cells, osteoblasts, and osteoclastic cells. J Bone Miner Metab 2005;23(4):275–279.
58. Schwartz AV, Sellmeyer DE, Vittinghoff E, et al. Thiazolidinedione (TZD) use and bone loss in older diabetic adults. J Clin Endocrinol Metab 2006.
59. Rosen J, Miner JN. The search for safer glucocorticoid receptor ligands. Endocr Rev 2005;26(3): 452–464.
60. Li X, Jin L, Cui Q, et al. Steroid effects on osteogenesis through mesenchymal cell gene expression. Osteoporos Int 2005;16(1):101–108.
61. Srouji S, Livne E. Bone marrow stem cells and biological scaffold for bone repair in aging and disease. Mech Ageing Dev 2005;126(2):281–287.
62. Bennett CN, Ross SE, Longo KA, et al. Regulation of Wnt signaling during adipogenesis. J Biol Chem 2002;277(34):30998–31004.
63. Ross SE, Hemati N, Longo KA, et al. Inhibition of adipogenesis by Wnt signaling. Science 2000; 289(5481):950–953.
64. Gong Y, Slee RB, Fukai N, et al. LDL receptor-related protein 5 (LRP5) affects bone accrual and eye development. Cell 2001;107(4):513–523.
65. Boyden LM, Mao J, Belsky J, et al. High bone density due to a mutation in LDL-receptor-related protein 5. N Engl J Med 2002;346(20):1513–1521.
66. Bennett CN, Longo KA, Wright WS, et al. Regulation of osteoblastogenesis and bone mass by Wnt10b. Proc Natl Acad Sci U S A 2005;102(9): 3324–3329.
67. Zhou S, Eid K, Glowacki J. Cooperation between TGF-beta and Wnt pathways during chondrocyte and adipocyte differentiation of human marrow

stromal cells. J Bone Miner Res 2004;19(3):463–470.
68. Tartaglia LA, Dembski M, Weng X, et al. Identification and expression cloning of a leptin receptor, OB-R. Cell 1995;83(7):1263–1271.
69. Hamrick MW, Ding KH, Pennington C, et al. Age-related loss of muscle mass and bone strength in mice is associated with a decline in physical activity and serum leptin. Bone 2006;39(4):845–853.
70. Crabbe P, Goemaere S, Zmierczak H, et al. Are serum leptin and the Gln223Arg polymorphism of the leptin receptor determinants of bone homeostasis in elderly men? Eur J Endocrinol 2006;154(5):707–714.
71. Hess R, Pino AM, Rios S, et al. High affinity leptin receptors are present in human mesenchymal stem cells (MSCs) derived from control and osteoporotic donors. J Cell Biochem 2005;94(1): 50–57.
72. Berner HS, Lyngstadaas SP, Spahr A, et al. Adiponectin and its receptors are expressed in bone-forming cells. Bone 2004;35(4):842–849.
73. Shinoda Y, Yamaguchi M, Ogata N, et al. Regulation of bone formation by adiponectin through autocrine/paracrine and endocrine pathways. J Cell Biochem 2006;99(1):196–208.
74. Steppan CM, Bailey ST, Bhat S, et al. The hormone resistin links obesity to diabetes. Nature 2001; 409(6818):307–312.
75. Thommesen L, Stunes AK, Monjo M, et al. Expression and regulation of resistin in osteoblasts and osteoclasts indicate a role in bone metabolism. J Cell Biochem 2006;99(3):824–834.
76. Oh KW, Lee WY, Rhee EJ, et al. The relationship between serum resistin, leptin, adiponectin, ghrelin levels and bone mineral density in middle-aged men. Clin Endocrinol (Oxf) 2005;63(2): 131–138.
77. Gimble JM, Robinson CE, Wu X, et al. The function of adipocytes in the bone marrow stroma: an update. Bone 1996;19(5):421–428.
78. Huggins C, Blocksom, BH. Changes in outlying bone marrow accompanying a local increase within physiological limits. J Exp Med 1936;64: 253–274.
79. Huggins C, Blocksom, BH, Noonan, WJ. Temperature conditions in bone marrow of rabbit, pigeon, and albino rat. Am J Physiol 1936;115:395–401.
80. Huggins C, Noonan, WJ. An increase in reticulo-endothelial cells in outlying bone marrow consequent upon a local increase in temperature. J Exp Med 1936;64:275–280.
81. Petrakis NL. Some physiological and developmental considerations of the temperature-gradient hypothesis of bone marrow distribution. Am J Phys Anthropol 1966;25(2):119–129.
82. Weiss LP, Wislocki, GB. Seasonal variations in hematopoiesis in the dermal bones of the nine-banded armidillo. Anat Rec 1956;123:143–163.
83. Tavassoli M. Marrow adipose cells and hemopoiesis: an interpretative review. Exp Hematol 1984;12(2):139–146.
84. Maniatis A, Tavassoli M, Crosby WH. Factors affecting the conversion of yellow to red marrow. Blood 1971;37(5):581–586.
85. Tavassoli M, Crosby WH. Bone marrow histogenesis: a comparison of fatty and red marrow. Science 1970;169(942):291–293.
86. Tavassoli M, Maniatis A, Crosby WH. Induction of sustained hemopoiesis in fatty marrow. Blood 1974;43(1):33–38.
87. Tavassoli M, Maniatis A, Crosby WH. The effects of phenylhydrazine-induced haemolysis on the behaviour of regenerating marrow stroma. Br J Haematol 1972;23(6):707–711.
88. Bathija A, Davis S, Trubowitz S. Marrow adipose tissue: response to erythropoiesis. Am J Hematol 1978;5(4):315–321.
89. Brookoff D, Weiss L. Adipocyte development and the loss of erythropoietic capacity in the bone marrow of mice after sustained hypertransfusion. Blood 1982;60(6):1337–1344.
90. Hussain MM, Mahley RW, Boyles JK, et al. Chylomicron-chylomicron remnant clearance by liver and bone marrow in rabbits. Factors that modify tissue-specific uptake. J Biol Chem 1989;264(16): 9571–9582.
91. Hussain MM, Mahley RW, Boyles JK, et al. Chylomicron metabolism. Chylomicron uptake by bone marrow in different animal species. J Biol Chem 1989;264(30):17931–17938.
92. Tavassoli M, Eastlund DT, Yam LT, et al. Gelatinous transformation of bone marrow in prolonged self-induced starvation. Scand J Haematol 1976; 16(4):311–319.
93. Gimble JM, Nuttall ME. Bone and fat: old questions, new insights. Endocrine 2004;23(2–3):183–188.
94. Little RD, Carulli JP, Del Mastro RG, et al. A mutation in the LDL receptor-related protein 5 gene results in the autosomal dominant high-bone-mass trait. Am J Hum Genet 2002;70(1): 11–19.
95. Hargrave KM, Li C, Meyer BJ, et al. Adipose depletion and apoptosis induced by trans-10, cis-12 conjugated linoleic acid in mice. Obes Res 2002;10(12):1284–1290.

96. Park Y, Albright KJ, Liu W, et al. Effect of conjugated linoleic acid on body composition in mice. Lipids 1997;32(8):853–858.
97. Rahman MM, Bhattacharya A, Fernandes G. Conjugated linoleic acid inhibits osteoclast differentiation of RAW264.7 cells by modulating RANKL signaling. J Lipid Res 2006;47(8):1739–1748.
98. Reid IR. Relationships among body mass, its components, and bone. Bone 2002;31(5):547–555.
99. Bolland MJ, Grey AB, Ames RW, et al. Fat mass is an important predictor of parathyroid hormone levels in postmenopausal women. Bone 2006; 38(3):317–321.
100. Hamrick MW, Della-Fera MA, Choi YH, et al. Leptin treatment induces loss of bone marrow adipocytes and increases bone formation in leptin-deficient ob/ob mice. J Bone Miner Res 2005; 20(6):994–1001.
101. Thomas T, Gori F, Khosla S, et al. Leptin acts on human marrow stromal cells to enhance differentiation to osteoblasts and to inhibit differentiation to adipocytes. Endocrinology 1999;140(4):1630–1638.
102. Takeda S, Elefteriou F, Levasseur R, et al. Leptin regulates bone formation via the sympathetic nervous system. Cell 2002;111(3):305–317.
103. Ducy P, Amling M, Takeda S, et al. Leptin inhibits bone formation through a hypothalamic relay: a central control of bone mass. Cell 2000;100(2): 197–207.
104. Lenchik L, Register TC, Hsu FC, et al. Adiponectin as a novel determinant of bone mineral density and visceral fat. Bone 2003;33(4):646–651.
105. Yokota T, Meka CS, Medina KL, et al. Paracrine regulation of fat cell formation in bone marrow cultures via adiponectin and prostaglandins. J Clin Invest 2002;109(10):1303–1310.
106. Oshima K, Nampei A, Matsuda M, et al. Adiponectin increases bone mass by suppressing osteoclast and activating osteoblast. Biochem Biophys Res Commun 2005;331(2):520–526.
107. Jurimae J, Rembel K, Jurimae T, et al. Adiponectin is associated with bone mineral density in perimenopausal women. Horm Metab Res 2005; 37(5):297–302.
108. Ahlborg HG, Johnell O, Turner CH, et al. Bone loss and bone size after menopause. N Engl J Med 2003;349(4):327–334.
109. Aloia JF, Vaswani A, Russo L, et al. The influence of menopause and hormonal replacement therapy on body cell mass and body fat mass. Am J Obstet Gynecol 1995;172(3):896–900.
110. Pacifici R, Brown C, Puscheck E, et al. Effect of surgical menopause and estrogen replacement on cytokine release from human blood mononuclear cells. Proc Natl Acad Sci U S A 1991;88(12): 5134–5138.
111. Pfeilschifter J, Koditz R, Pfohl M, et al. Changes in proinflammatory cytokine activity after menopause. Endocr Rev 2002;23(1):90–119.
112. Manolagas SC, Jilka RL. Bone marrow, cytokines, and bone remodeling. Emerging insights into the pathophysiology of osteoporosis. N Engl J Med 1995;332(5):305–311.
113. Jilka RL, Weinstein RS, Bellido T, et al. Osteoblast programmed cell death (apoptosis): modulation by growth factors and cytokines. J Bone Miner Res 1998;13(5):793–802.
114. Weinstein RS, Jilka RL, Parfitt AM, et al. Inhibition of osteoblastogenesis and promotion of apoptosis of osteoblasts and osteocytes by glucocorticoids. Potential mechanisms of their deleterious effects on bone. J Clin Invest 1998;102(2): 274–282.
115. Soroceanu MA, Miao D, Bai XY, et al. Rosiglitazone impacts negatively on bone by promoting osteoblast/osteocyte apoptosis. J Endocrinol 2004; 183(1):203–216.
116. Aguirre JI, Plotkin LI, Stewart SA, et al. Osteocyte apoptosis is induced by weightlessness in mice and precedes osteoclast recruitment and bone loss. J Bone Miner Res 2006;21(4):605–615.
117. Kume S, Kato S, Yamagishi S, et al. Advanced glycation end-products attenuate human mesenchymal stem cells and prevent cognate differentiation into adipose tissue, cartilage, and bone. J Bone Miner Res 2005;20(9):1647–1658.
118. Jilka RL, Weinstein RS, Bellido T, et al. Increased bone formation by prevention of osteoblast apoptosis with parathyroid hormone. J Clin Invest 1999;104(4):439–446.
119. Plotkin LI, Weinstein RS, Parfitt AM, et al. Prevention of osteocyte and osteoblast apoptosis by bisphosphonates and calcitonin. J Clin Invest 1999;104(10):1363–1374.
120. Duque G, El Abdaimi K, Henderson JE, Lomri A, Kremer R. Vitamin D inhibits Fas ligand-induced apoptosis in human osteoblasts by regulating components of both the mitochondrial and Fas-related pathways. Bone 2004;35(1):57–64.
121. Plotkin LI, Manolagas SC, Bellido T. Dissociation of the pro-apoptotic effects of bisphosphonates on osteoclasts from their anti-apoptotic effects on osteoblasts/osteocytes with novel analogs. Bone 2006;39(3):443–452.
122. Ahuja SS, Zhao S, Bellido T, et al. CD40 ligand blocks apoptosis induced by tumor necrosis factor alpha, glucocorticoids, and etoposide in osteo-

blasts and the osteocyte-like cell line murine long bone osteocyte-Y4. Endocrinology 2003;144(5): 1761–1769.
123. Miura M, Chen XD, Allen MR, et al. A crucial role of caspase-3 in osteogenic differentiation of bone marrow stromal stem cells. J Clin Invest 2004; 114(12):1704–1713.
124. Pantschenko AG, Zhang W, Nahounou M, et al. Effect of osteoblast-targeted expression of bcl-2 in bone: differential response in male and female mice. J Bone Miner Res 2005;20(8):1414–1429.
125. Byun CH, Koh JM, Kim DK, et al. Alpha-lipoic acid inhibits TNF-alpha-induced apoptosis in human bone marrow stromal cells. J Bone Miner Res 2005;20(7):1125–1135.
126. Zhao H, Ross FP, Teitelbaum SL. Unoccupied alpha(v)beta3 integrin regulates osteoclast apoptosis by transmitting a positive death signal. Mol Endocrinol 2005;19(3):771–780.
127. Sorisky A, Magun R, Gagnon AM. Adipose cell apoptosis: death in the energy depot. Int J Obes Relat Metab Disord 2000;24 Suppl 4:S3–S7.
128. Prins JB, Niesler CU, Winterford CM, et al. Tumor necrosis factor-alpha induces apoptosis of human adipose cells. Diabetes 1997;46(12): 1939–1944.
129. Niesler CU, Siddle K, Prins JB. Human preadipocytes display a depot-specific susceptibility to apoptosis. Diabetes 1998;47(8):1365–1368.
130. Kim HS, Hausman DB, Compton MM, et al. Induction of apoptosis by all-trans-retinoic acid and C2-ceramide treatment in rat stromal-vascular cultures. Biochem Biophys Res Commun 2000; 270(1):76–80.
131. Nelson-Dooley C, Della-Fera MA, Hamrick M, et al. Novel treatments for obesity and osteoporosis: targeting apoptotic pathways in adipocytes. Curr Med Chem 2005;12(19):2215–2225.

3
Calciotropic Hormones

E. Paul Cherniack and Bruce R. Troen

The calcium—vitamin D—parathyroid hormone (PTH) system plays a critical role in both health and disease. Despite longstanding acceptance of its importance in maintaining the skeleton, recent and accumulating data have significantly enhanced our understanding of the pathophysiology of calciotropic hormones in the setting of osteoporosis. Herein we review this information and make recommendations based on these studies.

Calcium

Calcium is one of the most abundant inorganic elements in the human body. The physiologic roles of calcium in the body are twofold. Firstly, calcium provides structural integrity to the skeleton. In addition, in the extracellular fluids and in the cytosol, the calcium concentration is critical to many biochemical processes, and these include hormone and enzyme secretion, neurotransmission, muscle contraction, blood clotting, and gene expression *(1)*. Therefore, calcium concentrations are tightly regulated.

Calcium is absorbed from the small intestine and kidney via both vitamin D-dependent and -independent pathways (Figure 3.1). When calcium is abundant, vitamin D-independent mechanisms are predominant. When calcium is scarce, vitamin D-dependent pathways are primarily utilized *(1,2)*. There is an age-related decrement in calcium absorption, and this appears in part to be caused by widespread vitamin D insufficiency and frank deficiency *(3)*. However, calcium absorption also declines in post-menopausal women independent of 25-hydroxycholecalciferol (25(OH) vitamin D) and PTH levels *(4)*.

Vitamin D

Vitamin D is an important multi-purpose steroid hormone that plays an essential role in humans in the maintenance of bone, muscle, immunity, metabolic signaling, and protection against cardiovascular disease and neoplasms. The action of vitamin D on bone is complex. Vitamin D regulates osteoblast differentiation and stimulates expression of alkaline phosphatase (AP) and bone matrix proteins *(1,2,5)*. Vitamin D also stimulates osteoclast formation via cellular interaction with osteoblasts and osteoclast cell precursors *(6)*. Whereas vitamin D indirectly stimulates osteoclast formation, it also enhances gastrointestinal calcium absorption, promotes mineralization, and inhibits PTH-induced bone resorption *(1,2,5)*.

In humans, sunlight exposure is necessary for the precursor of vitamin D, 7-dehydrocholesterol, which is obtained from the diet, to be converted into pre-vitamin D3, which is quickly isomerized into vitamin D3 (cholecalciferol) (Figure 3.2). Cholecalciferol is subsequently hydroxylated in the liver to 25-hydroxycholecalciferol (25(OH) vitamin D) by the mitochondrial enzyme CYP27A1 and again in the kidney to 1,25-dihydroxycholecalciferol (calcitriol) by the 1-α hydroxylase, CYP27B1 *(1,7)*. Calcitriol is the activated form of vitamin D and exerts its effects by directly binding to the vitamin D receptor *(3)*.

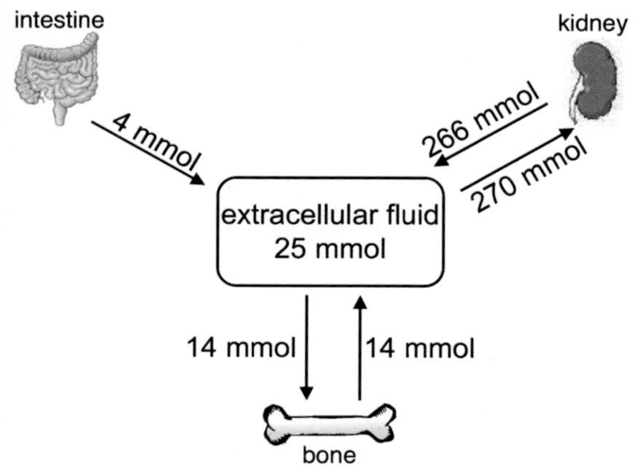

FIGURE 3.1. Calcium homeostasis *(1)*.

Low calcium stimulates the 1-α hydroxylation of 25-hydroxycholecalciferol by CYP27B1. Abundant calcium stimulates the enzymatic conversion of 25-hydroxycholecalciferol to 24,25-$(OH)_2D_3$ and 1,25-dihydroxycholecalciferol to 1,24,25-$(OH)_3D_3$ by CYP24. Conversely, increases in 1,25-dihydroxycholecalciferol inhibit and up-regulate the action of CYP27B1 and CYP24, respectively. Therefore, calcium and calcitriol work in opposition to regulate both the increased production of calcitriol and its metabolic degradation *(3,8)*.

The amount of sunlight capable of causing a mild sunburn stimulates the production and release into the circulation of 10,000 to 20,000 IU of vitamin D in the following 24 hours *(9)*. But this requires exposure of large parts of the body such as the thorax and legs, not just smaller surface areas such as the face, neck, and arms *(10)*. Because the production of vitamin D depends upon the extent of ultraviolet (UV) exposure, people with darker skin require longer exposure than do those with lighter skin *(11,12)*. Furthermore, the skin of older individuals (age 77–82) produces less than one-half of the cholecalciferol precursor, 7-dehydrocholesterol, than does the skin of younger individuals (age 8–18) *(13)*. Many elderly individuals consume suboptimal amounts of vitamin D and calcium *(14,15)*. There are relatively few dietary sources of vitamin D, and they include fortified milk and orange juice, and salmon and other fatty fish. Vitamin D is well absorbed from the small intestine through a bile-dependent mechanism. However, deficient consumption of dairy products, and high intake of high-protein, low calcium-containing foods has been implicated as factor for lack of calcium intake *(16,17)*. Lactose intolerance and low socioeconomic status also appears to contribute to poor calcium intake *(18,19)*. Therefore, decreased vitamin D production and consumption act in concert to predispose to hypovitaminosis D.

A surprisingly large percentage of the population has inadequate vitamin D levels *(20)*. Frank deficiency is below 10 ng/mL (25 nmol/L), but levels of 25(OH) vitamin D below 30 ng/mL (75 nmol/L) are now considered to be insufficient *(21)*. As many as 40–90% of the elderly have 25(OH) vitamin D levels below 30 ng/mL *(22–27)*. The level of 25(OH) vitamin D can vary as much as 40% between the summer and winter seasons, most likely owing to the seasonal changes in sun and UV exposure *(28)*. There is widespread vitamin D insufficiency even in climates with ample amounts of sunlight; however, cultural norms dictate clothing coverage, thereby diminishing UV radiation-induced production of vitamin D *(29–32)*. In one study, there was no difference between veiled and unveiled women *(33)*. However, approximately 80% in both groups had 25(OH) vitamin D levels below 40 nmol/L.

Lower vitamin D levels are more common among blacks, and blacks have lower bone mineral densities for given vitamin D levels than whites *(34–36)*. In the NHANES III, 53–76% of non-Hispanic blacks were found to have 25(OH) vitamin D levels below 50 nmol/L versus 8–33% of

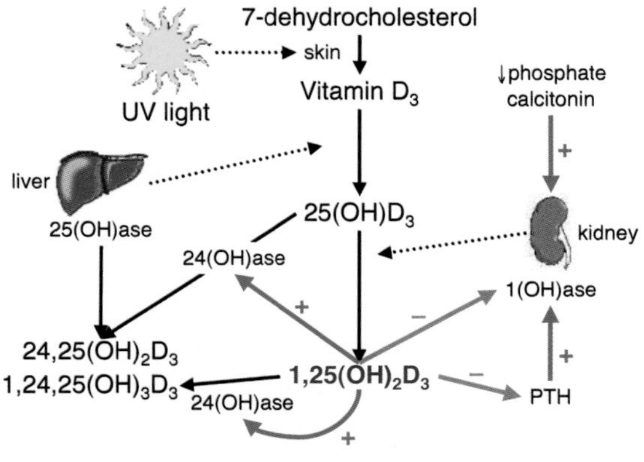

FIGURE 3.2. Vitamin D metabolism (Adapted from *[1]*).

non-Hispanic whites. Many African Americans do not achieve 25(OH) vitamin D levels of at least 30 ng/mL at any time of the year. Median vitamin D intakes are 6–31% lower than other racial groups, and there is decreased consumption of dairy products and fortified cereals. A recent study in which African American women were supplemented up to 2000 IU of vitamin D a day did not improve their bone mineral densities, although their mean 25(OH) vitamin D levels increased from 46.9 nmol/L to 70.8 nmol/L *(37)*.

The spectrum of vitamin D deficiency disease in the skeleton ranges from rickets, at the lowest vitamin D levels, to more insidiously developing disease, such as osteoporosis, at higher but still suboptimal levels. The entire range of pathology caused by hypovitaminosis D has been termed "hypovitaminosis D osteopathy (HVO)" *(38,39)*. Initially described by Michael Parfitt, there are three progressive stages *(38)*. In the least severe, lack of vitamin D results in calcium malabsorption, elevation of PTH level occurs to increase calcium absorption, and osteoporosis occurs, with bone remodeling and loss of osteoporosis. In a second and more severe stage, continued lack of calcium and bone remodeling create the histologic changes of osteomalacia. In the most extreme state of deficiency, bone remodeling ceases and the clinical manifestations of rickets are present *(39)*.

For over a decade, studies have reported that supplementation with vitamin D and calcium reduce fracture risk, falls, and improve balance *(40–42)*. Vitamin D is well known to play a role in maintaining skeletal integrity, regulating calcium entry via receptors in bone and small intestine *(43–45)*. In several studies in which vitamin D in community-dwelling elderly was supplemented, a 10–30% reduction in non-vertebral fracture incidence was noted over several years *(46,47)*. A study of 389 ambulatory elderly individuals supplemented daily with 700 IU of vitamin D and 500 mg of calcium observed an approximately 68% lower non-vertebral fracture risk after 3 years *(46)*. More than 3000 healthy older individuals (mean age 84) who received 800 IU of cholecalciferol and 1.2 g of calcium for 1.5 years experienced a 43% lower incidence of hip fracture and a 32% lower incidence of non-vertebral fractures *(48)*. These benefits were confirmed in a separate 2-year study of 583 ambulatory institutionalized women, showing that the same doses of calcium and vitamin D reduced hip fracture by 40% *(49)*. However, when 800 IU of cholecalciferol was provided to more than 8000 older individuals with a previous history of fracture or risk factors for fracture in two trials lasting 2–5 years, fracture incidence was not reduced *(50,51)*. However, compliance rates were 56 and 60%, and in only a small percentage of subjects were 25(OH) vitamin D levels assessed. Possible explanations for varying results include inadequate replacement of vitamin D, different baseline levels of vitamin D in the populations studied, and differences in the populations studied—particularly with respect to baseline bone mineral density, fall predisposition, and adherence to the regimen. Furthermore, neither study was powered sufficiently to detect decreases in fracture incidence less than 30%. A meta-analysis concluded that 700–800 IU of vitamin D per day significantly reduced vertebral, non-vertebral, and hip fractures, whereas 400 IU per day did not *(52)*. In the recent Women's Health Initiative study, 500 mg calcium and 400 IU of vitamin D per day was shown to reduce hip fracture in community-dwelling women (odds ratio [OR] 0.71: confidence interval [CI] 0.52–0.97) who took more than 80% of the doses *(53)*.

The role of vitamin D in fracture risk extends beyond bone; it appears to enhance physical performance through an effect on extraskeletal tissues *(54)*. Vitamin D receptors are found in muscle, although their expression decreases with age *(43)*. Higher serum levels of 25-OH vitamin D are correlated with better leg function as assessed by a timed walk test and a repeated sit-to-stand test *(54)*. Vitamin D supplementation reduces falls in subjects who maintain a minimum calcium intake *(40,41)*. A meta-analysis of the effect of vitamin D in 1237 subjects revealed a 22% reduced risk of falls, with a number needed to treat of only 15 *(40)*. A dose of 700–800 IU vitamin D per day significantly reduced falls, whereas 400 IU per day did not, although a study in community-dwelling Danish individuals demonstrated a fall reduction with 1000 mg of calcium carbonate and 400 IU vitamin D per day *(41)*. In elderly Australians in residential care, 1000 IU ergocalciferol (vitamin D2) per day significantly reduced falls, with a number needed to treat of only 12 *(55)*. This benefit was more pronounced in compliant individuals. Interestingly, fracture rates were not reduced.

Vitamin D supplementation also improves balance. When more than 100 subjects whose 25(OH) vitamin D levels were found to be less than 30 nmol/L were supplemented with a single dose of 600,000 IU of ergocalciferol, postural sway improved *(56)*. Furthermore, 242 disease-free elderly Germans who were supplemented with 800 IU vitamin D and 1000 mg calcium daily for 1 year exhibited less body sway than those who received calcium alone *(57)*. The subjects who received vitamin D also had greater quadriceps strength. In a survey of 4100 ambulatory individuals age 60 and higher, 25(OH) vitamin D levels below 60 nmol/L were correlated with reduced walking speed and increased time to stand from a seated position *(54)*. Vitamin D levels were also positively correlated with neuromuscular performance tasks in a longitudinal survey of 1300 elderly individuals *(58)*. However, the effect of vitamin D supplementation on parameters of physical performance is not unequivocal. A dose of 1000 U of cholecalciferol per day failed to improve upper and lower extremity strength and power in older men *(59)*, and a systematic review found no improvement in muscle strength with vitamin D supplementation using a variety of preparations and doses *(60)*. A recent trial observed no reduction in falls or fractures in nursing home residents given 100,000 IU of ergocalciferol orally every 3 months *(61)*. However, the serum 25(OH) vitamin D levels of one-half of the ergocalciferol recipients remained below 74–82 nmol/L. Again, possible explanations for the lack of effect of vitamin D in some investigations include inadequate dose of vitamin D used, variation in baseline vitamin D level, differences in medication compliance, and (in the case of measurements of muscle strength) inadequate choice of assessment parameters *(62)*.

A large and growing number of studies link vitamin D levels to many other physiological processes and pathologies beyond the musculoskeletal system (Figure 3.3). There is significant epidemiological evidence that implicates hypovitaminosis D in the development and progression of malignancies of the prostate, breast, colon, ovary, and hematopoietic system *(3,63,64)*. Many

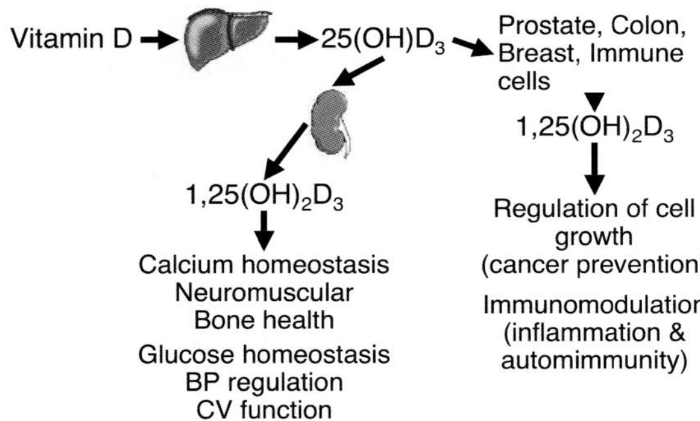

FIGURE 3.3. Biologic functions of vitamin D *(3)*.

of these observations are based upon the correlation between available levels of sunlight and UV exposure with the incidence and prevalence of cancer. As long ago as 1941, it was reported that overall death rates owing to cancer were greater in northern latitudes *(65)*. Garland et al. renewed interest in this phenomenon in 1980 when they showed that mortality owing to colon cancer was much greater in the northeastern United States than in southern states *(66)*. The risk of developing and dying from 17 cancers is related to living at higher latitudes, receiving less UV exposure, and being more at risk of vitamin D deficiency *(3,67,68)*. These cancers include bladder, breast, colon, esophageal, gastric, ovarian, prostate, rectal, renal, uterine cancer, non-Hodgkins lymphoma, cervical, gall bladder, laryngeal, oral, pancreatic, and Hodgkin's lymphoma.

The underlying pathophysiology of these malignancies is very likely related to expression of 1-α hydroxylase in many peripheral tissues and cells and their ability therefore to metabolize 25-hydroxy-vitamin D into 1,25-dihydroxy-vitamin D (calcitriol), which is the active form of vitamin D *(69,70)*. Consequently, vitamin D acts as an autocrine hormone in many extra-renal tissues *(71)*. Colon cancer cells, *in vitro*, metabolize vitamin D *(72)*. Vitamin D has been demonstrated to induce apoptosis in breast cancer cells *in vitro* *(73)*. Low vitamin D levels and vitamin D receptor polymorphisms have been associated with breast cancer *(74)*, and in one investigation, vitamin D intake was inversely correlated with the presence of densities found on mammograms *(75)*. Polymorphisms in the vitamin D receptor gene are also correlated with prostate cancer risk and melanoma *(76)*. Vitamin D may also be directly involved in the pathogenesis of skin cancer. Vitamin D induces the differentiation of keratinocytes, and neoplastic cells overexpress a coactivator induced by the binding of vitamin D to its receptor *(77)*. Interestingly, sun exposure may increase survival after diagnosis of melanoma and may also improve outcomes in cancers of the breast, colon, and prostate and in Hodkgins lymphoma *(78)*.

Vitamin D plays a role in insulin signaling, sarcopenia, inflammation, and the pathogenesis of diabetes and cardiovascular disease *(79,80)*. Serum levels of 25(OH) vitamin D are inversely correlated with glucose levels and are inversely correlated with insulin sensitivity *(81)*. Obese individuals exhibit decreased bioavailability of vitamin D as evidenced by diminished 25(OH) vitamin D levels in response to either UV exposure or oral supplementation *(82)*. Body fat percentage is inversely correlated with 25(OH) vitamin D levels and directly correlated with PTH levels *(83)*. Lower vitamin D levels increase the risk for metabolic syndrome and are inversely correlated with hyperglycemia, hypertension, hypertriglyceridemia, abdominal obesity, and low high-density lipoprotein (HDL) cholesterol *(79)*. Furthermore, low vitamin D levels and high PTH levels have been correlated with sarcopenia in a cohort of elderly individuals *(84)*, and low levels of 25(OH) vitamin D are a predictor of nursing home admission *(85)*. Immune cells such as T-lymphocytes, macrophages, and antigen-presenting cells express vitamin D receptors *(86,87)*. Vitamin D prevents antigen-induced progression in the T cell growth cycle, regulates T cell proliferation, and influences the expression of multiple cytokines that regulate immune cell signaling and responses, such as interleukin (IL)-2, IL-10, and interferon-γ *(87)*. Hypovitaminosis D also predisposes to the development of autoimmune diseases such as multiple sclerosis *(88)* and type I diabetes *(89)*. In addition, vitamin D plays a critical role in mediating antimicrobial responses of macrophages *(90)*.

Vitamin D also exerts cardiovascular effects. A group of 148 women (mean age 74) who had 25(OH) vitamin D levels below 50 nmol/L and blood pressures no greater than 180/95 were supplemented with 800 IU of vitamin D and 1200 mg of calcium for 8 weeks. Individuals who received both vitamin D and calcium experienced a 9.3% reduction in systolic blood pressure without a drop in diastolic blood pressure *(91)*. Low vitamin D levels and elevated PTH levels have been found to be higher in subjects with congestive heart failure than in controls *(92,93)*.

PTH

PTH is an 84 amino acid polypeptide that maintains normal extracellular calcium through its action on the bone, kidney, and the intestines (Figure 3.4). PTH is released from the parathyroid gland in response to insufficient calcium and estrogens, and its release is suppressed by vitamin D and phosphate loss *(1)*. Its action on bone is complex. PTH acts on osteoblasts to modulate the expression of a variety of growth factors, including insulin-like growth factor (IGF)-1, transforming growth factor (TGF)-β1 and TGF-β2, as well as IL-6 *(94,95)*. Persistent elevation of PTH stimulates osteoclast formation, in part via enhancing the expression of receptor activator of NFκB (RANK) ligand by osteoblasts, which plays a critical role in the differentiation and activation of osteoclasts *(96)*. This, in turn, leads to osteoclastic bone resorption, and the release of calcium from the skeleton *(97)*. Historically, PTH has long been conceived of as a catabolic agent that contributes to bone destruction and loss of bone mineral density. However, the normal physiologic role of PTH depends upon its intermittent secretion and subsequent action as an anabolic agent *(97)*. As long ago as 1980, Reeve et al. reported that intermittent injection of exogenous PTH in humans stimulated significant new bone formation *(98)*. Daily subcutaneous injection of PTH increases lumbar spinal and femoral bone mineral density both in post-menopausal women and in men with osteoporosis *(99,100)*. PTH reduces vertebral and non-vertebral fractures in post-menopausal women *(99)*. PTH treatment can also reverse the loss of bone in glucocorticoid-induced osteoporosis in post-menopausal women *(101)*. Unlike antiresorptive therapies such as estrogen, raloxifene, bisphosphonates, and calcitonin, which inhibit bone resorption, PTH stimulates new bone formation. PTH enhances bone quality and bone strength by increasing trabecular connectivity

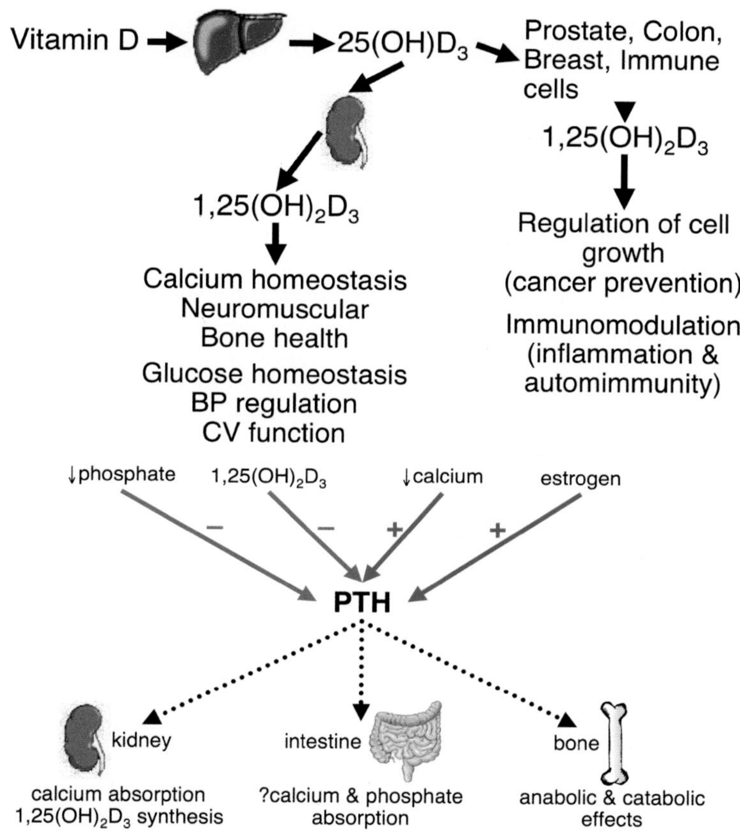

FIGURE 3.4. Parathyroid hormone (Adapted from *[1]*).

(102) and the cross-sectional area of the bone *(103)*. Furthermore, PTH stimulates deposition of bone in appropriate locations in the skeleton, on those surfaces that are subject to mechanical forces *(104)*. Therefore, new bone is formed where it is needed. PTH has multiple actions on the kidney. It causes retention of calcium by the cortical thick ascending limbs, and the distal convoluted collecting and connecting tubules. PTH also stimulates the 1-α hydroxylation of vitamin D, and excretion of phosphate *(1)*. In addition, PTH stimulates DNA synthesis in intestinal enterocytes and increases the influx of calcium.

The relationship between PTH and vitamin D is important in the pathogenesis of HVO, but complex. Numerous studies imply that individuals who have lower vitamin D levels have higher PTH levels *(20,23,105–107)*. With progressive increase in 25(OH) vitamin D levels, there appears to be a plateau in the suppression of PTH that occurs at approximately 75–90 nmol/L 25(OH) vitamin D *(20,23,107–109)*. This suggests that vitamin D is physiologically replete at these levels and above. However, Vieth et al. observed no plateau as 25(OH) vitamin D levels increased *(105)*. Kudlacek et al. found that 25(OH) vitamin D levels were inversely correlated with PTH levels and that PTH levels exhibited a significant age-related increase (27). For any given level of 25(OH) vitamin D, older subjects exhibit greater levels of PTH *(110)*. Older adults require 25(OH) vitamin D levels of greater than 100 nmol/L to suppress PTH to the same degree observed in younger subjects with 25(OH) vitamin D levels near 70 nmol/L *(105)*. Other causes of secondary hyperparathyroidism include declining renal function, estrogen deficiency, and low calcium intake *(111)*.

Sahota et al. found that only one-half of patients with hip fractures and a 25(OH) vitamin D level below 30 nmol/L exhibited secondary hyperparathyroidism *(112)*. They characterized the remaining patients with hypovitaminosis D and low or normal PTH levels as having "functional hypoparathyroidism," and these individuals had greater hip bone mineral density and fewer extracapsular fractures than did those with elevated PTH levels. In a second group of subjects with established vertebral osteoporosis, Sahota et al. found that of the 39% with 25(OH) vitamin D levels no greater than 30 nmol, only one-third exhibited secondary hyperparathyroidism *(113)*. The two-thirds of the vitamin D insufficient/deficient patients who did not have an elevated PTH had a lower mean serum calcium and reduced bone turnover than those with elevated PTH levels. Deplas et al. found that less than one-third of patients with hypovitaminosis D exhibited secondary hyperparathyroidism *(114)*. And in two additional investigations, less than one-half the patients who had both fractured their hip and were hypovitaminotic D had an elevated PTH *(115,116)*. In these subjects, PTH level did not inversely correlate with vitamin D level. Consequently, the feedback sensitivity of the vitamin D-PTH axis appears to be reduced with aging and/or disease. It is possible that a concomitant magnesium deficiency plays a role in altering the response of PTH to hypovitaminosis D *(117)*. It is unclear what the implications are for these two distinct populations of elderly patients with vitamin D deficiency (high and low PTH) regarding the pathogenesis of osteoporosis and its treatment.

These data suggest that caution may need to be exercised in using PTH as an indicator of vitamin D status, because the PTH response to hypovitaminosis and possibly even frank vitamin D deficiency may vary. Do these data mean that PTH is not a useful indicator of vitamin D status? No. It is widely accepted that PTH levels are, in general, inversely correlated with 25(OH) vitamin D levels. Instead, it may be prudent to assess the suppression in PTH in response to vitamin D supplementation by measuring both the pre- and post-treatment levels. However, controversy exists on the utility of measuring PTH to determine vitamin D repletion. Heaney strongly asserts that decreasing PTH levels will plateau when 25(OH) vitamin D levels begin to reach a physiologically optimal value *(118)*, whereas Vieth argues that PTH levels continue to decline as 25(OH) vitamin D levels increase *(119)*.

Calcium intake also influences the relationship between PTH and vitamin D at lower vitamin D levels. A study 2310 healthy individuals from Iceland observed that at very low serum 25(OH) vitamin D levels (<10 ng/mL), persons with lower calcium intakes had higher PTH levels *(120)*. However, at higher vitamin D levels, calcium intake did not significantly influence PTH. The action of PTH may exhibit gender-related differences. Both men and women experience age-related increases in PTH. However, there is evidence that the bones of elderly women are more sensitive to resorption-caused PTH than younger women. When elderly women receive an infusion of calcium, which suppresses their PTH, there is a greater increase in markers of bone turnover (urine n-telopeptide) than in younger women *(121)*. When calcium infusions are given to men, there is no difference in the response of the bones of younger and older men to the suppression of PTH *(122)*. These differences may be explained by the difference in sex steroid levels between men and women *(122)*. Nevertheless, after controlling for age, Blain et al. still found that an increased level of PTH was the most important predictor of bone loss in men *(123)*.

Calcitonin

The C cells of the thyroid manufacture and release calcitonin, which has multiple effects on body calcium *(1)*. Calcitonin is secreted when serum calcium is high, and suppressed when calcium is diminished *(124)*. Calcitonin may have actions on other systems such as the reproductive, central nervous, renal, respiratory, and gastrointestinal system, but not all its actions are known *(1,124)*. Calcitonin prevents bone resorption, and can be stimulated by PTH. It inhibits osteoclast action and can cause apoptosis *(125)*. One-half of all thyroidectomized men developed osteopenia in one study, and they exhibited lower serum calcium and higher PTH levels than control subjects *(126)*. However, the physiologic role of calcitonin is uncertain. There are no known pathologic states in humans that result from surplus or deficient calcitonin *(125)*. Recent data strongly implicate calcitonin in maintaining bone integrity during excessive resorption during lactation *(127)*. However, with that exception, calcitonin does not appear to significantly contribute to normal skeletal homeostasis or pathophysiology.

Conclusion

What is the best marker to assess adequate vitamin D supplementation? Thus far, studies have used 25-OH vitamin D and PTH. Is there a single marker or should several be assessed? Might other measures be needed? Potentially, these might include measurements of handgrip, hip or leg strength, mobility and balance tests, or quality of life instruments. Further investigation will determine what other markers might prove sensitive, specific, and cost-effective. Many important questions remain to be answered about the role of vitamin D in the preservation of health for the elderly. What should be the optimum recommended daily and maximum recommended vitamin D intake for elderly individuals? There is a growing consensus that vitamin D recommended daily intakes for the elderly are far too low, and that all individuals should take as much vitamin D as needed to raise levels to between 80 to 100 nmol/L *(3,68,128)*. Moreover, supplementation will be necessary, because diet and sunlight alone are inadequate sources of vitamin D *(9)*.

How much vitamin D (cholecalciferol) should be taken? The present Food and Drug Administration recommended daily intake of vitamin D is 400 IU for those age 51–70 and 600 IU for those over age 70, whereas the National Osteoporosis Foundation recommends between 400–800 IU per day. However, increasing evidence supports the necessity for daily doses significantly above these levels to achieve levels of vitamin D of 75 nmol/L and higher *(68)*. Cholecalciferol 100,000 IU orally every 4 months significantly reduced fractures *(47)*. A once-yearly intramuscular injection of 600,000 IU of cholecalciferol increased 25(OH) vitamin D levels to greater than 50 nmol/L in all subjects, raised average levels to 73 nmol/L after 12 months, normalized PTH levels in two-thirds of those with secondary hyperparathyroidism, and was well tolerated with only mild hypercalcemia in 4% of recipients *(129)*. Cholecalciferol supplementation is generally very safe and without toxicity in the absence of primary hyperparathyroidism, even with as much as 10,000 IU per day *(130)*. There are no adverse effects with concentration of 25(OH) vitamin D less than 140 nmol/L *(130)*, and there is evidence that increasing levels of 25(OH) vitamin D up to 120 nmol/L is correlated with increased bone mineral density in both non-Hispanic whites and in Mexican Americans *(35)*. Furthermore, it is possible that vitamin D repletion is necessary for optimal anti-resorptive therapy, as a preliminary report found poorer response to alendronate in post-menopausal vitamin D with 25(OH) vitamin D levels less than 37.5 nmol/L *(131)*. As much as 2600 IU per day of vitamin D may be necessary to insure that 97% of the population is vitamin D replete *(21)*, and more may be needed in the elderly. Indeed, two preliminary reports in the frail elderly show that doses of 1500–5000 IU per day of cholecalciferol are needed and can be administered without danger of hypercalcemia *(132,133)*. The key is to monitor the response to supplementation by obtaining 25-hydroxyvitamin D levels every 3–4 months.

Because the incidence of osteoporosis differs by gender, age, and race, future studies are needed to more clearly establish the best diagnostic and supplementation approaches to hypovitaminosis D for different populations. In the meantime, a heightened awareness of the widely prevalent vitamin D insufficiency will permit us to more actively intervene and to raise and maintain 25(OH) vitamin D levels at a minimum of 75 nmol/L.

References

1. Ramasamy I. Recent advances in physiological calcium homeostasis. Clin Chem Lab Med 2006; 44(3):237–273.
2. Lips P. Vitamin D physiology. Prog Biophys Mol Biol 2006;92(1):4–8.
3. Holick MF. The vitamin d epidemic and its health consequences. J Nutr 2005;135(11):2739S–2748S.
4. Nordin BE, Need AG, Morris HA, et al. Effect of age on calcium absorption in postmenopausal women. Am J Clin Nutr 2004;80(4):998–1002.

5. Dusso AS, Brown AJ, Slatopolsky E. Vitamin D. Am J Physiol Renal Physiol 2005;289(1):F8–F28.
6. Troen BR. The role of cathepsin K in normal bone resorption. Drug News Perspect 2004;17(1):19–28.
7. Anderson PH, O'Loughlin PD, May BK, et al. Determinants of circulating 1,25-dihydroxyvitamin D3 levels: the role of renal synthesis and catabolism of vitamin D. J Steroid Biochem Mol Biol 2004;89–90(1–5):111–113.
8. Holick MF. Resurrection of vitamin D deficiency and rickets. J Clin Invest 2006;116(8):2062–2072.
9. Hollis BW. Circulating 25-hydroxyvitamin D levels indicative of vitamin D sufficiency: implications for establishing a new effective dietary intake recommendation for vitamin D. J Nutr 2005;135(2):317–322.
10. Matsuoka LY, Wortsman J, Hollis BW. Use of topical sunscreen for the evaluation of regional synthesis of vitamin D3. J Am Acad Dermatol 1990;22(5 Pt 1):772–775.
11. Clemens TL, Adams JS, Henderson SL, et al. Increased skin pigment reduces the capacity of skin to synthesise vitamin D3. Lancet 1982; 1(8263):74–76.
12. Matsuoka LY, Wortsman J, Haddad JG, et al. Racial pigmentation and the cutaneous synthesis of vitamin D. Arch Dermatol 1991;127(4): 536–538.
13. MacLaughlin J, Holick MF. Aging decreases the capacity of human skin to produce vitamin D3. J Clin Invest 1985;76(4):1536–1538.
14. Grieger JA, Nowson CA. Nutrient intake and plate waste from an Australian residential care facility. Eur J Clin Nutr 2007;61(5):655–663.
15. Dumartheray EW, Krieg MA, Cornuz J, Whittamore DR, Lanham-New SA, Burckhardt P. Energy and nutrient intake of Swiss women aged 75–87 years. J Hum Nutr Diet 2006;19:431–435.
16. Avioli LV. Postmenopausal osteoporosis: prevention versus cure. Fed Proc 1981;40(9):2418–2422.
17. Gennari C. Calcium and vitamin D nutrition and bone disease of the elderly. Public Health Nutr 2001;4(2B):547–559.
18. Shahar D, Shai I, Vardi H, et al. Factors associated with low reported energy intake in the elderly. J Nutr Health Aging 2005;9(5):300–304.
19. French MR, Moore K, Vernace-Inserra F, et al. Factors that influence adherence to calcium recommendations. Can J Diet Pract Res 2005; 66(1):25–29.
20. Holick MF, Siris ES, Binkley N, et al. Prevalence of vitamin D inadequacy among postmenopausal North American women receiving osteoporosis therapy. J Clin Endocrinol Metab 2005;90(6): 3215–3224.
21. Heaney RP. The vitamin D requirement in health and disease. J Steroid Biochem Mol Biol 2005; 97(1–2):13–19.
22. Harinarayan CV. Prevalence of vitamin D insufficiency in postmenopausal south Indian women. Osteoporos Int 2005;16(4):397–402.
23. Chapuy MC, Preziosi P, Maamer M, et al. Prevalence of vitamin D insufficiency in an adult normal population. Osteoporos Int 1997;7(5):439–443.
24. Vecino-Vecino C, Gratton M, Kremer R, et al. Seasonal variance in serum levels of vitamin d determines a compensatory response by parathyroid hormone: study in an ambulatory elderly population in Quebec. Gerontology 2006;52(1):33–39.
25. Nakamura K, Nishiwaki T, Ueno K, et al. Serum 25-hydroxyvitamin D levels and activities of daily living in noninstitutionalized elderly Japanese requiring care. J Bone Miner Metab 2005;23(6): 488–494.
26. Levis S, Gomez A, Jimenez C, et al. Vitamin D deficiency and seasonal variation in an adult South Florida population. J Clin Endocrinol Metab 2005;90(3):1557–1562.
27. Kudlacek S, Schneider B, Peterlik M, et al. Assessment of vitamin D and calcium status in healthy adult Austrians. Eur J Clin Invest 2003;33(4): 323–331.
28. Meier C, Woitge HW, Witte K, et al. Supplementation with oral vitamin D3 and calcium during winter prevents seasonal bone loss: a randomized controlled open-label prospective trial. J Bone Miner Res 2004;19(8):1221–1230.
29. Dawodu A, Absood G, Patel M, et al. Biosocial factors affecting vitamin D status of women of childbearing age in the United Arab Emirates. J Biosoc Sci 1998;30(4):431–437.
30. Dawodu A, Dawson KP, Amirlak I, et al. Diet, clothing, sunshine exposure and micronutrient status of Arab infants and young children. Ann Trop Paediatr 2001;21(1):39–44.
31. Gannage-Yared MH, Chemali R, Yaacoub N, et al. Hypovitaminosis D in a sunny country: relation to lifestyle and bone markers. J Bone Miner Res 2000;15(9):1856–1862.
32. Guzel R, Kozanoglu E, Guler-Uysal F, et al. Vitamin D status and bone mineral density of veiled and unveiled Turkish women. J Womens Health Gend Based Med 2001;10(8):765–770.
33. Islam MZ, Akhtaruzzaman M, Lamberg-Allardt C. Hypovitaminosis D is common in both veiled and nonveiled Bangladeshi women. Asia Pac J Clin Nutr 2006;15(1):81–87.

34. Harris SS. Vitamin D and African Americans. J Nutr 2006;136(4):1126–1129.
35. Bischoff-Ferrari HA, Dietrich T, Orav EJ, et al. Positive association between 25-hydroxy vitamin D levels and bone mineral density: a population-based study of younger and older adults. Am J Med 2004;116(9):634–639.
36. Dawson-Hughes B. Racial/ethnic considerations in making recommendations for vitamin D for adult and elderly men and women. Am J Clin Nutr 2004;80(6 Suppl):1763S–1766S.
37. Aloia JF, Talwar SA, Pollack S, et al. A randomized controlled trial of vitamin D3 supplementation in African American women. Arch Intern Med 2005;165(14):1618–1623.
38. Parfitt AM. Osteomalacia and related disorders. In: *Metabolic bone disease and clinical related disorders, 2nd edition.* Avioli LV, Krane SM, eds. Philadelphia: Saunders, 1990; 329–396.
39. Heaney RP. Lessons for nutritional science from vitamin D. Am J Clin Nutr 1999;69(5):825–826.
40. Bischoff-Ferrari HA, Dawson-Hughes B, Willett WC, et al. Effect of vitamin D on falls: a meta-analysis. JAMA 2004;291(16):1999–2006.
41. Larsen ER, Mosekilde L, Foldspang A. Vitamin D and calcium supplementation prevents severe falls in elderly community-dwelling women: a pragmatic population-based 3-year intervention study. Aging Clin Exp Res 2005;17(2):125–132.
42. Wilkins CH, Birge SJ. Prevention of osteoporotic fractures in the elderly. Am J Med 2005;118(11): 1190–1195.
43. Bischoff-Ferrari HA, Borchers M, Gudat F, et al. Vitamin D receptor expression in human muscle tissue decreases with age. J Bone Miner Res 2004;19(2):265–269.
44. Kitazawa R, Kitazawa S. Vitamin D(3) augments osteoclastogenesis via vitamin D-responsive element of mouse RANKL gene promoter. Biochem Biophys Res Commun 2002;290(2): 650–655.
45. Liang CT, Barnes J, Imanaka S, et al. Alterations in mRNA expression of duodenal 1,25-dihydroxyvitamin D3 receptor and vitamin D-dependent calcium binding protein in aged Wistar rats. Exp Gerontol 1994;29(2):179–186.
46. Dawson-Hughes B, Harris SS, Krall EA, et al. Effect of calcium and vitamin D supplementation on bone density in men and women 65 years of age or older. N Engl J Med 1997;337(10):670–676.
47. Trivedi DP, Doll R, Khaw KT. Effect of four monthly oral vitamin D3 (cholecalciferol) supplementation on fractures and mortality in men and women living in the community: randomised double blind controlled trial. BMJ 2003;326(7387): 469.
48. Chapuy MC, Arlot ME, Duboeuf F, et al. Vitamin D3 and calcium to prevent hip fractures in the elderly women. N Engl J Med 1992;327(23): 1637–1642.
49. Chapuy MC, Pamphile R, Paris E, et al. Combined calcium and vitamin D3 supplementation in elderly women: confirmation of reversal of secondary hyperparathyroidism and hip fracture risk: the Decalyos II study. Osteoporos Int 2002; 13(3):257–264.
50. Porthouse J, Cockayne S, King C, et al. Randomised controlled trial of calcium and supplementation with cholecalciferol (vitamin D3) for prevention of fractures in primary care. BMJ 2005;330(7498): 1003.
51. Grant AM, Avenell A, Campbell MK, et al. Oral vitamin D3 and calcium for secondary prevention of low-trauma fractures in elderly people (Randomised Evaluation of Calcium Or vitamin D, RECORD): a randomised placebo-controlled trial. Lancet 2005;365(9471):1621–1628.
52. Bischoff-Ferrari HA, Willett WC, Wong JB, et al. Fracture prevention with vitamin D supplementation: a meta-analysis of randomized controlled trials. JAMA 2005;293(18):2257–2264.
53. Jackson RD, LaCroix AZ, Gass M, et al. Calcium plus vitamin D supplementation and the risk of fractures. N Engl J Med 2006;354(7):669–683.
54. Bischoff-Ferrari HA, Dietrich T, Orav EJ, et al. Higher 25-hydroxyvitamin D concentrations are associated with better lower-extremity function in both active and inactive persons aged > or = 60 y. Am J Clin Nutr 2004;80(3):752–758.
55. Flicker L, MacInnis RJ, Stein MS, et al. Should older people in residential care receive vitamin D to prevent falls? Results of a randomized trial. J Am Geriatr Soc 2005;53(11):1881–1888.
56. Dhesi JK, Jackson SH, Bearne LM, et al. Vitamin D supplementation improves neuromuscular function in older people who fall. Age Ageing 2004;33(6):589–595.
57. Pfeifer M, Dobnig H, Begerow B, Suppan K. Effects of vitamin D and calcium supplementation on falls and parameters of muscle function—a prospective, randomized, double-blind, multi-center study. J Bone Miner Res 2004.
58. Wicherts IS, Schoor van NM, Boeke AJP, Lips P. Vitamin D deficiency and neuromuscular performance in the Longitudinal Aging Study Amsterdam (LASA). J Bone Miner Res 2005.
59. Kenny AM, Biskup B, Robbins B, et al. Effects of vitamin D supplementation on strength, physical

function, and health perception in older, community-dwelling men. J Am Geriatr Soc 2003;51(12):1762–1767.
60. Latham NK, Anderson CS, Lee A, et al. A randomized, controlled trial of quadriceps resistance exercise and vitamin D in frail older people: the Frailty Interventions Trial in Elderly Subjects (FITNESS). J Am Geriatr Soc 2003;51(3):291–299.
61. Law M, Withers H, Morris J, et al. Vitamin D supplementation and the prevention of fractures and falls: results of a randomised trial in elderly people in residential accommodation. Age Ageing 2006;35(5):482–486.
62. Judge JO, Kenny A. Vitamin D and quadriceps exercise—got milk? Got a chair? J Am Geriatr Soc 2003;51(3):427–428.
63. Garland CF, Garland FC, Gorham ED, et al. The role of vitamin D in cancer prevention. Am J Public Health 2006;96(2):252–261.
64. Grant WB. Epidemiology of disease risks in relation to vitamin D insufficiency. Prog Biophys Mol Biol 2006;92(1):65–79.
65. Apperly FL. The relation of solar radiation to cancer mortality in North America. Cancer Res 1941;1:191–195.
66. Garland CF, Garland FC. Do sunlight and vitamin D reduce the likelihood of colon cancer? Int J Epidemiol 1980;9(3):227–231.
67. Grant WB, Garland CF. The association of solar ultraviolet B (UVB) with reducing risk of cancer: multifactorial ecologic analysis of geographic variation in age-adjusted cancer mortality rates. Anticancer Res 2006;26(4A):2687–2699.
68. Grant WB, Holick MF. Benefits and requirements of vitamin D for optimal health: a review. Altern Med Rev 2005;10(2):94–111.
69. Howard GA, Turner RT, Sherrard DJ, et al. Human bone cells in culture metabolize 25-hydroxyvitamin D3 to 1,25-dihydroxyvitamin D3 and 24,25-dihydroxyvitamin D3. J Biol Chem 1981;256(15):7738–7740.
70. Hewison M, Zehnder D, Bland R, et al. 1alpha-Hydroxylase and the action of vitamin D. J Mol Endocrinol 2000;25(2):141–148.
71. Zehnder D, Bland R, Williams MC, et al. Extrarenal expression of 25-hydroxyvitamin d(3)-1 alpha-hydroxylase. J Clin Endocrinol Metab 2001;86(2):888–894.
72. Bareis P, Bises G, Bischof MG, et al. 25-hydroxy-vitamin d metabolism in human colon cancer cells during tumor progression. Biochem Biophys Res Commun 2001;285(4):1012–1017.
73. Zinser GM, Tribble E, Valrance M, et al. 1,24(S)-dihydroxyvitamin D2, an endogenous vitamin D2 metabolite, inhibits growth of breast cancer cells and tumors. Anticancer Res 2005;25(1A):235–241.
74. Lowe LC, Guy M, Mansi JL, et al. Plasma 25-hydroxy vitamin D concentrations, vitamin D receptor genotype and breast cancer risk in a UK Caucasian population. Eur J Cancer 2005;1(8):1164–1169.
75. Berube S, Diorio C, Verhoek-Oftedahl W, et al. Vitamin D, calcium, and mammographic breast densities. Cancer Epidemiol Biomarkers Prev 2004;13(9):1466–1472.
76. Moon S, Holley S, Bodiwala D, et al. Associations between G/A1229, A/G3944, T/C30875, C/T48200 and C/T65013 genotypes and haplotypes in the vitamin D receptor gene, ultraviolet radiation and susceptibility to prostate cancer. Ann Hum Genet 2006;70(Pt 2):226–236.
77. Bikle DD. Vitamin D regulated keratinocyte differentiation. J Cell Biochem 2004;92(3):436–444.
78. Kricker A, Armstrong B. Does sunlight have a beneficial influence on certain cancers? Prog Biophys Mol Biol 2006;92(1):132–139.
79. Ford ES, Ajani UA, McGuire LC, et al. Concentrations of serum vitamin D and the metabolic syndrome among U.S. adults. Diabetes Care 2005;28(5):1228–1230.
80. Mathieu C, Gysemans C, Giulietti A, et al. Vitamin D and diabetes. Diabetologia 2005;48(7):1247–1257.
81. Chiu KC, Chu A, Go VL, et al. Hypovitaminosis D is associated with insulin resistance and beta cell dysfunction. Am J Clin Nutr 2004;79(5):820–825.
82. Wortsman J, Matsuoka LY, Chen TC, et al. Decreased bioavailability of vitamin D in obesity. Am J Clin Nutr 2000;72(3):690–693.
83. Snijder MB, van Dam RM, Visser M, et al. Adiposity in relation to vitamin D status and parathyroid hormone levels: a population-based study in older men and women. J Clin Endocrinol Metab 2005;90(7):4119–4123.
84. Visser M, Deeg DJ, Lips P. Low vitamin D and high parathyroid hormone levels as determinants of loss of muscle strength and muscle mass (sarcopenia): the Longitudinal Aging Study Amsterdam. J Clin Endocrinol Metab 2003;88(12):5766–5772.
85. Visser M, Deeg DJ, Puts MT, et al. Low serum concentrations of 25-hydroxyvitamin D in older persons and the risk of nursing home admission. Am J Clin Nutr 2006;84(3):616–622; quiz 671–672.
86. Hayes CE, Nashold FE, Spach KM, et al. The immunological functions of the vitamin D endo-

crine system. Cell Mol Biol (Noisy-le-grand) 2003;49(2):277–300.

87. van Etten E, Mathieu C. Immunoregulation by 1,25-dihydroxyvitamin D3: basic concepts. J Steroid Biochem Mol Biol 2005;97(1–2):93–101.
88. Cantorna MT. Vitamin D and its role in immunology: multiple sclerosis, and inflammatory bowel disease. Prog Biophys Mol Biol 2006;92(1):60–64.
89. Harris SS. Vitamin D in type 1 diabetes prevention. J Nutr 2005;135(2):323–325.
90. Gombart AF, Borregaard N, Koeffler HP. Human cathelicidin antimicrobial peptide (CAMP) gene is a direct target of the vitamin D receptor and is strongly up-regulated in myeloid cells by 1,25-dihydroxyvitamin D3. FASEB J 2005;19(9): 1067–1077.
91. Pfeifer M, Begerow B, Minne HW, et al. Effects of a short-term vitamin D(3) and calcium supplementation on blood pressure and parathyroid hormone levels in elderly women. J Clin Endocrinol Metab 2001;86(4):1633–1637.
92. Shane E, Mancini D, Aaronson K, et al. Bone mass, vitamin D deficiency, and hyperparathyroidism in congestive heart failure. Am J Med 1997;103(3): 197–207.
93. Zittermann A, Schleithoff SS, Tenderich G, et al. Low vitamin D status: a contributing factor in the pathogenesis of congestive heart failure? J Am Coll Cardiol 2003;41(1):105–112.
94. Sanders JL, Stern PH. Protein kinase C involvement in interleukin-6 production by parathyroid hormone and tumor necrosis factor-alpha in UMR-106 osteoblastic cells. J Bone Miner Res 2000;15(5):885–893.
95. Wu Y, Kumar R. Parathyroid hormone regulates transforming growth factor beta1 and beta2 synthesis in osteoblasts via divergent signaling pathways. J Bone Miner Res 2000;15(5):879–884.
96. Troen BR. Molecular mechanisms underlying osteoclast formation and activation. Exp Gerontol 2003;38(6):605–614.
97. Hodsman AB, Bauer DC, Dempster DW, et al. Parathyroid hormone and teriparatide for the treatment of osteoporosis: a review of the evidence and suggested guidelines for its use. Endocr Rev 2005;26(5):688–703.
98. Reeve J, Meunier PJ, Parsons JA, et al. Anabolic effect of human parathyroid hormone fragment on trabecular bone in involutional osteoporosis: a multicentre trial. Br Med J 1980;280(6228): 1340–1344.
99. Neer RM, Arnaud CD, Zanchetta JR, et al. Effect of parathyroid hormone (1–34) on fractures and bone mineral density in postmenopausal women with osteoporosis. N Engl J Med 2001;344(19): 1434–1441.
100. Orwoll ES, Scheele WH, Paul S, et al. The effect of teriparatide [human parathyroid hormone (1–34)] therapy on bone density in men with osteoporosis. J Bone Miner Res 2003;18(1):9–17.
101. Lane NE, Sanchez S, Modin GW, et al. Parathyroid hormone treatment can reverse corticosteroid-induced osteoporosis. Results of a randomized controlled clinical trial. J Clin Invest 1998;102(8): 1627–1633.
102. Dempster DW, Cosman F, Kurland ES, et al. Effects of daily treatment with parathyroid hormone on bone microarchitecture and turnover in patients with osteoporosis: a paired biopsy study. J Bone Miner Res 2001;16(10): 1846–1853.
103. Uusi-Rasi K, Semanick LM, Zanchetta JR, et al. Effects of teriparatide [rhPTH (1–34)] treatment on structural geometry of the proximal femur in elderly osteoporotic women. Bone 2005;36(6): 948–958.
104. Hagino H, Okano T, Akhter MP, et al. Effect of parathyroid hormone on cortical bone response to in vivo external loading of the rat tibia. J Bone Miner Metab 2001;19(4):244–250.
105. Vieth R, Ladak Y, Walfish PG. Age-related changes in the 25-hydroxyvitamin D versus parathyroid hormone relationship suggest a different reason why older adults require more vitamin D. J Clin Endocrinol Metab 2003;88(1):185–191.
106. Souberbielle JC, Cormier C, Kindermans C, et al. Vitamin D status and redefining serum parathyroid hormone reference range in the elderly. J Clin Endocrinol Metab 2001;86(7):3086–3090.
107. Mosekilde L, Hermann AP, Beck-Nielsen H, et al. The Danish Osteoporosis Prevention Study (DOPS): project design and inclusion of 2000 normal perimenopausal women. Maturitas 1999; 31(3):207–219.
108. Thomas MK, Lloyd-Jones DM, Thadhani RI, et al. Hypovitaminosis D in medical inpatients. N Engl J Med 1998;338(12):777–783.
109. Tangpricha V, Pearce EN, Chen TC, et al. Vitamin D insufficiency among free-living healthy young adults. Am J Med 2002;112(8):659–662.
110. Maggio D, Cherubini A, Lauretani F, et al. 25(OH)D Serum levels decline with age earlier in women than in men and less efficiently prevent compensatory hyperparathyroidism in older adults. J Gerontol A Biol Sci Med Sci 2005;60(11): 1414–1419.
111. Lips P. Vitamin D deficiency and secondary hyperparathyroidism in the elderly: consequences for

bone loss and fractures and therapeutic implications. Endocr Rev 2001;22(4):477–501.
112. Sahota O, Gaynor K, Harwood RH, Hosking DJ. Hypovitaminosis D and "functional hypoparathyroidism"—the NoNoF (Nottingham Neck of Femur) study. Age Ageing 2001;30(6):467–472.
113. Sahota O, Mundey MK, San P, et al. The relationship between vitamin D and parathyroid hormone: calcium homeostasis, bone turnover, and bone mineral density in postmenopausal women with established osteoporosis. Bone 2004;35(1):312–319.
114. Deplas A, Debiais F, Alcalay M, et al. Bone density, parathyroid hormone, calcium and vitamin D nutritional status of institutionalized elderly subjects. J Nutr Health Aging 2004;8(5):400–404.
115. Sakuma M, Endo N, Oinuma T, et al. Vitamin D and intact PTH status in patients with hip fracture. Osteoporos Int 2006;17(11):1608–1614.
116. Fisher AA, Davis MW. Calcium-PTH-vitamin D axis in older patients with hip fracture. Osteoporos Int 2007;18(5):693–695.
117. Sahota O, Mundey MK, San P, et al. Vitamin D insufficiency and the blunted PTH response in established osteoporosis: the role of magnesium deficiency. Osteoporos Int 2006;17(7):1013–1021.
118. Heaney RP. Serum 25-hydroxyvitamin D and parathyroid hormone exhibit threshold behavior. J Endocrinol Invest 2005;28(2):180–182.
119. Vieth R, El-Hajj Fuleihan G. There is no lower threshold level for parathyroid hormone as 25-hydroxyvitamin D concentrations increase. J Endocrinol Invest 2005;28(2):183–186.
120. Steingrimsdottir L, Gunnarsson O, Indridason OS, et al. Relationship between serum parathyroid hormone levels, vitamin D sufficiency, and calcium intake. JAMA 2005;294(18):2336–2341.
121. Ledger GA, Burritt MF, Kao PC, et al. Role of parathyroid hormone in mediating nocturnal and age-related increases in bone resorption. J Clin Endocrinol Metab 1995;80(11):3304–3310.
122. Kennel KA, Riggs BL, Achenbach SJ, et al. Role of parathyroid hormone in mediating age-related changes in bone resorption in men. Osteoporos Int 2003;14(8):631–636.
123. Blain H, Vuillemin A, Blain A, et al. Age-related femoral bone loss in men: evidence for hyperparathyroidism and insulin-like growth factor-1 deficiency. J Gerontol A Biol Sci Med Sci 2004; 59(12):1285–1289.
124. Findlay DM, Sexton PM. Calcitonin. Growth Factors 2004;22(4):217–224.
125. Miller S. Calcitonin—guardian of the Mammalian skeleton or is it just a fish story? Endocrinology 2006;147(9):4007–4009.
126. Cappelli C, Cottarelli C, Cumetti D, et al. [Bone density and mineral metabolism in calcitonin-deficiency patients]. Minerva Endocrinol 2004; 29(1):1–10.
127. Woodrow JP, Sharpe CJ, Fudge NJ, et al. Calcitonin plays a critical role in regulating skeletal mineral metabolism during lactation. Endocrinology 2006;147(9):4010–4021.
128. Grant WB, Gorham ED. Commentary: time for public health action on vitamin D for cancer risk reduction. Int J Epidemiol 2006;35(2):224–225.
129. Diamond TH, Ho KW, Rohl PG, et al. Annual intramuscular injection of a megadose of cholecalciferol for treatment of vitamin D deficiency: efficacy and safety data. Med J Aust 2005;183(1): 10–12.
130. Hathcock JN, Shao A, Vieth R, et al. Risk assessment for vitamin D. Am J Clin Nutr 2007;85(1): 6–18.
131. Ishijima M, Yamanaka M, Sakamoto Y, et al. Vitamin D insufficiency impairs the effect of alendronate for the treatment of osteoporosis in postmenopausal women. J Bone Miner Res 2005; 20(Suppl 1):S296.
132. Ish-Shalom S, Salganik T, Segal E, et al. Daily, weekly or monthly protocols to reach the desired serum 25-hydroxyvitamin D concentration for the elderly. J Bone Miner Res 2005;20(Suppl 1): S288.
133. Mocanu V, Stitt PA, Costan A, et al. Safety and bone mineral density effects of bread fortified with 125 mcg vitamin D3/day in romanian nursing-home residents. J Bone Miner Res 2005;20 (Suppl 1):S288.

4
Sex Steroids and Aging Bone

Jane A. Cauley

Introduction

Sex steroids play key roles in the development and maintenance of the skeleton in both men and women. Historically, it was thought that sex steroids were gender-specific: estrogen was important for women and testosterone for men. However, research over the past decade has demonstrated a key role for estrogen in maintaining skeletal integrity in men. Thus, a unitary model for involutional osteoporosis has been proposed *(1)* that identifies estrogen deficiency as a cause of the accelerated phase of bone loss in women and the slower age-related phase of bone loss in both men and women. It is also likely that androgens play a role, although evidence supporting their role is stronger in laboratory and clinical experiments than in population studies.

In this chapter, the evidence supporting a role for sex steroids in maintaining the skeleton into old age is reviewed. The focus is on both estrogen and testosterone in men and women from an epidemiologic perspective.

Methodologic Issues

It is important to acknowledge the difficulty in evaluating this literature. Older hormone assays lacked sufficient sensitivity to be reliable. Most estradiol assays were originally developed for pre-menopausal women and lack the sensitivity to measure the very low levels that are typical of post-menopausal women. These assays could discriminate pre-from post-menopausal women, but could not discriminate between post-menopausal women with very low levels. Measurements in pre-menopausal need to be standardized across the menstrual cycle. In the Study of Women's Health Across the Nation (SWAN), we used a standard protocol that specified that the blood be obtained in the 2- to 5-day window of the early follicular phase of the menstrual cycle. However, in women with irregular menstrual cycles or in women who were beginning to transition into menopause, this standardization was increasingly difficult. Whether or not the sample was drawn according to the protocol influenced our results *(2)*.

Two major methods are used to measure estradiol: indirect and direct immunoassays. Indirect assays typically include an initial extraction step before the radioimmunoassay (RIA). In contrast, direct assays do not involve extraction. A recent study compared four direct assay and three indirect assay methods and found that indirect estradiol assays correlated more highly with mass spectrometry *(3)*. The extraction step in indirect assays removes cross-reacting substances that interfere with the assay. Mass spectrometry is the reference standard for measuring both male and female sex hormones *(4,5)*. Newer approaches to the assessment of sex steroids specifically using mass spectrometry have been developed to reduce or eliminate interfering substances and now serve as the reference methods for sex steroid assays *(6,7)*. However, until these methods are widely available, extraction-based indirect methods are preferable.

In addition, the biosynthesis of androgens and estrogens is complex, and it differs in men and women, as well as in pre-and post-menopausal women. Many enzymes are involved in the production and metabolism of steroid hormones *(8)*. Androgens and estrogens are correlated. In post-menopausal women and men, androgens serve as the major precursor to estradiol. Free unbound and bioavailable hormone levels (the portion loosely bound to albumin) are highly correlated with each other and to the total hormone concentration. Nevertheless, most findings are generally stronger for the bioavailable hormone. Finally, in most studies, a single concentration of estrogen or testosterone is available and the within-person variability in the hormone concentration will lead to some misclassification and weaken the findings.

Sex Steroids and Age

Testosterone and estradiol levels, especially the free or bioavailable fractions, decline with increasing age in both men and women. This decline may lead to some of the most important sequels of aging. In addition to skeletal strength, the decline in sex steroids could relate to declines in physical function, as well as changes in cognition and quality of life.

Using sex steroid data from the Mayo Clinic, (data chosen because results are derived from the same laboratory), differences in total and bioavailable testosterone and estradiol by gender across ages is shown in Figures 4.1 and 4.2 *(9,10)*. Testosterone levels are higher in men than women at every age group. As expected, younger pre-menopausal women have higher estradiol levels than younger men, but this trend is reversed among the older women. Total estradiol levels are 76% higher, and bioavailable estradiol levels are almost three-fold higher on average, in older men than in older women. In these data, the greatest declines were observed in the bioavailable fraction and not the total hormone. Nevertheless, there may be substantial individual variability in the age-related decline in sex steroid hormones *(11)*, suggesting that targeting risk factors that contribute to the decline could prevent fractures.

Sex Steroids and Bone Mineral Density (BMD)

Serum estrogen measures have been consistently linked with appendicular and axial BMD measures in post-menopausal women *(12–21)*. The strongest associations were observed for bioavailable estradiol. However, in pre-menopausal women, total estradiol and bioavailable estradiol were unrelated to BMD at the hip *(13)* or spine *(22)*. The strongest hormonal predictor of BMD in pre- and early peri-menopausal women was follicle-stimulating hormone (FSH) levels.

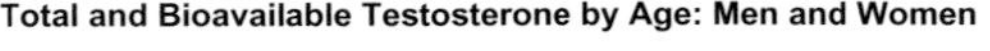

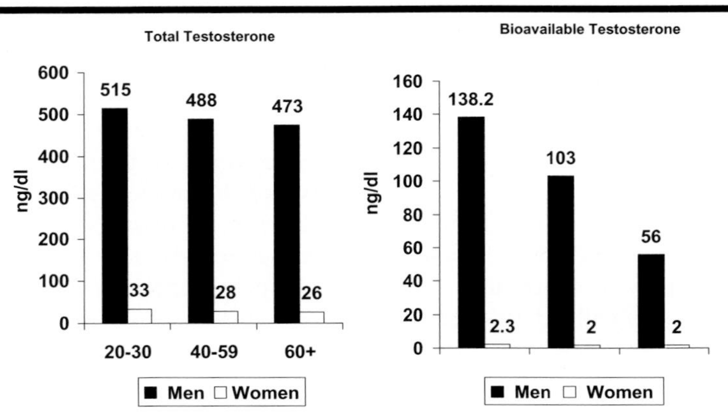

FIGURE 4.1. Total and bioavailable testosterone by age: men and women.

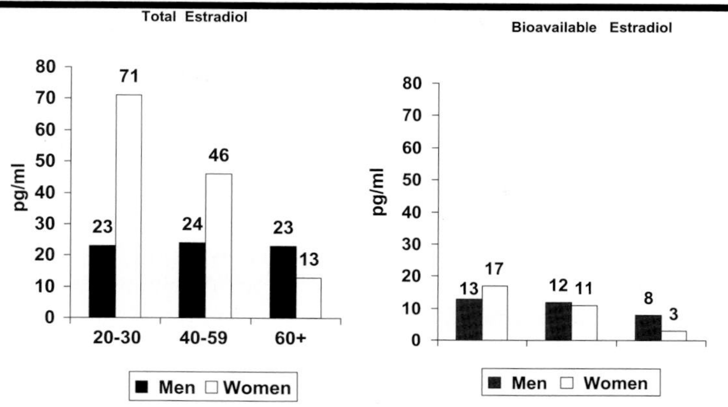

FIGURE 4.2. Total and bioavailable estradiol by age: men and women.

The association between testosterone and BMD in older post-menopausal women is less consistent, with some reports showing associations with one BMD site and not others *(14,17,18)* or free testosterone and not total testosterone *(14,16)*. In contrast to findings with respect to estradiol, total bioavailable testosterone levels were positively correlated with BMD in pre-menopausal women *(13)*.

Longitudinally, low estradiol concentrations are associated with faster rates of bone loss in older post-menopausal women *(19,23,24)* but not in pre-menopausal women *(2,22,23,25–27)*. Nevertheless, within a group of pre-menopausal women, those with lower estrogens experienced faster rates of bone loss *(28)*. Follow-up in most of these studies was less than 4 years, and it's possible that over longer periods of time, estrogen levels could predict rates of bone loss. In the 12-year study of Rannevik et al., after approximately 3 years post-menopausally, estradiol correlated with rates of bone loss *(29)*. Testosterone was not correlated with changes in BMD *(2,26,27)*, except for a single study (23). Bone loss over a 2- to 8-year follow-up was related to lower androgens in pre-menopausal women, but to both lower androgens and estrogens in post-menopausal women *(23)*.

Men

Two "Experiments of Nature" *(30)* have provided essential information about the importance of estrogen to the male skeleton. An alpha-estrogen receptor-deficient male was found to have high circulating estrogens, normal testosterone levels, but very low BMD *(31)*. Three men with an aromatase deficiency rendering them estrogen-deficient were found to have very low BMD, and all responded well to estrogen replacement *(32,33)*.

Population studies of older men have reported positive correlations between total estradiol and/or bioavailable estradiol in both older and younger men *(13,34–39)*. The relationships tended to be stronger for bioavailable estradiol than total *(13,36)*. In contrast, there is little evidence that total or bioavailable testosterone is correlated with BMD in older or younger men, at least in the range of normal testosterone *(13,35,39–41)*. In the Framingham Study, BMD at any site did not differ in hypogonadal men compared to eugonadal men *(38)*.

The relative contribution of testosterone and estrogen in regulating bone resorption and formation in men was examined by eliminating endogenous testosterone and estrogen production in 59 older men, average age 68 years *(42)*, and then replacing either testosterone, estradiol, or both. Bone resorption markers increased significantly in the absence of both testosterone and estradiol. Administration of estradiol alone prevented the increase in bone resorption, but administration of testosterone had no effect. In contrast, both testosterone and estradiol individually maintained levels of bone formation. Thus, although correlations between BMD and testosterone levels are usually not apparent, testosterone may influence bone formation.

Cross-sectional studies have consistently shown an important role for estrogen in determining the skeleton, but it is unclear whether estrogen contributes to peak skeletal mass or affects bone loss in men. Low total bioavailable estradiol concentrations were associated with faster rates of bone loss in older men *(43–45)*. There was no association between total or bioavailable testosterone concentrations and change in BMD *(44)*. Similarly, the rate of increase in BMD in younger men (age 22–39) was correlated with total and bioavailable estradiol, but not with total or bioavailable testosterone *(43)*. Of importance, a threshold level for bioavailable estradiol below which aging men begin to lose bone was suggested *(43)*. Elderly men with bioavailable estradiol below the median (40 pmol/L) had significantly higher rates of bone loss and levels of bone resorption markers than men with higher bioavailable estradiol levels. This subset of older men may be the most likely to benefit from preventive efforts.

Sex Steroids, Volumetric BMD and Skeletal Structure

All previous studies used areal BMD measures and were unable to examine the associations between sex steroids and trabecular and cortical bone separately or to structural parameters. Khosla et al. have recently published three key papers *(9,10,46)*. As shown in Figure 4.3 (women) and Figure 4.4 (men), the "threshold" theory exists only for cortical bone. At all cortical sites, volumetric BMD was associated with bioavailable estradiol at low but not high levels. Trabecular bone, on the other hand, was correlated with

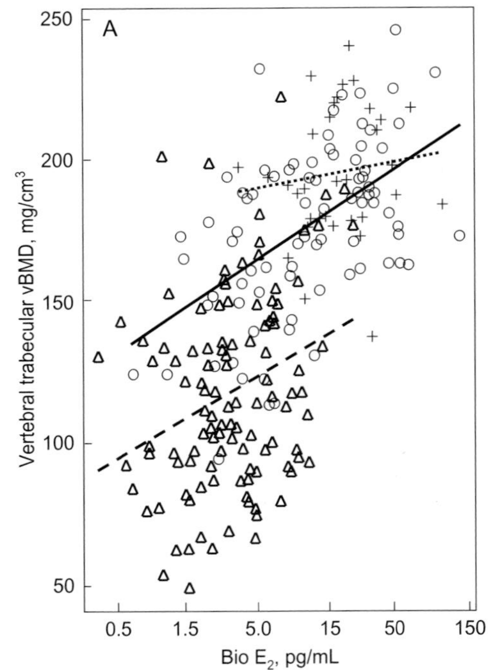

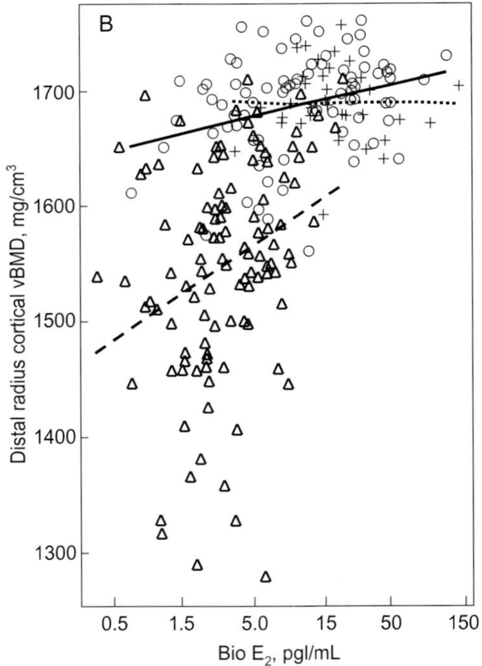

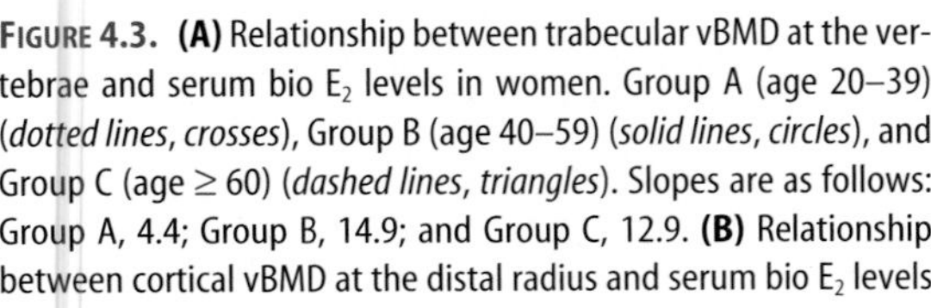

FIGURE 4.3. **(A)** Relationship between trabecular vBMD at the vertebrae and serum bio E_2 levels in women. Group A (age 20–39) (*dotted lines, crosses*), Group B (age 40–59) (*solid lines, circles*), and Group C (age ≥ 60) (*dashed lines, triangles*). Slopes are as follows: Group A, 4.4; Group B, 14.9; and Group C, 12.9. **(B)** Relationship between cortical vBMD at the distal radius and serum bio E_2 levels in women. Group A (age 20–39) (*dotted lines, crosses*), Group B (age 40–59) (*solid lines, circles*), and Group C (age ≥ 60) (*dashed lines, triangles*). Slopes are as follows: Group A, –0.01; Group B, 12.4; and Group C, 36.3. Note that bio E_2 levels are on a log scale. See text for details (From 9 by permission of The Endocrine Society).

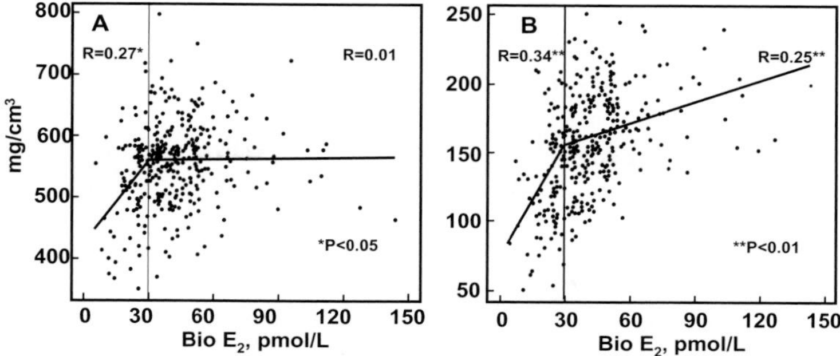

FIGURE 4.4. **(A)** Femur neck cortical vBMD and **(B)** vertebral trabecular vBMD as a function of bio E_2 levels below and above 30 pM in Rochester, MN, men (From 10 by permission of Journal of Bone Mineral Research).

bioavailable estradiol both above and below the median. The authors speculate that reductions in bioavailable estradiol levels to below the threshold will result in greater decreases in trabecular bone than cortical bone. But cortical bone is not sensitive to declining bioavailable estradiol levels until they decline past the threshold. This theory is consistent with the observation that menopause-related bone loss primarily affects trabecular and not cortical bone. Further studies are needed to confirm this observation. Improved assays are needed to identify the specific cutpoint. In the papers described previously, the "cutpoint" was the median level and it differed in both men and women.

None of the structural parameters (vertebral area, bone area, subendocortical area, cortical area, and trabecular microstructural measures) were related to bioavailable estradiol or bioavailable testosterone in young men or pre-menopausal women. In older men and women, both bioavailable estradiol and bioavailable testosterone were related to many of these structural parameters and to trabecular microstructure.

In a longitudinal study of 108 women followed over the menopause for 15 years, there was an increase in periosteal apposition, leading to an increase in skeletal size *(47)*. This increase in size in part compensates for the loss in bone strength caused by post-menopausal bone loss. Of importance, post-menopausal serum estradiol levels were highly correlated with changes in the periosteal diameter. Taken together, these results support a role for both estrogens and androgens in maintaining bone size parameters and trabecular microarchitecture.

Sex Steroids and Fractures

Women

Early case control studies comparing sex steroids in women with and without a fracture were conflicting *(48–51)*. These contradictory results may have reflected the small sample size, biased selections of cases and controls, alterations in hormones resulting from the fracture itself, and use of low-sensitivity assays. Prevalent vertebral fractures were less common among women who had an estradiol level greater than 5 pg/mL (18 pmol/L): The multiple adjusted odds ratio was 0.4 (95% confidence intervals, 0.2–0.8) *(15)*. In contrast, in the Rancho Bernardo Study, the prevalence of vertebral fractures was not related to either total or bioavailable estradiol or bioavailable testosterone in older women *(52)*, although earlier reports from this cohort showed a relationship between estimated bioavailable testosterone (but not estradiol) and height loss *(53)*.

The prospective studies of endogenous hormones and fracture are summarized in Table 4.1 *(54–59)*. In the Study of Osteoporotic Fractures (SOF), women with estradiol below the sensitivity of the assay (<5 pg/mL [18 pmol/L]), had a 2.5-fold increased risk of a hip fracture (Relative Risk (RR) = 2.5; 1.4–4.2) even after adjusting for age and body weight *(54)*. Adjustment for BMD attenuated

Table 4.1. Summary of Prospective Studies of Endogenous Sex Steroid Hormones and Fracture in Women

Author	Design	Study Population	Outcomes	Hormones	Results
Cummings (1998) USA	case-cohort	SOF cohort $n = 9704$; age 65+ mean age = 73 yr; exclude hormone users 274 controls randomly selected from cohort	133 hip fx; 138 vertebral fx, mean follow-up 5.9 yrs	E2, Free T, SHBG	vertebral fx (adj for age and weight) RR (95% CI) E2 (<18 pmol/L): 2.5 (1.4–4.2) SHBG (<34.7 nmol/L): 2.3 (1.2–4.4) T (≤2.4 pmol/L): 1.4 (08–2.4) hip fx (adj for age and weight) RR (95% CI) E2 (<18 pmol/L): 2.5 (1.4–4.6) SHBG (<34.7 nmol/L): 2.0 (1.1–3.9) T (≤2.4 pmol/L): 1.6 (1.0–2.7)
Garnero (1998) France	nested case-control	OFELY cohort $n = 1039$; mean age 64 yr excluded if pre-menopausal; excluded if on active bone agents; 380 controls	30 vertebral fx 35 peripheral fx, mean follow-up: 5 yr	E2, T, SHBG	any fx (adj age, prevalent vertebral fx, and activity) RR (95% CI) E2 (<39.6 pmol/L): 2.2 (1.2–4.0) SHBG (>40.2 nmol/L): 1.6 (0.9–2.9) T (lowest Quartile[a]) 1.4 (0.7–2.8)
Chapurlat (2000) France	nested case-control	EPIDOS cohort $n = 7598$; mean age 82 yr; 636 controls	212 hip fx, mean follow-up 3.3 yrs	E2 SHBG	RR (95% CI) E2 (<18 pmol/L): 1.07 (0.6–1.87) E2 (>36 pmol/L): 0.66 (0.44–0.98) SHBG (<25.8 mg/L): 0.75 (0.49, 1.12)
Goderie-Plomp (2004) Netherlands	nested case-control	Rotterdam cohort $n = 4878$; age 55+ mean age = 68 yr; age-matched 339 controls	115 vertebral fx, mean follow-up 6.5 yr	E2, T, SHBG	RR (95% CI) E2 (≤15.5 pmol/L) = 2.09 (1.26–3.46) SHBG (<42.9 nmol/L) = 0.51 (0.30–0.87) T no association (results not shown)
Devine (2005) Australia	prospective cohort	1499 women mean age = 75 yr	151 Incident fx mean follow-up 3 yr	E2, SHBG, FEI	cases mean / control mean / *p*-value E2 (pmol/L): 24.0 / 25.0 / 0.08 SHBG (nmol/L): 54.5 / 50.0 / 0.02 FEI: 0.40 / 0.49 / 0.002
Sipila (2006) Finland	prospective cohort	175 women age 75+	121 incident fx, mean follow-up 10 yr	E2, T, SHBG	E2 (nmol/L) — RR (95% CI) >0.066: 1.0 0.022–0.066: 2.24 (0.97–5.19) <0.022: 3.05 (1.26–7.36) SHBG (nmol/L) >91.5: 1.0 42.6–91.5: 0.79 (0.35–1.81) <42.6: 1.10 (0.57–2.13)

[a] Lowest quartile cutpoint: NOT available.

SOF, Study of Osteoporotic Fractures; adj, adjusted; fx, fracture; E2 estradiol; T, testosterone, SHBG, sex hormone binding globulin; RR, relative risk; CI, confidence intervals; EPIDOS, French Epidemiology of Osteoporosis; FEL, free eatrogen index.

the RR slightly to 1.9 (1.0–3.6), suggesting that at least part of this association reflected the higher BMD among women with higher endogenous concentrations of estradiol. Of importance, the RR remained significant, suggesting that estradiol may have other effects, which contribute to their effect on fractures.

Women with low free testosterone had an increased risk of hip but not vertebral fracture, but this was not significant after adjusting for estradiol *(54)*. The risk of hip fracture increased with increasing serum concentrations of sex hormone binding globulin (SHBG), but this association appeared to be slightly dependent upon body weight. The combination of low estradiol and high SHBG was associated with an age-adjusted 14-fold increase in hip and 12-fold increase in vertebral fractures.

The OFELY cohort of French women were approximately 10 years younger on average than women in SOF *(55)*. In this study, low estradiol (defined as lowest Quartile (<39.6 pmol/L) was associated with an increased risk of fracture (Table 4.1). Neither SHBG nor testosterone were significantly related to fracture, although there was a trend of increasing fracture with increasing SHBG. Adjustment for BMD or bone turnover had little effect. The authors estimated that women with both high resorption markers and low estradiol had a threefold increased risk of fracture.

In the French Epidemiology of Osteoporosis (EPIDOS) Study, low concentrations of estradiol were unrelated to hip fractures, even after exploring various cutoffs from less than 10.8 pmol/L (2% of subjects) to less than 25.2 pmol/L (38% of subjects) *(56)*. However, women with *high* (>36 pmol/L) concentrations were protected (RR = 0.71; 0.47–1.06). Women with the highest levels of SHBG (Quartile IV) had a 2.5-fold (1.4–4.6) increased risk of hip fracture in comparison to women with the lowest SHBG (Quartile 1).

In the Rotterdam Study of vertebral fractures, mean age of 68 years, low estradiol was associated with an increased risk and low SHBG with a decreased risk of vertebral fractures, independent of BMD *(57)*. Women with a combination of both low estradiol and high SHBG had a 7.8-fold (2.7–22.5) increased risk of vertebral fractures. Testosterone was not related to fractures in this study.

Finally, two studies examined the association of endogenous hormones to any type of incident fractures *(58,59)*. In these studies, low estradiol, or a measure of free estrogen index, were associated with increased fractures. In the Finnish Study, SHBG was unrelated to fracture risk.

Taken together, these studies suggest an association between estradiol and fracture. Of importance, these associations were found across several different cohorts, representing women with an average age ranging from 64 to 82 years, recruited from several different countries. Nevertheless, the results are confined to Caucasian women, and little is known about sex steroids and fracture in other ethnic groups. Asian women have a high rate of hip fracture *(60)*, and it will be important to study whether estradiol predicts fracture in these women, especially because their body weight tends to be lower than Caucasians *(61)*. Overall, testosterone was not related to fractures in women and the association between SHBG was inconsistent. Future studies should use state of the art assays for testosterone and include the free or bioavailable testosterone.

Men

To my knowledge, seven case control or cross-sectional studies have examined the association of sex steroids to fractures in older men (Table 4.2) *(52,62–67)*. The prevalence of testosterone deficiency was reported to be higher among men with hip fracture *(62,63)* in comparison to controls. Estradiol levels were lower and SHBG higher in two small studies of men with idiopathic osteoporosis *(64,66)*, but not in other studies *(65)*. In the Rancho Bernardo cohort, men with a prevalent vertebral fracture had lower total and bioavailable estradiol, but there was no difference in testosterone *(52)*. Finally, estradiol and testosterone levels were similar in men with and without a vertebral fracture, but SHBG levels were higher in the fracture group *(67)*. These retrospective studies are limited by their small sample size (ranging from 12 to 81) and their highly select nature of the cases and controls.

There is limited longitudinal data on sex steroid hormones and fractures in older men (Table 4.3) *(41,57,68,69)*. The number of cases of fractures was extremely small, ranging from 22–54. The

Table 4.2. Summary of Case-Control or Cross-Sectional Studies of Endogenous Sex Steroid Hormones and Fractures in Men

Author	Cases	Controls	Hormones	Results Cases	Results controls	*p*-Value
Stanley (1991) USA	19 hip fx mean age = 77 yr, VA long term care facility	65 controls; matched on age and facility	%T (<9 pg/mL)	58.9% OR = 6.5 (2.0–20.6)	18%	0.002
Jackson (1992) USA	17 incident hip fx, 11 prevalent hip fx; 28 total	28 controls; matched on age, race and living facility	%T (<10.4 nmol/L)	71% OR = 5.3 (1.7–16.5)	32%	0.003
Gillberg (1999) Sweden	12 men idiopathic osteoporosis	12 controls matched on age	E2 (pmol/L)	71 ± 13	85 ± 15	0.03
			SHBG (mg/L)	3.7 ± 1.6	2.5 ± 1.0	0.04
Barrett-Connor (2000) USA	prevalent vertebral fx ($n = 28$) median age = 66 yr	no vertebral fx ($n =$ 324) median age = 65 yr	total E2 (pmol/L)	64.1	75.4	<0.05
			total bio E2 (pmol/L)	43.0	51.4	<0.05
			total T (nmol/L)	10.1	10.9	NS
			total bioT (nmol/L)	3.5	3.8	NS
				Controls	1^0 Osteo	2^0 Osteo
Legrand (2001) France	80 men BMD T score <–2.5 $n = 40$: 1^0 osteoporosis $n = 40$: 2^0 osteoporosis, mean age 49–51 yr	40 controls matched on age	E2 (ng/L)	23.9	27.2	25.3
			T (lg/L)	5.0	5.9	4.9
			SHBG (nmol/L)	24.4	32.7	36.6
Pietschmann (2001) Austria	31 men, idiopathic osteoporosis mean age = 60.6 yr	35 matched on age mean age = 56.1 yr	E2 (pmol/L)	91.3	114.6	0.04
			SHBG (nmol/L)	31.5	24.2	0.03
			FAI	42.6	56.4	0.02
Evans (2002) United Kingdom	81 men, vertebral fx mean age = 62.6 yr	68 volunteers mean age = 59.3 yr	E2 (pmol/L)	37.9	36.8	NS
			T (nmol/L)	19.5	14.9	NS
			FAI	32.1	33.9	NS
			FEI	73.5	88.8	NS
			SHBG(log) (nmol/L)	1.80	1.65	0.01

Fx, fractures; E2 estradiol; T, testosterone, SHBG, sex hormone binding globulin; FEI, free estrogen index; FAI, free androgen index; NS, not significant; VA, Veterans Affairs; OR, odds ratio; 1°, primary; 2°, secondary.

Table 4.3. Summary of Prospective Studies of Endogenous Sex Steroid Hormones and Fracture in Older Men

Author	Design	Population 1	Outcomes	Hormones		Results fx	Results No fx
Nyquist *(68)* (1998) Sweden	prospective	242 men, mean age = 67 yr	all fx ($n = 22$) mean follow-up 7 yr	T (nmol/L)		16.7	17.2
				SHBG (mg/L)		2.3	2.6
					No fx	Minor fx	Major fx
Center (2000) Australia	prospective	Dubbo cohort ($n = 437$) mean age = 72 yr	all fx ($n = 54$) mean follow-up = 1.7 yr, minor fx = 30, major fx = 24	E2 (pmol/L)	70	65	71
				Free T (pmol/L)	40	42	36
				SHBG (nmol/L)	40	41	54+
							$+p < 0.05$ vs no fx
							Adj age and weight
Gonderie-Plomp (2004) (Netherlands	nested case-control	Rotterdam cohort ($n = 3105$) mean age = 66 yr age-matched controls, $n = 133$	45 incident vertebral fx, mean follow-up = 6.5 yr	E2 (pmol/L)	⩽40.5		1.37 (0.6–3.1)
					40.6–53.8		1.33 (0.6–3.0)
					⩾53.9		Referent
				Bio E2 (pmol/L)	<28.5		1.10 (0.3–3.7)
					28.6–38.7		1.66 (0.6–4.7)
					38.8–72.9		Referent
				SHBG (nmol/L)	⩽34.2		0.75 (0.3–1.7)
					34.3–47.7		0.86 (0.4–1.8)
					>47.8		Referent

Fx, fracture; E2, estradiol; T, testosterone, SHBG, sex hormone binding globulin; adj, adjusted.

results of these studies primarily show no association, but these results are difficult to interpret. Clearly, more prospective information is needed on the relationship of sex steroid hormones and fracture in older men.

Summary

This review clearly supports a key role for estradiol in the maintenance of skeletal integrity in both men and women. Testosterone is also important, especially in older men and in maintaining bone formation, although the epidemiologic data do not support a strong independent role for testosterone in women. Most of the available research has focused on correlations with areal BMD. More information is needed on other aspects of skeletal strength including bone size, geometry, and the micro-architecture of bone. The possibility of a "threshold" level of estradiol in both men and women and differential effects on trabecular and cortical bone needs to be confirmed. Prospective studies of sex hormones and fracture in women generally show a strong relationship between serum estradiol and subsequent fracture risk. Nevertheless, until mass spectrometry is routinely available, clinical use of estradiol as a marker of risk is not recommended. There is a paucity of data on sex hormones and fracture in men. Because fractures are the most important clinical consequence of osteoporosis, these data are needed.

Individual differences in sex hormones contribute to areal BMD and to fractures, at least in older women. Generally, sex steroids decline with age. But of importance, there is considerable individual variability in the absolute levels of sex hormones and in the decline in sex steroids. The heritability of testosterone and SHBG was substantial and much higher than the genetic effects on serum estradiol *(70)*, suggesting that identification of both the genetic and non-genetic influences on hormone concentrations may help to improve our understanding of the factors that contribute to the individual variability in sex hormones and disease risk.

References

1. Riggs BL, Khosla S, Melton LJ III. A unitary model for involutional osteoporosis: estrogen deficiency causes both type I and type II osteoporosis in postmenopausal women and contributes to bone loss in aging men. J Bone Miner Res 1998;13(5):763–773.
2. Sowers MR, Jannausch M, McConnell D, et al. Hormone predictors of bone mineral density changes during the menopausal transition. J Clin Endocrinol Metab 2006;91(4):1261–1267.
3. Lee JS, Ettinger B, Stanczyk FZ, et al. Comparison of methods to measure low serum estradiol levels in postmenopausal women. J Clin Endocrinol Metab 2006;91(10):3791–3797.
4. Thienpont LM, De Leenheer AP. Efforts by industry toward standardization of serum estradiol-17 beta measurements. Clin Chem 1998;44(3):671–674.
5. Taieb J, Mathian B, Millot F, et al. Testosterone measured by 10 immunoassays and by isotope-dilution gas chromatography-mass spectrometry in sera from 116 men, women, and children. Clin Chem 2003;49(8):1381–1395.
6. Siekmann L. Determination of steroid hormones by the use of isotope dilution–mass spectrometry: a definitive method in clinical chemistry. J Steroid Biochem 1979;11(1A):117–123.
7. Lawson AM, Gaskell SJ, Hjelm M. International Federation of Clinical Chemistry (IFCC), Office for Reference Methods and Materials (ORMM). Methodological aspects on quantitative mass spectrometry used for accuracy control in clinical chemistry. J Clin Chem Clin Biochem 1985;23(7):433–441.
8. Norman A, Litwack, G. Steroid hormones: chemistry, biosynthesis, and metabolism. In: *Hormones, 2nd edition*. San Diego: Academic; 1997, 49–85.
9. Khosla S, Riggs BL, Robb RA, et al. Relationship of volumetric bone density and structural parameters at different skeletal sites to sex steroid levels in women. J Clin Endocrinol Metab 2005;90(9):5096–5103.
10. Khosla S, Melton LJ III, Robb RA, et al. Relationship of volumetric BMD and structural parameters at different skeletal sites to sex steroid levels in men. J Bone Miner Res 2005;20(5):730–740.
11. Orwoll E, Lambert LC, Marshall LM, et al. Testosterone and estradiol among older men. J Clin Endocrinol Metab 2006;91(4):1336–1344.
12. Cauley JA, Gutai JP, Sandler RB, et al. The relationship of endogenous estrogen to bone density and bone area in normal postmenopausal women. Am J Epidemiol 1986;124(5):752–761.
13. Khosla S, Melton LJ III, Atkinson EJ, et al. Relationship of serum sex steroid levels and bone turnover markers with bone mineral density in men and women: a key role for bioavailable estrogen. J Clin Endocrinol Metab 1998;83(7):2266–2274.
14. Greendale GA, Edelstein S, Barrett-Connor E. Endogenous sex steroids and bone mineral density

in older women and men: the Rancho Bernardo Study. J Bone Miner Res 1997;12(11):1833–1843.
15. Ettinger B, Pressman A, Sklarin P, et al. Associations between low levels of serum estradiol, bone density, and fractures among elderly women: the study of osteoporotic fractures. J Clin Endocrinol Metab 1998;83(7):2239–2243.
16. Murphy S, Khaw KT, Sneyd MJ, et al. Endogenous sex hormones and bone mineral density among community-based postmenopausal women. Postgrad Med J 1992;68(805):908–913.
17. Lambrinoudaki I, Christodoulakos G, Aravantinos L, et al. Endogenous sex steroids and bone mineral density in healthy Greek postmenopausal women. J Bone Miner Metab 2006;24(1):65–71.
18. Tok EC, Ertunc D, Oz U, et al. The effect of circulating androgens on bone mineral density in postmenopausal women. Maturitas 2004;48(3):235–242.
19. Rapuri PB, Gallagher JC, Haynatzki G. Endogenous levels of serum estradiol and sex hormone binding globulin determine bone mineral density, bone remodeling, the rate of bone loss, and response to treatment with estrogen in elderly women. J Clin Endocrinol Metab 2004;89(10):4954–4962.
20. Bagur A, Oliveri B, Mautalen C, et al. Low levels of endogenous estradiol protect bone mineral density in young postmenopausal women. Climacteric 2004;7(2):181–188.
21. Rogers A, Saleh G, Hannon RA, et al. Circulating estradiol and osteoprotegerin as determinants of bone turnover and bone density in postmenopausal women. J Clin Endocrinol Metab 2002;87(10):4470–4475.
22. Sowers MR, Finkelstein JS, Ettinger B, et al. The association of endogenous hormone concentrations and bone mineral density measures in pre- and perimenopausal women of four ethnic groups: SWAN. Osteoporos Int 2003;14(1):44–52.
23. Slemenda C, Longcope C, Peacock M, et al. Sex steroids, bone mass, and bone loss. A prospective study of pre-, peri-, and postmenopausal women. J Clin Invest 1996;97(1):14–21.
24. Stone K, Bauer DC, Black DM, et al. Hormonal predictors of bone loss in elderly women: a prospective study. The Study of Osteoporotic Fractures Research Group. J Bone Miner Res 1998;13(7):1167–1174.
25. Yoshimura N, Kasamatsu T, Sakata K, et al. The relationship between endogenous estrogen, sex hormone-binding globulin, and bone loss in female residents of a rural Japanese community: the Taiji Study. J Bone Miner Metab 2002;20(5):303–310.
26. Guthrie JR, Lehert P, Dennerstein L, et al. The relative effect of endogenous estradiol and androgens on menopausal bone loss: a longitudinal study. Osteoporos Int 2004;15(11):881–886.
27. Keen RW, Nguyen T, Sobnack R, et al. Can biochemical markers predict bone loss at the hip and spine?: a 4-year prospective study of 141 early postmenopausal women. Osteoporos Int 1996;6(5):399–406.
28. Hui SL, Perkins AJ, Zhou L, et al. Bone loss at the femoral neck in premenopausal white women: effects of weight change and sex-hormone levels. J Clin Endocrinol Metab 2002;87(4):1539–1543.
29. Rannevik G, Jeppsson S, Johnell O, et al. A longitudinal study of the perimenopausal transition: altered profiles of steroid and pituitary hormones, SHBG and bone mineral density. Maturitas 1995;21(2):103–113.
30. Khosla S, Bilezikian JP. The role of estrogens in men and androgens in women. Endocrinol Metab Clin North Am 2003;32(1):195–218.
31. Smith EP, Boyd J, Frank GR, et al. Estrogen resistance caused by a mutation in the estrogen-receptor gene in a man. N Engl J Med 1994;331(16):1056–1061.
32. Morishima A, Grumbach MM, Simpson ER, et al. Aromatase deficiency in male and female siblings caused by a novel mutation and the physiological role of estrogens. J Clin Endocrinol Metab 1995;80(12):3689–3698.
33. Carani C, Qin K, Simoni M, et al. Effect of testosterone and estradiol in a man with aromatase deficiency. N Engl J Med 1997;337(2):91–95.
34. Center JR, Nguyen TV, Sambrook PN, Eisman JA. Hormonal and biochemical parameters in the determination of osteoporosis in elderly men. J Clin Endocrinol Metab 1999;84(10):3626–3635.
35. Szulc P, Hofbauer LC, Heufelder AE, et al. Osteoprotegerin serum levels in men: correlation with age, estrogen, and testosterone status. J Clin Endocrinol Metab 2001;86(7):3162–3165.
36. van den Beld AW, de Jong FH, Grobbee DE, et al. Measures of bioavailable serum testosterone and estradiol and their relationships with muscle strength, bone density, and body composition in elderly men. J Clin Endocrinol Metab 2000;85(9):3276–3282.
37. Ravaglia G, Forti P, Maioli F, et al. Body composition, sex steroids, IGF-1, and bone mineral status in aging men. J Gerontol A Biol Sci Med Sci 2000;55(9):M516–M521.
38. Amin S, Zhang Y, Sawin CT, et al. Association of hypogonadism and estradiol levels with bone mineral density in elderly men from the Framing-

ham study. Ann Intern Med 2000;133(12):951–963.

39. Slemenda CW, Longcope C, Zhou L, et al. Sex steroids and bone mass in older men. Positive associations with serum estrogens and negative associations with androgens. J Clin Invest 1997;100(7):1755–1759.
40. Martinez Diaz-Guerra G, Hawkins F, Rapado A, Ruiz Díaz MA, Díaz-Curiel M. Hormonal and anthropometric predictors of bone mass in healthy elderly men: major effect of sex hormone binding globulin, parathyroid hormone and body weight. Osteoporos Int 2001;12(3):178–184.
41. Rapado A, Hawkins F, Sobrinho L, et al. Bone mineral density and androgen levels in elderly males. Calcif Tissue Int 1999;65(6):417–421.
42. Falahati-Nini A, Riggs BL, Atkinson EJ, et al. Relative contributions of testosterone and estrogen in regulating bone resorption and formation in normal elderly men. J Clin Invest 2000;106(12):1553–1560.
43. Khosla S, Melton LJ III, Atkinson EJ, et al. Relationship of serum sex steroid levels to longitudinal changes in bone density in young versus elderly men. J Clin Endocrinol Metab 2001;86(8):3555–3561.
44. Gennari L, Merlotti D, Martini G, et al. Longitudinal association between sex hormone levels, bone loss, and bone turnover in elderly men. J Clin Endocrinol Metab 2003;88(11):5327–5333.
45. Van Pottelbergh I, Goemaere S, Kaufman JM. Bioavailable estradiol and an aromatase gene polymorphism are determinants of bone mineral density changes in men over 70 years of age. J Clin Endocrinol Metab 2003;88(7):3075–3081.
46. Khosla S, Melton LJ III, Achenbach SJ, et al. Hormonal and biochemical determinants of trabecular microstructure at the ultradistal radius in women and men. J Clin Endocrinol Metab 2006;91(3):885–891.
47. Ahlborg HG, Johnell O, Turner CH, et al. Bone loss and bone size after menopause. N Engl J Med 2003;349(4):327–334.
48. Marshall DH, Crilly RG, Nordin BE. Plasma androstenedione and oestrone levels in normal and osteoporotic postmenopausal women. Br Med J 1977;2(6096):1177–1179.
49. Longcope C, Baker RS, Hui SL, et al. Androgen and estrogen dynamics in women with vertebral crush fractures. Maturitas 1984;6(4):309–318.
50. Davidson BJ, Riggs BL, Wahner HW, et al. Endogenous cortisol and sex steroids in patients with osteoporotic spinal fractures. Obstet Gynecol 1983;61(3):275–278.
51. Riggs BL, Ryan RJ, Wahner HW, et al. Serum concentrations of estrogen, testosterone, and gonadotropins in osteoporotic and nonosteoporotic postmenopausal women. J Clin Endocrinol Metab 1973;36(6):1097–1099.
52. Barrett-Connor E, Mueller JE, von Muhlen DG, Laughlin GA, Schneider DL, Sartoris DJ. Low levels of estradiol are associated with vertebral fractures in older men, but not women: the Rancho Bernardo Study. J Clin Endocrinol Metab 2000;85(1):219–223.
53. Jassal SK, Barrett-Connor E, Edelstein SL. Low bioavailable testosterone levels predict future height loss in postmenopausal women. J Bone Miner Res 1995;10(4):650–654.
54. Cummings SR, Browner WS, Bauer D, et al. Endogenous hormones and the risk of hip and vertebral fractures among older women. Study of Osteoporotic Fractures Research Group. N Engl J Med 1998;339(11):733–738.
55. Garnero P, Sornay-Rendu E, Claustrat B, et al. Biochemical markers of bone turnover, endogenous hormones and the risk of fractures in postmenopausal women: the OFELY study. J Bone Miner Res 2000;15(8):1526–1536.
56. Chapurlat RD, Garnero P, Breart G, et al. Serum estradiol and sex hormone-binding globulin and the risk of hip fracture in elderly women: the EPIDOS study. J Bone Miner Res 2000;15(9):1835–1841.
57. Goderie-Plomp HW, van der Klift M, de Ronde W, et al. Endogenous sex hormones, sex hormone-binding globulin, and the risk of incident vertebral fractures in elderly men and women: the Rotterdam Study. J Clin Endocrinol Metab 2004;89(7):3261–3269.
58. Devine A, Dick IM, Dhaliwal SS, et al. Prediction of incident osteoporotic fractures in elderly women using the free estradiol index. Osteoporos Int 2005;16(2):216–221.
59. Sipila S, Heikkinen E, Cheng S, et al. Endogenous hormones, muscle strength, and risk of fall-related fractures in older women. J Gerontol A Biol Sci Med Sci 2006;61(1):92–96.
60. Cummings SR, Melton LJ. Epidemiology and outcomes of osteoporotic fractures. Lancet 2002;359(9319):1761–1767.
61. Finkelstein JS, Sowers M, Greendale GA, et al. Ethnic variation in bone turnover in pre- and early perimenopausal women: effects of anthropometric and lifestyle factors. J Clin Endocrinol Metab 2002;87(7):3051–3056.
62. Stanley HL, Schmitt BP, Poses RM, et al. Does hypogonadism contribute to the occurrence of a minimal

trauma hip fracture in elderly men? J Am Geriatr Soc 1991;39(8):766–771.
63. Jackson JA, Riggs MW, Spiekerman AM. Testosterone deficiency as a risk factor for hip fractures in men: a case-control study. Am J Med Sci 1992;304(1):4–8.
64. Gillberg P, Johansson AG, Ljunghall S. Decreased estradiol levels and free androgen index and elevated sex hormone-binding globulin levels in male idiopathic osteoporosis. Calcif Tissue Int 1999; 64(3):209–213.
65. Legrand E, Hedde C, Gallois Y, et al. Osteoporosis in men: a potential role for the sex hormone binding globulin. Bone 2001;29(1):90–95.
66. Pietschmann P, Kudlacek S, Grisar J, et al. Bone turnover markers and sex hormones in men with idiopathic osteoporosis. Eur J Clin Invest 2001;31 (5):444–451.
67. Evans SF, Davie MW. Low body size and elevated sex-hormone binding globulin distinguish men with idiopathic vertebral fracture. Calcif Tissue Int 2002;70(1):9–15.
68. Nyquist F, Gardsell P, Sernbo I, et al. Assessment of sex hormones and bone mineral density in relation to occurrence of fracture in men: a prospective population-based study. Bone 1998;22(2): 147–151.
69. Center JR, Nguyen TV, Sambrook PN, et al. Hormonal and biochemical parameters and osteoporotic fractures in elderly men. J Bone Miner Res 2000;15(7):1405–1411.
70. Ring HZ, Lessov CN, Reed T, et al. Heritability of plasma sex hormones and hormone binding globulin in adult male twins. J Clin Endocrinol Metab 2005;90(6):3653–3658.

5 Animal Models for Senile Osteoporosis

Ken Watanabe

Age-related decline in bone mass is a universal phenomenon among laboratory mammals. Research on aging has been conducted using various models from yeast and nematode to mouse and non-human primates, and has rapidly progressed because of the recent development of forward and reverse genetics, as well as functional genomics. A number of mouse models bearing artificially or naturally modified genes develop bone phenotypes with various pathologies. Among those mice, some are considered to be potent models for understanding the pathophysiology of senile osteoporosis in humans. Here, available models for the study of senile osteoporosis, and mouse models in particular, are introduced and discussed.

General Animal Models of Senile Osteoporosis

Besides mice and rats, studies of osteoporosis in guinea pigs, rabbits, cats, dogs, and pigs have been reported. And although some of those evaluated are generally considered to be better models relative to humans in terms of similarity in estrus cycles or Haversian remodeling compared to mice and rats, the number of studies is quite limited. Studies in non-human primates, such as monkeys, have been conducted and are considered to be the best and most relevant in terms of human skeletal structure and metabolism *(1–6)*. Although breeding cost and ethical consideration are the highest compared to other animal models, therapeutic trials in non-human primate models are considered the most informative, relative to humans. Age-dependent bone loss in these animals has also been well described. On the other hand, primary screening of candidate anti-osteoporotic compounds has been tested more often in rat than mouse models, probably because they have relatively more bone mass and an overall better response to ovariectomy (OVX). As observed in humans, decreased bone marrow cellularity and increased adiposity, as well as age-related decline of bone mass, are apparent in rodent models of aging. However, the relatively recent trend of using genetic approaches, which are more easily applied to mouse models and include the targeted manipulation and ablation *in vivo* of genes, have been instrumental to our rapidly expanding knowledge of the molecular and cellular mechanisms underlying both normal and pathological bone biology.

Laboratory mice usually live for 2–3 years and show a peak bone mass at 4–8 months of age, followed by declining bone mass as they age. A popular laboratory mouse strain, C57BL/6, develops a senile osteoporosis-like bone phenotype with decreased bone mass and quality *(7–11)*. Both trabecular and cortical bones suffer dynamic changes upon aging in these mice. Whereas the cancellous bone volume fraction (BV/TV) is significantly decreased as these mice age from 6 weeks to 24 months, cortical thickness is increased until reaching peak bone mass (approximately 6 months), followed by a progressive decline thereafter *(9)*. Interestingly, expression of receptor activator of NFκB ligand (RANKL), also known as osteoclast differentiation factor, is increased upon aging, correlating with cancellous bone volume *(7,11)*. In another common strain, BALB/c, osteogenic stem cells from 24-month-old mice exhibit a decrease in proliferative potential upon aging *(12)*. It is suggested that the age-related bone loss is caused by decreased osteogenic potential caused by both quantitative and qualitative declines, especially in stem cell function *(12)*. On the other hand, bone marrow hematopoiesis is often affected by aging *(13)*. C57BL/6 is known to develop clonal B cell expansion and lymphoma frequently in this aging mouse strain *(14,15)*, suggesting that age-related, strain-specific hematopoietic disorganization, such as lymphoma, largely affects bone metabolism, and bone resorption in particular.

Senescence-accelerated mice (SAM) have been established by Takeda et al., and accepted as suitable models for aging *(16)*. The SAM lines, derived from a mouse strain AKR/J, are divided into two classes; SAM-P lines exhibit an accelerated aging phenotype with shortened life-span, and SAM-R lines, which show a less accelerated phenotype than that of SAM-P. The aging phenotype of SAM-P lines becomes apparent at 6–8 months of age. Among the SAM lines, SAM-P6 has been demonstrated to be a correlative model for senile osteoporosis in humans *(17–20)*, and its bone phenotype has been well described. For example, Jilka et al. *(17)* demonstrated that the osteopenic phenotype in SAM-P6 is caused by reduced osteoblastogenesis and that their bone metabolism is resistant to gonadectomy. Furthermore, increased adipogenesis and myelopoiesis are observed in the bone marrow of these mice *(19)*. In addition, the long bones in SAM-P6 are longer but more fragile than controls *(18)*. This line is among the best studied as a model for senile osteoporosis, not only in terms of skeletal morphology and pathology, but also in terms of its application for therapeutic-targeting experiments, such as drug testing and bone marrow transplantation *(21–23)*. Other numerous *in vivo* and *ex vivo* reports of SAM-P6 have been published whose observations are thought to be consistent between these aged mice and humans, but also include some controversial observations or interpretations, probably owing to their complicated genetic backgrounds. Because the SAM strains are polygenic, the specific genetic factors accounting for their bone phenotype remain to be elucidated.

The observed differences in bone metabolism resulting from the various genetic backgrounds of these different mouse strains have been studied by quantitative trait locus (QTL) analyses. For example, whereas C57BL/6 mice have relatively low bone mineral density (BMD) and reduced bone mass, C3H/HeJ have high BMD and are resistant to bone loss in response to OVX *(24,25)*. These studies indicate that usage of wild-type inbred strains of mice, as well as rats, need to be well-characterized and given strong consideration in studies of bone metabolism and pathophysiology.

The Premature Aging Phenotype With Decreased Bone Mass

Given the potential pitfalls with mouse models of aging as described, such animals remain reasonably good models for studies of senile osteoporosis. However, aging is a complex phenomenon and difficult to understand at the molecular level. Some of the genetically modified mice recently developed by knockout or transgenic techniques show premature aging phenotypes. The clearest conclusion to be drawn from these models is that single gene mutations cause multiple aging phenotypes. This advantage is useful in defining the mechanisms regulating bone metabolism *(26)*.

Mouse models for human progeroid syndromes have been reported *(27–31)*. These genetically modified mice develop multiple aging phenotypes and exhibit a shortened life span (Table 5.1). For example, Werner syndrome is caused by a loss-of-function mutation in *WRN*, encoding the RecQ family DNA helicase, which plays a role in genome stability including telomere maintenance *(32)*. Unexpectedly, knockout mice for the Wrn gene are essentially normal and exhibit no characteristics of premature aging *(33)*. Mice have long telomeres and relatively high telomerase activity, suggesting that the aging phenotype is latent in these mice and results from residual activity surrounding telomere maintenance. Evidently, double knockout mice for Wrn and Terc, which

Table 5.1. Genetically Modified Mice With Premature Aging Phenotype and/or Short Life Span

Gene	Function	Modification	Bone phenotype	Characterization of bone	Related human case
Atm	cell cycle checkpoint	KO	osteopenia	microCT, histological analysis, *ex vivo* cell culture	Ataxia telangiectasia
BubR1	spindle assembly checkpoint	hypomorph	Normal (kyphosis)	DXA	
DNA-PKcs	DNA repair	KO	osteopenia	X-ray analysis	
klotho	hormone/growth factor stimulating, mineral metabolism	hypomorph	osteopenia	SXA, microCT, histological analysis, *ex vivo* cell culture	
Ku86	DNA repair, transcription	KO	(not indicated)		
Lmna	Nuclear architecture	knock-in	osteopenia	DXA	Hutchinson-Golford progeria syndrome
mTR	telomere maintenance	KO	normal[a]	X-ray analysis, histological analysis	
PASG	DNA methylation	hypomorph	osteopenia	X-ray analysis, histological analysis	
PolgA	mitochondrial DNA replication	knock-in	osteoporosis	X-ray analysis	
Recql4	DNA replication and repair	KO	osteopenia	X-ray analysis, histological analysis	Rothmund-Thomson syndrome
Sirt6	DNA repair	KO	osteopenia	X-ray analysis, DXA	
TRp53	cell cycle checkpoint	deletion mutant	osteopenia	X-ray analysis, histological analysis	
		mutant Tg	osteopenia	X-ray analysis	
		short isoform Tg	osteopenia	X-ray analysis, histological analysis	
XPD	DNA replication and repair	knock-in	osteoporosis	X-ray analysis, DXA	Xeroderma pigmentosum
Wrn/Terc	telomere maintenance	double KO	osteopenia	microCT	Werner syndrome

[a] The phenotype was observed in the 6th generation from mTR knockout mouse matings.

encodes the RNA component of telomerase activity, show a Werner-like phenotype with osteoporosis *(34,35)*. RecQ like-4 (Recql4) is a gene mutated in a subset of Rothmund-Thomson syndrome, recognized as a premature aging syndrome *(36,37)*. Although Reql4 null mice are embryonic lethal, targeted deletion of exon 13 results in a form of aging phenotype that includes osteopenia *(38)*. Yang et al. showed that osteoprogenitors are significantly decreased in heterozygous Recql4 (+/–) mice compared to wild-type controls *(39)*. In addition, mutated Recql4 has also been reported in Baller-Gerold syndrome, a rare autosomal recessive disorder with radial aplasia/hypoplasia and craniosynostosis *(40)*.

Recently, a gene encoding lamin A has been identified to be responsible for human progeria, Hutchinson-Gilford syndrome *(41,42)*. Mice carrying an autosomal recessive point mutation in the lamin A gene, corresponding to that identified in humans, also develop a progeria-like phenotype with osteoporotic symptoms *(43)*. Interestingly, Duque and Rivas found that expression of lamin A/C in osteoblasts and chondrocytes of C57BL/6 mice is decreased in an age-related manner, suggesting that lamin A/C in osteoblasts may play a role in physiological aging and senile osteoporosis *(44)*.

Mice presenting with multiple aging phenotypes have also been reported. Null mutation of a gene, Ku86 (also known as Ku80), which plays roles in DNA repair and transcription, exhibits a shortened life span and elicits a premature aging phenotype including osteopenia *(45)*. The aging phenotype has also been observed in mice lacking PASG, an SNF-like molecule that functions in DNA methylation *(46)*. Mutant mice show decreased BMD and a delay in the secondary ossification of the tibial epiphyses *(46)*. In addition to mutations in genes involved in genomic stability and nuclear organization, mice carrying mitochondrial DNA polymerase mutations that exclude a region responsible for its proofreading activity also present the osteoporotic phenotype together with other premature aging symptoms *(47)*. A sir2/SIRT family of NAD-dependent histone deacetylase has been reported to be implicated in life span. Knockout mice for Sirt6 exhibit genomic instability and an aging-like phenotype with osteopenia *(48)*; particularly decreased bone mass, now considered a hallmark of premature aging phenotypes. However, most observations of the skeletal phenotype were examined by X-ray analysis. The pathophysiology, including histology, of the bone phenotype in these models for premature aging has not yet been fully described.

Errors in cell duplication, such as those misprogrammed by the previously mentioned mutations, can be detected and corrected by arresting cell cycle. A system of cell cycle checkpoints has been shown to play a critical mechanistic role *(49,50)*. Checkpoint kinase cascades are involved in DNA replication and other cell cycle events. ATM is a PI3K family kinase involved in DNA repair and oxidative response *(51)*. The gene encoding the protein kinase has been identified as a gene mutated in ataxia telangiectasia, recognized as one of the human premature aging syndromes *(52)*. Knockout mice for ATM exhibit a similar phenotype to the human disease, including hyper-radiosensitivity and ataxic defects *(53–55)*. It has been shown that the self-renewal capacity of hematopoietic stem cells in Atm knockout mice is significantly impaired with elevated reactive oxygen species (ROS), and that treatment with anti-oxidative agents rescues the bone marrow failure *(56)*. An osteopenic phenotype has also been observed in these knockout mice. Colony formation assays revealed that the phenotype was mainly caused by a proliferative defect in bone marrow mesenchymal stem cells or its progenitors *(57)*.

Gain-of-function mutations in p53, a downstream effector of ATM kinase, also exhibit premature aging with an osteoporotic phenotype *(58,59)*. Among them, p44 transgenic mice show a low progenitor turnover with significant decreases in osteoblast number and a slight reduction of osteoclasts *(59)*. Although further characterization of the models is required, these data suggest that the stem cell defect caused by cell cycle arrest upon DNA damage or other cell cycle abnormalities, at least in part, may account for the decreased bone formation and subsequent osteopenia observed in these premature aging models.

In addition to stem cell defects in p53 and other checkpoint deficiencies, recent evidence indicates that p53 can directly regulate osteoblast differentiation *(60,61)*. Wang et al. showed that mice lacking p53 exhibit increased bone mass because of accelerated osteoblast differentiation caused by elevated Osterix levels. Lengner et al. examined osteoblast-specific ablation of Mdm2, a negative regulator of p53, and found reduced proliferation and decreased levels of Runx2 in the osteoblasts. Furthermore, they also described elevated Runx2 levels in p53-null osteoblasts, suggesting that p53 negatively regulates bone development and growth by inhibition of Runx2. Defects in osteoblast differentiation caused by dysregulation of Osterix was also recently reported in Atm knockout mice *(62)*. Thus, not only stem cell defects, but also cell autonomous differentiation defects of osteoblasts may be associated with the osteopenic phenotype in mouse models of premature aging.

Osteopenia Caused By Decrease in Bone Formation

Low turnover rates or uncoupling between bone resorption and formation in aged bones is often associated with decline in osteoblast function *(63)*. Reduced bone formation is one of the features observed in models for senile osteoporosis. A number of genes playing critical roles in bone formation have been described using genetically modified mice *(64–67)*. Several typical models are listed in Table 5.2. Sca1/Ly6A is a GPI-anchored membrane protein expressed in hematopoietic stem cells and a subset of bone marrow stromal cells *(68,69)*. Whereas Sca1 knockout mice have normal bone development, the aged animals (15 months of age) show significant bone loss *(70)*. Progenitor and differentiation assays of bone marrow cells in these mice reveal that decreased bone mass is caused by impaired self-renewal of mesenchymal progenitors. Stem cell defects in

TABLE 5.2. Osteopenic Mice With Altered Bone Formation

Gene	Phenotype (knockout)	Osteoprogenitor (incl. stem cells)	Number of osteoblasts	Number of osteoclasts	Ex vivo osteoblast differentiation
Kl (klotho)	osteopenia	↓	↓	↓	↓
Ly6a (Sca1)	osteopenia	↓	↓	↓	↔
Irs1	osteopenia	n.d.	↓	↓	↔
Lrp5	osteopenia	↓	↓	↔	↔
Fhl2	osteopenia	n.d.	↔	↔	↓
Abl1 (Abl)	osteopenia	↓	↓	↔	↓

n.d., not described.

hematopoietic lineages have also been reported in Sca1 knockout mice *(71)*. Although multiple aging phenotypes in Sca1 knockout mice have not been reported, this is a good model for senile osteoporosis in humans, supporting the stem cell hypothesis in the pathogenesis of senile osteoporosis *(72)*.

IRS1, a major substrate of insulin receptor (IR) and insulin-like growth factor-1 receptor (IGF1R) that transduces signals by interacting with signaling molecules in a phosphorylation-dependent manner, is expressed in osteoblasts but not in osteoclasts. IRS1 knockout mice exhibit low bone mass compared with wild-type controls, and cultured osteoblasts from the knockout mice are impaired in IGF-induced proliferation and differentiation, whereas bone morphogenetic protein (BMP)-induction is not altered *(73)*. Reduced osteoclast formation is the result of defective osteoblasts, resulting in low turnover osteopenia *(73)*.

Wnt signaling regulates bone mass through the osteoblastic lineage. It has been revealed that an autosomal recessive disorder, osteoporosis-pseudoglioma syndrome (OPPG), is caused by mutations in the gene encoding LRP5, a cell surface co-receptor for Wnt *(74)*. It has also been independently shown that Val171 mutation of LRP5 causes high bone density in humans *(75)*. These correlative findings indicate a role for the Wnt pathway in bone development and remodeling. Kato et al. generated mice deficient in Lrp5, and showed that Lrp5 knockout mice also develop osteopenia caused by reduced osteoblast proliferation and function *(76)*. A significant decrease in the number of bone marrow stromal progenitor cell (colony-forming unit fibroblastoids [CFU-F]) colonies was observed in the knockout mice. Inhibition of GSK3, a negative regulator of Wnt/β-catenin signaling, stimulates osteoblastic differentiation of the progenitors *(77,78)*. The ligands, such as Wnt10b, specifically activate the canonical pathway, and constitutively activate β-catenin-stimulated osteoblast differentiation *(79)*. These finding support the idea that the canonical pathway via β-catenin signaling of Wnt plays a role in the regulation of osteoblasts. It should be noted that the canonical pathway also inhibits adipogenic differentiation of progenitor cells *(80)*, suggesting that the pathway is also important in lineage commitment between osteoblastic and adipogenic fates. This observation may be associated with age-related alterations of bone marrow, resulting in decreased bone formation and increased adipogenesis to what is described as "fatty marrow."

On the other hand, some models presenting with osteopenia exhibit defects in osteoblast differentiation. Mice lacking a transcriptional cofactor, *four and a half LIM domains 2 (Fhl2)*, also present with a significant decrease in bone mass *(81)*. Although numbers of osteoblasts and osteoclasts were comparable to littermate controls, bone formation rate was markedly reduced. Furthermore, transgenic mice overexpressing Fhl2 in osteoblasts exhibited enhanced bone formation and increased bone mass. Fhl2 interacts with Runx2 to increase its transcriptional activity and stimulates osteoblast maturation, suggesting that the Fhl2 knockout is a unique model for osteopenia caused by osteoblast activation deficiency *(81)*.

c-Abl, a downstream protein kinase of ATM, functions in DNA repair and oxidative stress response *(82,83)*. Mice deficient for the Abl gene also develop osteopenia with reduced bone formation *(84)*. *Ex vivo* assays of osteoclastogenesis were not affected, and the number of osteoclasts in the Abl-deficient mice was similar to that of wild-type controls. Whereas the number of progenitors in bone marrow is significantly decreased, the differentiation of osteoblasts from Abl knockout mice is also impaired *(84)*. Using osteoblast culture, distinct roles in the oxidative stress response between c-Abl and ATM have been proposed *(85)*. Although decreased expression of peroxiredoxin 1 (Prdx1) caused by down-regulation of PKCδ was observed on arsenate-induced oxidative stress in osteoblasts from Atm knockout mice, expression of the redox protein, through the upregulation of PKCδ, was increased in the cells derived from Abl knockouts. The opposite roles in the oxidative stress response may cause similar bone phenotypes in the knockout mice of Abl and Atm genes through distinct mechanisms. Life-span shortening and age-related defects have been reported in mice lacking Prdx1 or MsrA, which encodes methionine sulfoxide reductase *(86,87)*. Both genes play important roles in the oxidative stress response through anti-ROS activity. Whereas the bone phenotype in these mutant mice has not yet been described, it will be interesting to see the potential pathogenic phenotype in bone from these mice. Oxidative stress, such as that caused by ROS, often causes damage in DNA, suggesting that the genomic stability and oxidative stress response may share some common pathways in the aging phenotype (Figures 5.1 and 5.2). As mentioned with Atm mice, an antioxidant also partially rescues perinatal lethality of Ku86 knockout mice *(88)*. In addition to DNA damage, ROS is important in signal transduction and

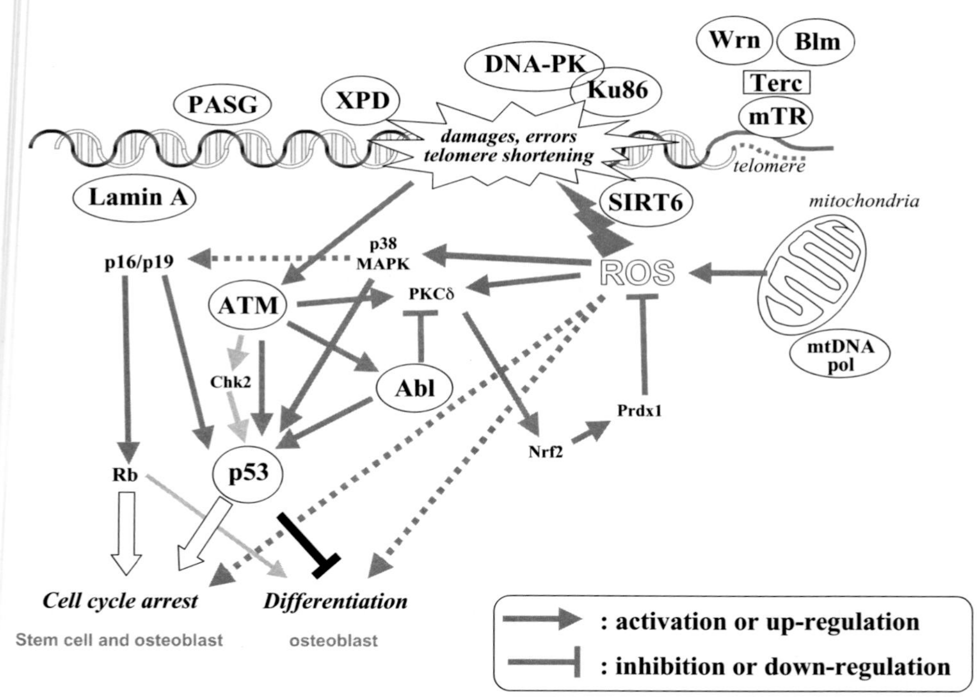

FIGURE 5.1. Predicted pathways connecting the gene products responsible for the premature aging mutant phenotype.
Most of the mouse models for premature aging described by now are caused by mutations in the genes involved in genomic integrity and subsequent cell cycle regulation. Errors and damage to the genome or telomere shortening, which also affects DNA integrity could, in theory, be detected and corrected. Mutations in the genes responsible for genomic stability cause accumulation of phenotypic abnormalities. Genomic disorganization activates cell cycle-regulating pathways involving checkpoint kinases and p53. Oxidative stress is among the triggers that elicit genomic instability via DNA damage. Elevation and excess of ROS affect downstream signaling, including PKCδ, which subsequently stimulates the anti-ROS pathway, including transcriptional activation of Prdx1.

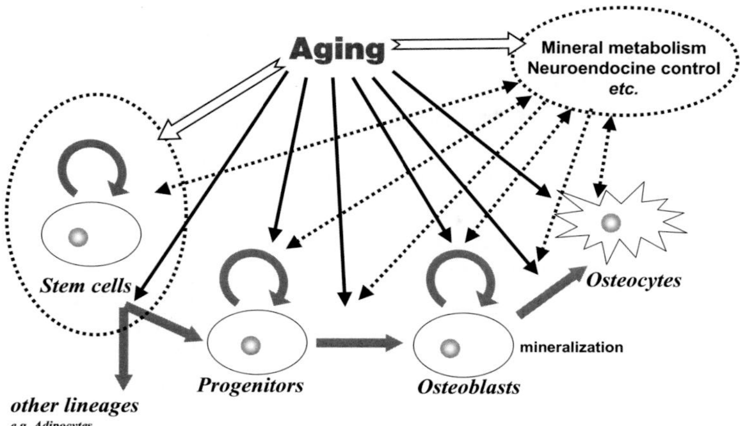

FIGURE 5.2. Osteogenesis and aging. Observations in naturally aged laboratory animals and mutant mice with aging phenotypes suggest that one of the keys to understanding aging and premature aging pathogenesis may be self-renewing stem cells. In these models, the pathway involving p53 (Figure 5-1) up-regulates the genes responsible for cell cycle arrest and/or apoptosis, lowering the regenerative potential necessary for homeostasis and tissue repair. Although the mechanisms responsible for aging are largely unknown, the existing models suggest that there are common pathways, which may help in our understanding of the aging phenotype.

pathogenesis of diseases as well. For example, anti-oxidative agents reverse insulin resistance in diabetic models *(89,90)*. Although it remains unclear whether ROS targets are part of the mechanistic pathways affected by aging, management of ROS may be significantly implicated in osteoblast function and aging.

The Aging Phenotype and Defects in Mineral Metabolism

Other models for accelerated aging phenotypes, where the responsible genes are apparently not directly involved in genomic integrity, also exist. Mice carrying hypomorphic mutations of the gene, Klotho, show multiple aging phenotypes *(91)*. In klotho mice (kl/kl), both bone formation and resorption are reduced, indicating a low turnover of bone metabolism resembling human osteoporosis *(92)*. Although neither osteoblasts nor osteoclasts express the kl gene, *ex vivo* cultures of osteoblastogenesis and osteoclastogenesis show reduced differentiation independently in both lineages. This is a unique model for senile osteoporosis in humans, in contrast to the canonical progeroid models. Recently, the molecular functions of KL protein have been reported. The protein, which is structurally similar to β-glucosidase, possesses β-glucuronidase activity (93). KL protein acts as a co-receptor for IGF and is also required for FGF23 signaling through FGFR1 *(94,95,96)*. FGF23 has been identified as a gene responsible for autosomal dominant hypophosphatemic rickets and is suggested to play an important role in phosphate metabolism as a hormone, a candidate for phosphatonin *(97)*. FGF23 knockout mice also exhibit a premature aging-like phenotype *(98)*. Interestingly, the mice have elevated serum levels of vitamin D and hyperphosphatemia, and a part of the aging phenotype was rescued by lowering the vitamin D levels *(98–100)*. It is therefore suggested that control of the phosphate-regulating system by FGF23-KL is associated with the aging phenotype including osteoporosis. Notably, PHEX (phosphate-regulating gene with homology to endopeptidases on the X chromosome) is highly expressed in osteocytes *(101–104)*, of which number declines with age as well as with post-OVX and mechanical unloading *(105–107)*. Conceivably, osteocytes may be implicated in phosphate metabolism and senile osteoporosis, although the model directly demonstrating its function is not yet described.

What Mouse Models Teach

It has been recently described that mice deficient for molecular clock genes, such as Per1/2, Cry1/2, and BMAL1, exhibit increased bone mass with elevated bone formation *(108)*. The clock components inhibit osteoblast proliferation triggered by CREB activation responding to signals from sympathetic neurons. In contrast, it has also been reported that BMAL1 knockout mice have impaired circadian rhythms and display a premature aging phenotype, including decreased bone mass (109). Although these apparently opposite observations might be owing to age differences (increased bone mass at 2 months; decreased at 40 weeks of age, compared to wild-type controls), bone phenotype is largely affected by many factors including mobility. Thus, the same mouse can tell different stories. Whereas decreased bone mass is a major indication of the aging phenotype as mentioned, age-related structural and functional alterations are seen not only in bone, but also in other tissues and organs as well. Senile osteoporosis has been recognized as a secondary osteoporosis and not essentially caused by cell autonomous effects of age-related bone cell dysfunction, but may be secondary to age-related decline of mineral metabolism or hormonal regulation, as well as neuronal and/or gonadal dysregulation. Nevertheless, these models inform us of the molecular mechanisms involved in bone biology, especially the molecular and cellular basis of bone pathophysiology, and include the possibility that cell autonomous bone defects may be implicated, at least in part, in the pathogenesis of senile osteoporosis. Furthermore, the described genetically defined models can be useful for elucidation of the underlying mechanisms in pharmacological and other therapeutic-targeting studies.

References

1. Aufdemorte TB, Fox WC, Miller D, Buffum K, Holt GR, Carey KD. A non-human primate model for the study of osteoporosis and oral bone loss. Bone 1993;14(3):581–586.
2. Champ JE, Binkley N, Havighurst T, Colman RJ, Kemnitz JW, Roecker EB. The effect of advancing age on bone mineral content of female rhesus monkeys. Bone 1996;19(5):485–492.
3. Colman RJ, Kemnitz JW, Lane MA, Abbott DH, Binkley N. Skeletal effects of aging and menopausal status in female rhesus macaques. J Clin Endocrinol Metab 1999;84(11):4144–4148.
4. Colman RJ, Lane MA, Binkley N, Wegner FH, Kemnitz JW. Skeletal effects of aging in male rhesus monkeys. Bone 1999;24(1):17–23.
5. Jayo MJ, Rankin SE, Weaver DS, Carlson CS, Clarkson TB. Accuracy and precision of lumbar bone mineral content by dual-energy X-ray absorptiometry in live female monkeys. Calcif Tissue Int 1991;49(6):438–440.
6. Jayo MJ, Weaver DS, Rankin SE, Kaplan JR. Accuracy and reproducibility of lumbar bone mineral status determined by dual photon absorptiometry in live male cynomolgus macaques (Macaca fascicularis). Lab Anim Sci 1990;40(3): 266–269.
7. Ikeda T, Utsuyama M, Hirokawa K. Expression profiles of receptor activator of nuclear factor kappaB ligand, receptor activator of nuclear factor kappaB, and osteoprotegerin messenger RNA in aged and ovariectomized rat bones. J Bone Miner Res 2001;16(8):1416–1425.
8. Perkins SL, Gibbons R, Kling S, Kahn AJ. Age-related bone loss in mice is associated with an increased osteoclast progenitor pool. Bone 1994; 15(1):65–72.
9. Halloran BP, Ferguson VL, Simske SJ, Burghardt A, Venton LL, Majumdar S. Changes in bone structure and mass with advancing age in the male C57BL/6J mouse. J Bone Miner Res 2002; 17(6):1044–1050.
10. Ferguson VL, Ayers RA, Bateman TA, Simske SJ. Bone development and age-related bone loss in male C57BL/6J mice. Bone 2003;33(3):387–398.
11. Cao J, Venton L, Sakata T, Halloran BP. Expression of RANKL and OPG correlates with age-related bone loss in male C57BL/6 mice. J Bone Miner Res 2003;18(2):270–277.
12. Bergman RJ, Gazit D, Kahn AJ, Gruber H, McDougall S, Hahn TJ. Age-related changes in osteogenic stem cells in mice. J Bone Miner Res 1996; 11(5):568–577.
13. Morrison SJ, Wandycz AM, Akashi K, Globerson A, Weissman IL. The aging of hematopoietic stem cells. Nat Med 1996;2(9):1011–1016.
14. Ghia P, Melchers F, Rolink AG. Age-dependent changes in B lymphocyte development in man and mouse. Exp Gerontol 2000;35(2):159–165.
15. LeMaoult J, Manavalan JS, Dyall R, Szabo P, Nikolic-Zugic J, Weksler ME. Cellular basis of B cell clonal populations in old mice. J Immunol 1999;162(11):6384–6391.

16. Takeda T, Matsushita T, Kurozumi M, Takemura K, Higuchi K, Hosokawa M. Pathobiology of the senescence-accelerated mouse (SAM). Exp Gerontol 1997;32(1–2):117–127.
17. Jilka RL, Weinstein RS, Takahashi K, Parfitt AM, Manolagas SC. Linkage of decreased bone mass with impaired osteoblastogenesis in a murine model of accelerated senescence. J Clin Invest 1996;97(7):1732–1740.
18. Silva MJ, Brodt MD, Ettner SL. Long bones from the senescence accelerated mouse SAMP6 have increased size but reduced whole-bone strength and resistance to fracture. J Bone Miner Res 2002;17(9):1597–1603.
19. Kajkenova O, Lecka-Czernik B, Gubrij I, et al. Increased adipogenesis and myelopoiesis in the bone marrow of SAMP6, a murine model of defective osteoblastogenesis and low turnover osteopenia. J Bone Miner Res 1997;12(11):1772–1779.
20. Matsushita M, Tsuboyama T, Kasai R, et al. Age-related changes in bone mass in the senescence-accelerated mouse (SAM). SAM-R/3 and SAM-P/6 as new murine models for senile osteoporosis. Am J Pathol 1986;125(2):276–283.
21. Takada K, Inaba M, Ichioka N, et al. Treatment of senile osteoporosis in SAMP6 mice by intra-bone marrow injection of allogeneic bone marrow cells. Stem Cells 2006;24(2):399–405.
22. Duque G, Macoritto M, Dion N, Ste-Marie LG, Kremer R. 1,25(OH)2D3 acts as a bone-forming agent in the hormone-independent senescence-accelerated mouse (SAM-P/6). Am J Physiol Endocrinol Metab 2005;288(4):E723–E730.
23. Ichioka N, Inaba M, Kushida T, et al. Prevention of senile osteoporosis in SAMP6 mice by intrabone marrow injection of allogeneic bone marrow cells. Stem Cells 2002;20(6):542–551.
24. Li CY, Schaffler MB, Wolde-Semait HT, Hernandez CJ, Jepsen KJ. Genetic background influences cortical bone response to ovariectomy. J Bone Miner Res 2005;20(12):2150–2158.
25. Beamer WG, Shultz KL, Donahue LR, et al. Quantitative trait loci for femoral and lumbar vertebral bone mineral density in C57BL/6J and C3H/HeJ inbred strains of mice. J Bone Miner Res 2001; 16(7):1195–1206.
26. Hishiya A, Watanabe K. Progeroid syndrome as a model for impaired bone formation in senile osteoporosis. J Bone Miner Metab 2004;22(5): 399–403.
27. Warner HR, Sierra F. Models of accelerated ageing can be informative about the molecular mechanisms of ageing and/or age-related pathology. Mech Ageing Dev 2003;124(5):581–587.
28. Hasty P, Vijg J. Accelerating aging by mouse reverse genetics: a rational approach to understanding longevity. Aging Cell 2004;3(2):55–65.
29. Hasty P, Campisi J, Hoeijmakers J, van Steeg H, Vijg J. Aging and genome maintenance: lessons from the mouse? Science 2003;299(5611):1355–1359.
30. Kuro-o M. Disease model: human aging. Trends Mol Med 2001;7(4):179–181.
31. Kipling D, Davis T, Ostler EL, Faragher RG. What can progeroid syndromes tell us about human aging? Science 2004;305(5689):1426–1431.
32. Yu CE, Oshima J, Fu YH, et al. Positional cloning of the Werner's syndrome gene. Science 1996; 272(5259):258–262.
33. Lombard DB, Beard C, Johnson B, et al. Mutations in the WRN gene in mice accelerate mortality in a p53-null background. Mol Cell Biol 2000;20(9): 3286–3291.
34. Du X, Shen J, Kugan N, et al. Telomere shortening exposes functions for the mouse werner and bloom syndrome genes. Mol Cell Biol 2004; 24(19):8437–8446.
35. Chang S, Multani AS, Cabrera NG, et al. Essential role of limiting telomeres in the pathogenesis of Werner syndrome. Nat Genet 2004;36(8):877–882.
36. Mohaghegh P, Hickson ID. DNA helicase deficiencies associated with cancer predisposition and premature ageing disorders. Hum Mol Genet 2001;10(7):741–746.
37. Kitao S, Shimamoto A, Goto M, et al. Mutations in RECQL4 cause a subset of cases of Rothmund-Thomson syndrome. Nat Genet 1999;22(1):82–84.
38. Hoki Y, Araki R, Fujimori A, et al. Growth retardation and skin abnormalities of the Recql4-deficient mouse. Hum Mol Genet 2003;12(18): 2293–2299.
39. Yang J, Murthy S, Winata T, et al. Recql4 haploinsufficiency in mice leads to defects in osteoblast progenitors: implications for low bone mass phenotype. Biochem Biophys Res Commun 2006; 344(1):346–352.
40. Van Maldergem L, Siitonen HA, Jalkh N, et al. Revisiting the craniosynostosis-radial ray hypoplasia association: Baller-Gerold syndrome caused by mutations in the RECQL4 gene. J Med Genet 2006;43(2):148–152.
41. Eriksson M, Brown WT, Gordon LB, et al. Recurrent de novo point mutations in lamin A cause Hutchinson-Gilford progeria syndrome. Nature 2003;423(6937):293–298.

42. De Sandre-Giovannoli A, Bernard R, Cau P, et al. Lamin a truncation in Hutchinson-Gilford progeria. Science 2003;300(5628):2055.
43. Mounkes LC, Kozlov S, Hernandez L, Sullivan T, Stewart CL. A progeroid syndrome in mice is caused by defects in A-type lamins. Nature 2003;423(6937):298–301.
44. Duque G, Rivas D. Age-related changes in lamin A/C expression in the osteoarticular system: laminopathies as a potential new aging mechanism. Mech Ageing Dev 2006;127(4):378–383.
45. Vogel H, Lim DS, Karsenty G, Finegold M, Hasty P. Deletion of Ku86 causes early onset of senescence in mice. Proc Natl Acad Sci U S A 1999; 96(19):10770–10775.
46. Sun LQ, Lee DW, Zhang Q, et al. Growth retardation and premature aging phenotypes in mice with disruption of the SNF2-like gene, PASG. Genes Dev 2004;18(9):1035–1046.
47. Trifunovic A, Wredenberg A, Falkenberg M, et al. Premature ageing in mice expressing defective mitochondrial DNA polymerase. Nature 2004; 429(6990):417–423.
48. Mostoslavsky R, Chua KF, Lombard DB, et al. Genomic instability and aging-like phenotype in the absence of mammalian SIRT6. Cell 2006; 124(2):315–329.
49. Hartwell L. Defects in a cell cycle checkpoint may be responsible for the genomic instability of cancer cells. Cell 1992;71(4):543–546.
50. Nurse P. Checkpoint pathways come of age. Cell 1997;91(7):865–867.
51. Rotman G, Shiloh Y. ATM: from gene to function. Hum Mol Genet 1998;7(10):1555–1563.
52. Lavin MF, Shiloh Y. The genetic defect in ataxia-telangiectasia. Annu Rev Immunol 1997;15:177–202.
53. Barlow C, Hirotsune S, Paylor R, et al. Atm-deficient mice: a paradigm of ataxia telangiectasia. Cell 1996;86(1):159–171.
54. Xu Y, Ashley T, Brainerd EE, Bronson RT, Meyn MS, Baltimore D. Targeted disruption of ATM leads to growth retardation, chromosomal fragmentation during meiosis, immune defects, and thymic lymphoma. Genes Dev 1996;10(19):2411–2422.
55. Elson A, Wang Y, Daugherty CJ, et al. Pleiotropic defects in ataxia-telangiectasia protein-deficient mice. Proc Natl Acad Sci U S A 1996;93(23): 13084–13089.
56. Ito K, Hirao A, Arai F, et al. Regulation of oxidative stress by ATM is required for self-renewal of haematopoietic stem cells. Nature 2004;431(7011):997–1002.
57. Hishiya A, Ito M, Aburatani H, Motoyama N, Ikeda K, Watanabe K. Ataxia telangiectasia mutated (Atm) knockout mice as a model of osteopenia due to impaired bone formation. Bone 2005;37(4):497–503.
58. Tyner SD, Venkatachalam S, Choi J, et al. p53 mutant mice that display early ageing-associated phenotypes. Nature 2002;415(6867):45–53.
59. Maier B, Gluba W, Bernier B, et al. Modulation of mammalian life span by the short isoform of p53. Genes Dev 2004;18(3):306–319.
60. Lengner CJ, Steinman HA, Gagnon J, et al. Osteoblast differentiation and skeletal development are regulated by Mdm2-p53 signaling. J Cell Biol 2006;172(6):909–921.
61. Wang X, Kua HY, Hu Y, et al. p53 functions as a negative regulator of osteoblastogenesis, osteoblast-dependent osteoclastogenesis, and bone remodeling. J Cell Biol 2006;172(1):115–125.
62. Rasheed N, Wang X, Niu QT, Yeh J, Li B. Atm-deficient mice: an osteoporosis model with defective osteoblast differentiation and increased osteoclastogenesis. Hum Mol Genet 2006;15(12): 1938–1948.
63. Manolagas SC, Jilka RL. Bone marrow, cytokines, and bone remodeling. Emerging insights into the pathophysiology of osteoporosis. N Engl J Med 1995;332(5):305–311.
64. Davey RA, MacLean HE, McManus JF, Findlay DM, Zajac JD. Genetically modified animal models as tools for studying bone and mineral metabolism. J Bone Miner Res 2004;19(6):882–892.
65. Chien KR, Karsenty G. Longevity and lineages: toward the integrative biology of degenerative diseases in heart, muscle, and bone. Cell 2005; 120(4):533–544.
66. Karsenty G. The complexities of skeletal biology. Nature 2003;423(6937):316–318.
67. Karsenty G. The genetic transformation of bone biology. Genes Dev 1999;13(23):3037–3051.
68. Yeh ET, Reiser H, Benacerraf B, Rock KL. The expression, function, and ontogeny of a novel T cell-activating protein, TAP, in the thymus. J Immunol 1986;137(4):1232–1238.
69. Stanford WL, Haque S, Alexander R, et al. Altered proliferative response by T lymphocytes of Ly-6A (Sca-1) null mice. J Exp Med 1997;186(5): 705–717.
70. Bonyadi M, Waldman SD, Liu D, Aubin JE, Grynpas MD, Stanford WL. Mesenchymal progenitor self-renewal deficiency leads to age-dependent osteoporosis in Sca-1/Ly-6A null mice. Proc Natl Acad Sci U S A 2003;100(10): 5840–5845.

71. Ito CY, Li CY, Bernstein A, Dick JE, Stanford WL. Hematopoietic stem cell and progenitor defects in Sca-1/Ly-6A-null mice. Blood 2003;101(2):517–523.
72. Oreffo RO, Bord S, Triffitt JT. Skeletal progenitor cells and ageing human populations. Clin Sci (Lond) 1998;94(5):549–555.
73. Ogata N, Chikazu D, Kubota N, et al. Insulin receptor substrate-1 in osteoblast is indispensable for maintaining bone turnover. J Clin Invest 2000;105(7):935–943.
74. Gong Y, Slee RB, Fukai N, et al. LDL receptor-related protein 5 (LRP5) affects bone accrual and eye development. Cell 2001;107(4):513–523.
75. Boyden LM, Mao J, Belsky J, et al. High bone density due to a mutation in LDL-receptor-related protein 5. N Engl J Med 2002;346(20):1513–1521.
76. Kato M, Patel MS, Levasseur R, et al. Cbfa1-independent decrease in osteoblast proliferation, osteopenia, and persistent embryonic eye vascularization in mice deficient in Lrp5, a Wnt coreceptor. J Cell Biol 2002;157(2):303–314.
77. Kulkarni NH, Onyia JE, Zeng Q, et al. Orally bioavailable GSK-3alpha/beta dual inhibitor increases markers of cellular differentiation in vitro and bone mass in vivo. J Bone Miner Res 2006;21(6):910–920.
78. Clement-Lacroix P, Ai M, Morvan F, et al. Lrp5-independent activation of Wnt signaling by lithium chloride increases bone formation and bone mass in mice. Proc Natl Acad Sci U S A 2005;102(48):17406–17411.
79. Bennett CN, Longo KA, Wright WS, et al. Regulation of osteoblastogenesis and bone mass by Wnt10b. Proc Natl Acad Sci U S A 2005;102(9):3324–3329.
80. Ross SE, Hemati N, Longo KA, et al. Inhibition of adipogenesis by Wnt signaling. Science 2000;289(5481):950–953.
81. Gunther T, Poli C, Muller JM, et al. Fhl2 deficiency results in osteopenia due to decreased activity of osteoblasts. Embo J 2005;24(17):3049–3056.
82. Kharbanda S, Yuan ZM, Weichselbaum R, Kufe D. Functional role for the c-Abl protein tyrosine kinase in the cellular response to genotoxic stress. Biochim Biophys Acta 1997;1333(2):O1–O7.
83. Hantschel O, Superti-Furga G. Regulation of the c-Abl and Bcr-Abl tyrosine kinases. Nat Rev Mol Cell Biol 2004;5(1):33–44.
84. Li B, Boast S, de los Santos K, et al. Mice deficient in Abl are osteoporotic and have defects in osteoblast maturation. Nat Genet 2000;24(3):304–308.
85. Li B, Wang X, Rasheed N, et al. Distinct roles of c-Abl and Atm in oxidative stress response are mediated by protein kinase C delta. Genes Dev 2004;18(15):1824–1837.
86. Moskovitz J, Bar-Noy S, Williams WM, Requena J, Berlett BS, Stadtman ER. Methionine sulfoxide reductase (MsrA) is a regulator of antioxidant defense and lifespan in mammals. Proc Natl Acad Sci U S A 2001;98(23):12920–12925.
87. Neumann CA, Krause DS, Carman CV, et al. Essential role for the peroxiredoxin Prdx1 in erythrocyte antioxidant defence and tumour suppression. Nature 2003;424(6948):561–565.
88. Reliene R, Goad ME, Schiestl RH. Developmental cell death in the liver and newborn lethality of Ku86 deficient mice suppressed by antioxidant N-acetyl-cysteine. DNA Repair (Amst) 2006;5(11):1392–1397.
89. Furukawa S, Fujita T, Shimabukuro M, et al. Increased oxidative stress in obesity and its impact on metabolic syndrome. J Clin Invest 2004;114(12):1752–1761.
90. Houstis N, Rosen ED, Lander ES. Reactive oxygen species have a causal role in multiple forms of insulin resistance. Nature 2006;440(7086):944–948.
91. Kuro-o M, Matsumura Y, Aizawa H, et al. Mutation of the mouse klotho gene leads to a syndrome resembling ageing. Nature 1997;390(6655):45–51.
92. Kawaguchi H, Manabe N, Miyaura C, Chikuda H, Nakamura K, Kuro-o M. Independent impairment of osteoblast and osteoclast differentiation in klotho mouse exhibiting low-turnover osteopenia. J Clin Invest 1999;104(3):229–237.
93. Tohyama O, Imura A, Iwano A, et al. Klotho is a novel beta-glucuronidase capable of hydrolyzing steroid beta-glucuronides. J Biol Chem 2004;279(11):9777–9784.
94. Kurosu H, Ogawa Y, Miyoshi M, et al. Regulation of fibroblast growth factor-23 signaling by klotho. J Biol Chem 2006;281(10):6120–6123.
95. Kurosu H, Yamamoto M, Clark JD, et al. Suppression of aging in mice by the hormone Klotho. Science 2005;309(5742):1829–1833.
96. Urakawa I, Yamazaki Y, Shimada T, et al. Klotho converts canonical FGF receptor into a specific receptor for FGF23. Nature 2006;444(7120):770–774.
97. ADHR-Consortium. Autosomal dominant hypophosphataemic rickets is associated with mutations in FGF23. Nat Genet 2000;26(3):345–348.
98. Razzaque MS, Sitara D, Taguchi T, St-Arnaud R, Lanske B. Premature aging-like phenotype in fibroblast growth factor 23 null mice is a vitamin D-mediated process. FASEB J 2006;20:720–722.

99. Tsujikawa H, Kurotaki Y, Fujimori T, Fukuda K, Nabeshima Y. Klotho, a gene related to a syndrome resembling human premature aging, functions in a negative regulatory circuit of vitamin D endocrine system. Mol Endocrinol 2003;17(12):2393–2403.
100. Yoshida T, Fujimori T, Nabeshima Y. Mediation of unusually high concentrations of 1,25-dihydroxyvitamin D in homozygous klotho mutant mice by increased expression of renal 1alpha-hydroxylase gene. Endocrinology 2002;143(2):683–689.
101. Liu S, Zhou J, Tang W, Jiang X, Rowe DW, Quarles LD. Pathogenic role of Fgf23 in Hyp mice. Am J Physiol Endocrinol Metab 2006;291(1):E38–E49.
102. Thompson DL, Sabbagh Y, Tenenhouse HS, et al. Ontogeny of Phex/PHEX protein expression in mouse embryo and subcellular localization in osteoblasts. J Bone Miner Res 2002;17(2):311–320.
103. Westbroek I, De Rooij KE, Nijweide PJ. Osteocyte-specific monoclonal antibody MAb OB7.3 is directed against Phex protein. J Bone Miner Res 2002;17(5):845–853.
104. Miao D, Bai X, Panda D, McKee M, Karaplis A, Goltzman D. Osteomalacia in hyp mice is associated with abnormal phex expression and with altered bone matrix protein expression and deposition. Endocrinology 2001;142(2):926–939.
105. Aguirre JI, Plotkin LI, Stewart SA, et al. Osteocyte apoptosis is induced by weightlessness in mice and precedes osteoclast recruitment and bone loss. J Bone Miner Res 2006;21(4):605–615.
106. Jilka RL, Weinstein RS, Bellido T, Roberson P, Parfitt AM, Manolagas SC. Increased bone formation by prevention of osteoblast apoptosis with parathyroid hormone. J Clin Invest 1999;104(4):439–446.
107. Tomkinson A, Gevers EF, Wit JM, Reeve J, Noble BS. The role of estrogen in the control of rat osteocyte apoptosis. J Bone Miner Res 1998;13(8):1243–1250.
108. Fu L, Patel MS, Bradley A, Wagner EF, Karsenty G. The molecular clock mediates leptin-regulated bone formation. Cell 2005;122(5):803–815.
109. Kondratov RV, Kondratova AA, Gorbacheva VY, Vykhovanets OV, Antoch MP. Early aging and age-related pathologies in mice deficient in BMAL1, the core componentof the circadian clock. Genes Dev 2006;20(14):1868–1873.

6
Senile Osteoporosis as a Geriatric Syndrome

Rujuta H. Patel and Kenneth W. Lyles

Introduction

With the rise in the aging population, osteoporosis has become a major health burden. From 50 years of age onward, 4 in 10 women will have a hip, vertebral, or forearm fracture. And in the years to come, they are more likely to die from complications as a consequence of fracture rather than from breast cancer. Although osteoporosis is viewed as a disease occurring in post-menopausal women, men account for 30% of hip fractures worldwide *(1)*. More importantly, osteoporosis causes a greater health burden in older people. Billions of dollars are spent each year in the US on acute and long-term care required for people who sustain osteoporosis-related fractures *(2)*. Globally, osteoporotic fractures caused an estimated 5.8 million disability adjusted life years in the year 2000 *(3)*. This figure is expected to increase worldwide as the population ages.

Fractures, as a result of osteoporosis, consume a significant proportion of healthcare resources. Recently, the annual cost of all osteoporotic fractures in the US has been estimated to be $20 billion *(2)*. In 1995, more than 400,000 hospitalizations, 3.4 million outpatient visits, and 179,000 nursing home admissions were a direct consequence of osteoporotic fractures *(1)*. Hip fractures have the highest morbidity and mortality. Almost all of the hip fractures occur after a fall; 80% occur amongst women and 90% occur in people over the age of 50 *(2)*. People with hip fractures have 12–39% higher mortality in the immediate following year compared to the same age population; 13–50% of survivors are not able to walk after the event and 12–20% of the survivors need nursing home placement *(2)*. Vertebral fractures are the most common osteoporotic fractures. Many are not recognized clinically. Whether recognized clinically or not, they cause pain, height loss, deformity, and increased risk for further fractures *(4)*.

Osteoporosis in older persons should be distinguished from the typical post-menopausal, hormone-deficient increase in bone turnover, which is the primary focus of most of the literature in the field. First, with advanced aging there are clear changes in the ability of the aged marrow such that mesenchymal stem cells are more likely to differentiate into adipocytes, rather than osteoblasts or even myoblasts. This leads to the accumulation of fat in the marrow with less bone formation during skeletal remodeling *(5)*. Second, the loss of muscle mass with aging ("sarcopenia"), and the relative decrease in physical activity, leads to reduced loading of the aged skeleton, and ultimately reduced bone formation and increased resorption *(6)*. Furthermore, as falls increase dramatically with aging, trauma to an already fragile skeleton is the formula for the extremely high risk for osteoporotic fracture with aging *(7)*.

Epidemiology

Fractures in the spine, hip, and distal forearm are considered typically osteoporotic fractures. But there is a changing trend in such notions

Table 6.1. Fractures That Should Be Included as Osteoporotic, in Descending Anatomical Order (4)

Proximal humerus	Femoral diaphysis
Distal humerus	Patella distal femur
Olecranon	Bi-malleolar ankle
Proximal radius and ulna	Tri-malleolar ankle
Distal radius	Thoracolumbar vertebrae
Proximal femoral	Pelvis
Sub-trochanteric	Multiple fractures

that is supported by recent studies indicating that numerous other fracture sites need to be considered under the umbrella of osteoporosis *(8)*. Table 6.1 lists fracture sites that fall within the osteoporotic realm. Among these fractures, hip fractures are more prevalent in older populations with incidence rising from 22.5 and 23.9 per 100,000 population at age 50 to 630.2 and 1289.3 per 100,000 population by age 80, for men and women respectively *(9–11)*.

Low skeletal bone mass at any location is associated with an increased incidence of fracture. Other risk factors increasing fracture risk include advanced age, low body mass index (BMI), history of osteoporosis from the maternal side, smoking, rheumatoid, arthritis, glucocorticoid use, more than 3 alcohol drinks daily, and most importantly previous history of fractures *(12)*. Recent studies also implicate a reduction in leg muscle mass as an additional contributor to fractures in older persons *(6)*. Glucocorticoid-induced osteoporosis (GIOP) is a predictable complication of prolonged steroid use. The loss in bone mass, as an outcome of chronic steroid use, occurs in the first 6 months of treatment, and the risk of fracture increases in the first 3 months of steroid therapy.

Oral glucocorticoids are taken by 1% of the population and 2.5% of those over age 75 years, thus elderly patients on glucocorticoids amplify their increased risk of fractures *(13)*. Current guidelines for the treatment of GIOP indicate that all patients who require more than 5 mg/day of glucocorticoid for a period of longer than 3 months should be treated with 1500 mg/day of calcium, 800 IU/day of vitamin D, and an oral bisphosphonate. These patients should have a dual-energy X-ray absorptiometry (DXA) scan prior to beginning steroid treatment to establish a baseline *(14)*.

Pathophysiology

The National Institute of Health (NIH) defines osteoporosis as a disease of increased bone frailty in addition to low bone mineral density (BMD) (a T score below −2.5) and micro-architectural decline *(15)*. Certain physical signs maybe useful in recognizing patients with osteoporosis (Table 6.2). However, osteoporotic fractures result from a combination of decreased bone strength and falls. Several measures, in addition to the BMD, affect the skeletal fracture rate. These include macro-architecture (form and geometry), micro-architecture of trabecular and cortical bone, amount of mineralization, bone turnover, and sequential micro-damage *(2)*.

The bone mass acquired during intrauterine life signifies the peak bone mass built in childhood and puberty stages with contrast to the simultaneous rate of bone loss. Even though genetic elements have a strong influence in achieving peak bone mass, environmental factors alter the pattern of bone growth determined by genes *(2)*.

At the cell level, a disparity between the activity of osteoclasts and osteoblasts contributes to bone loss. There is continuous remodeling in an adult skeleton where bone resorption is followed by bone formation. If these two processes are not coordinated, there may be remodeling discrepancy exaggerated by an increase in the rate of new bone remodeling cycles (activation frequency)

Table 6.2. Physical Signs Suggesting the Presence of Osteoporosis or Vertebral Fractures (54)

Loss of height greater than 2 inches
Wall-occiput distance greater than 0 inches[a]
Rib-pelvis distance less than 2 fingerbreaths
Fewer than 20 teeth
Weight less than 51 kg (112 lb)

[a] While standing with back and heels to the wall, the distance between the occiput and wall in a horizontal plane.

(2). With aging the rate of bone resorption increases, but the bone formation rate is not increased, and in fact, declines, so there is no bone loss over time.

Estrogen deficiency, in post-menopausal women, facilitates bone loss. Estrogen has a vital role in physiological remodeling and estrogen deficiency in the post-menopausal state results in plasticity, inequity of remodeling, and significant increase in bone turnover. This divergence leads to a progressive loss of trabecular bone. Estrogen negatively regulates osteoclastogenic proinflammatory cytokines, such as interleukin (IL)-1 and tumor necrosis factor (TNF). Thereby, an estrogen-deficient setting enhances elaboration of these osteoclastogenic proinflammatory cytokines, which in turn encourage osteoclastogenesis *(2)* (Figure 1.3).

Age-related bone loss is a complex phenomenon with multiple factors involved in the pathogenesis. Studies show a slow and consistent decline in BMD after the third decade of approximately 0.5% per year. Women experience accelerated bone loss of approximately 3–5% per year during menopause. In men the decline in bone mass is gradual until quite late in life, when the risk for fractures increases rapidly. Age-related bone loss is a mixture of several factors such as changes at the cellular level, including diminished osteoblastogenesis, shortened osteoblast life span, and increased adipogenesis *(16)*. In addition to this there are hormonal alterations, including decreased levels and activity of sex steroid hormones, reduced vitamin D level, declining renal function leading to lower level of active form of vitamin D3, and increased levels of parathyroid hormone (PTH) *(16)*. Osteoporosis in men appears to result from cellular and hormonal changes that include lower levels of testosterone, dehydroepiandrosterone (DHEA), and insulin-like growth factor (IGF)-1, with subsequent lower osteoblast activity and higher osteoblast apoptosis. Recent evidence suggests that estrogen is essential for bone health in men as well as women. Further exploration is required to explain the precise roles of these factors in the decline of BMD and high fracture rates in men after the seventh decade of life *(17)*.

Research in the last several years lends valuable insight into the cellular basis of bone remodeling. The key regulators of osteoclastic bone resorption are receptor activator of NFκB (RANK), its ligand (RANKL), and the decoy receptor osteoprotegerin. The osteoblasts express RANKL on their cell surface; RANKL interacts with its corresponding receptors. RANK is present on osteoclast precursors and facilitates osteoclast maturation. The interface between RANKL and RANK on mature osteoclasts stimulates the activation and prolonged survival (Figure 1.3). Osteoprotegerin is present in the skeletal milieu and generated by osteoblasts and stromal cells. Osteoprotegerin inhibits the interaction between RANK and RANKL, thus acting as a regulator of bone turnover. Estrogen exerts part of its anti-resorptive effect on bone by exciting osteoprotegerin expression in osteoblasts *(2)*. More recently, a new system of osteoblast-osteoclast coupling has been reported. This system, which is known as Ephrin signaling *(18)*, involves a bidirectional signaling between osteoblasts, which express EphrinB4, and the osteoclasts which express EphrinB2. The interaction between Ephrin 2 and 4 activates a signaling from osteoclasts to osteoblasts that is responsible for driving the formation of the new bone packet (Figure 6.1). Additionally, this interaction is responsible for the cessation of continued bone resorption. Since this interaction is not as dependent on the presence of estrogens as the RANK-RANKL system, a new role of the Ephrin interaction is being assessed in the pathogenesis of age-related bone loss.

A common feature seen in both males and females with osteoporosis is a deficit in osteoblastogenesis and osteoblastic activity *(16)*. This deficit is known to be caused by several factors including a reduced number of stromal precursors in the bone marrow, a decreased osteoblastogenesis at the expense of adipogenesis, and increased osteoblast/osteocyte apoptosis *(19)*. The end result of these age-related changes is that a lower number of osteoblasts will be available at the bone-remodeling unit to replace the bone that has been resorbed by active osteoclasts, which explains the constant deficit in bone formation observed in age-related bone loss *(16,19)*.

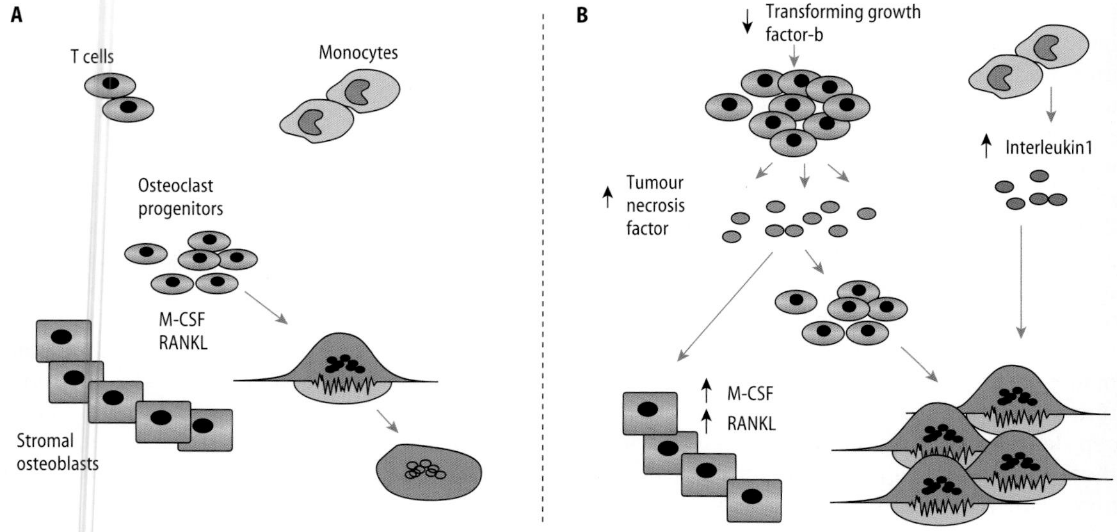

FIGURE 6.1. Ephrin signaling regulates osteoclast-osteoblast bi-directional interaction *(18)*.

Diagnosis

With aging, the burden of chronic diseases increases, and this contributes to the observed reduction in function that occurs. Although there has been an increased awareness of the need for screening for osteoporosis in addition to attending to all of the other chronic diseases that affect older persons, generally speaking, osteoporosis is under-diagnosed and under-treated in elderly individuals *(20)*. Screening for the risk of osteoporosis in seniors has been facilitated by the improved access to bone densitometry that resulted from Medicare approval for this procedure. However, fracture risk may also be assessed without the need for BMD testing *(21)*. In fact, the Rotterdam Study showed that although the incidence of hip fracture increased 13-fold from the age of 60 to 80 years, the reduction in BMD accounted only for a small part of this increase *(22)*. Additionally, fall risk assessments should be done in concert with fracture risk assessments in older persons *(23)*, as demonstrated in several studies *(24)* where the risk of fracture was determined not only by BMD and other skeletal risk factors, but also by factors associated with physical frailty and an increased risk of falls *(21)*.

Treatment

Vitamin D is recognized as a critical factor in maintaining normal serum calcium levels by enhancing gastrointestinal absorption of calcium and phosphorus. Low serum 25 hydroxyvitamin D levels (the measure of vitamin D status) are low in all segments of the population, students, hospitalized patients, hip fracture subjects, and residents of long-term care facilities. Vitamin D insufficiency causes secondary hyperparathyroidism, bone loss, and muscle weakness *(25)*. There are studies showing that the traditional 400 IU of vitamin supplementation is inadequate to bring serum 25 hydroxyvitamin D level into the recommended range *(26)*. A complete review on the rationale for the use of vitamin D in osteoporosis and falls is included in Chapter 3 of this book.

The prevention of falls is crucial because most fractures occur after a fall. This is especially true for the geriatric population, which is the fastest-growing age group and the group with the greatest fall risk. Recent studies indicate that calcitriol [1,25-dihydroxyvitamin D, 1,25 $(OH)_2D$] may be useful in preventing falls in older women with a glomerular filtration rate (GFR) less than 60 mL/minute *(27)*. Furthermore, correction of vitamin

D deficiency with standard cholecalciferol has been shown to reduce the risk of falls in older individuals *(28)*. Higher doses may be required than traditionally considered *(29)*. Medications should be reviewed to avoid those that increase the risk of falls. Homes need to be evaluated for unstable hazards such as throw rugs and smooth surfaces. Some studies have shown that hip protectors can reduce the risk of fracture from a fall; however, patient compliance remains an issue *(30)*.

Physical activity early in the formative years of life contributes to the peak bone mass. Regular exercise and weight-bearing activities may help improve gait, thus diminishing the risk of falls *(31)*. Research shows that exercise can reduce the risk of falls by approximately 25% in frail older persons. Studies indicate that load-bearing exercises are valuable in increasing bone mass when compared to other activities. The high-impact exercises boost the BMD by 1–2% at some but not all the sites in the skeleton. The augmentation in the bone density is maintained after stopping the exercise. Some evidence has been accumulating that loading the skeleton with low-magnitude stimuli at high frequency may increase bone density *(32)*. After a vertebral fracture, an organized exercise program is recommended in older individuals to preserve the strength and elasticity of the spine. However, no organized studies show that exercise programs lessen the fracture risk, at any age *(33)*.

The drugs used for the treatment of osteoporosis may be classified based on their mechanisms as anti-resorptive agents (reduce bone resorption) and anabolic agents (stimulate bone formation). The majority of approved therapies for osteoporosis target bone resorption, rather than bone formation. As such, although fracture reduction has been demonstrated with many anti-resorptive agents, perhaps a more logical approach to drug therapy in older persons would be to stimulate bone formation, as is the case for teriparatide *(34)* and possibly strontium *(35)*.

The anti-resorptive medications include calcium, vitamin D, hormone therapy, bisphosphonates, selective estrogen-receptor modulators, and calcitonin *(36)*. Although the active form of vitamin D ($1,25(OH)_2D_3$) has been recently reported to have an anabolic effect in bone *(37)*, the only currently approved anabolic agent is PTH. Clinical trials have employed intact PTH (hPTH 1–84) and a 34 amino acid peptide (hPTH 1–34) commonly known as teriparatide *(34)*. Table 6.3 lists the frequently used medications for osteoporosis treatment in the United States.

Although several clinical trials have tested the effectiveness of anti-resorptives in osteoporosis in

Table 6.3. Commonly Used Medications for Osteoporosis Treatment in the United States (2)

Drug Type	Route of Administration	Dosage	Average Wholesale Price per 30-Day Supply[a]
Estrogen	Oral	0.3 mg/day	$8.49 (multi-pack)
		0.45 mg/day	$34.60 (multi-pack)
		0.625 mg/day	$36.41
		0.9 mg/day	$14.00 (multi-pack)
		1.25 mg/day	$40.05
SERM Raloxifene	Oral	60 mg/day	$96.00
Salmon calcitonin	Intranasal	200 IU/day in alternating nostrils	$77.95
Bisphosphonates			
Alendronate	Oral	5–10 mg/day	$82.63 (5 mg) $107.51 (10 mg)
		35–70 mg/week	$82.65 (35 mg) $86.09 (70 mg)
Risedronate	Oral	5 mg/day	$82.63
		35 mg /week	$86.09
Ibandronate	Oral	2.5 mg/day	$80.50
		150 mg/month	$78.50
Anabolic therapy PTH 1–34	Intravenous injection	20 mg/day	$543.60
Strontium	Oral	2 gm/day	$55.60

[a] Correct as of October 2005.
SERM, selective estrogen-receptor modulator; PTH, parathyroid hormone.

the elderly, very few have been tested in the very old and frail population older than 75 years of age. Additionally, most of the clinical trials have focused on the prevention of vertebral fractures, which are more common in "younger" post-menopausal patients in contrast with non-vertebral fractures, which are more prevalent in older populations and in osteoporotic men. Here, we will review some evidence that has come out of these trials with emphasis on the prevention of fractures in older populations.

The first and most remarkable study that showed the efficacy of calcium and vitamin D included a high-risk group of 3270 elderly women in residential care. These women were treated with 1200 mg calcium and 800 IU of vitamin D for 18 months. The trial showed a 43% reduction in hip fractures and 32% decrease in total non-vertebral fractures *(38)*. A successive trial involved 2686 people living in the community. This study examined the role of oral cholecalciferol 1,000,000 IU given every 4 months for a total of 5 years. The results showed a reduction in the risk of hip, wrist, forearm, or vertebral fractures by 33% when compared with a placebo. The RECORD trial included 5292 ambulatory patients who had sustained a recent low trauma fracture. These patients were randomized to calcium alone, vitamin D (800 IU alone), combined calcium and vitamin D, or a placebo. The results did not show a significant difference in fracture rates between the four groups; however, the analysis was limited by the low compliance and lack of baseline vitamin D levels. A meta-analysis later concluded that the vitamin D decreased the risk of hip fractures by 26% and non-vertebral fractures by 23% in subjects who were deficient in vitamin D *(39)*. Vitamin D in an 800 IU daily dose should be provided to all patients with osteoporosis and those at risk for developing it.

The role of post-menopausal hormone replacement therapy in the treatment of osteoporosis is controversial after the publication of Women's Health Initiative (WHI) study *(40)*. The WHI trial showed an increased incidence of cardiovascular events with combined hormone therapy, especially if the women were older than 70 years at the time of initiation of therapy. The study also showed a higher event of breast cancer and stroke in patients who were using the combined hormone therapy. Currently, estrogen therapy is approved for osteoporosis treatment only in women who are experiencing menopausal symptoms such as hot flashes. If estrogen is used, it must be given at the lowest possible dose for the shortest time, usually 2 years *(2)*.

Selective estrogen receptor modulators are structured based on their ability to attach to the estrogen receptor, thus modifying the action in the cell by affecting the cellular transcription. The selective nature of these drugs results in mimicking the effects of estrogen in the body but avoiding the adverse effects of estrogen, such as increased risk of breast cancer and endometrial hyperplasia. At present, raloxifene is the only selective estrogen receptor modulator approved for treatment of osteoporosis in postmenopausal women *(41)*. In the phase III study of 7705 post-menopausal women, raloxifene 60 mg daily decreased the rate of vertebral fractures by approximately 50% in people without prior fractures and by 34% in women with previous vertebral fractures. Raloxifene is associated with a threefold increment in the risk of deep vein thrombosis, pulmonary embolism, and retinal venous clots. Raloxifene also increases hot flashes *(42)*.

Salmon calcitonin has been studied in a double-blinded randomized controlled trial. The minimum dose of calcitonin required to produce a noteworthy effect on BMD is 200 IU intranasally daily. Calcitonin is less efficient in prevention of cortical bone loss compared to cancellous bone loss. A small controlled study in women with osteoporosis showed a decline in new fractures in persons taking calcitonin. In the PROOF (Prevent Recurrence Of Osteoporotic Fractures) study, which was a 5-year double-blinded randomized placebo controlled study of 1255 post-menopausal women with osteoporosis, intranasal calcitonin 200 IU per day decreased the threat of vertebral but not peripheral fractures by approximately 30% when compared to the placebo *(42)*. Salmon calcitonin is well tolerated, with minimal side effects such as rhinitis and rarely epistaxis. There is ongoing research to develop long-acting oral salmon calcitonin. The evidence for salmon calcitonin as an anti-resorptive agent is not strong and does not compare to the efficacy of bisphosphonates *(43)*.

Bisphosphonates have become the mainstay for the treatment of osteoporosis in the last decade. Clinical trials involving bisphosphonates have shown a reduction in vertebral fractures by 40–50% and non-vertebral fractures by 20–40% (44). Bisphosphonates are pyrophosphate analogs that act as bone-specific anti-resorptive agents. Bisphosphonates reduce osteoclast-mediated bone resorption by inhibiting farnesyl diphosphate synthase in the cholesterol mevalonic acid pathway, which is vital in protein prenylation (Figure 6.2). This process affects multiple intracellular functions, including membrane integrity at the ruffled border in the osteoclasts and arrangement of the cytoskeleton.

Bisphosphonates are poorly absorbed from the gastrointestinal tract; approximately 0.6–0.7% of the total dose is absorbed through the gastric mucosa. Bisphosphonates have to be administered on an empty stomach for best results. After absorption, they are either taken up by the active resorbing surfaces on the bone (50%) or are excreted in the urine (50%). Current bisphosphonates approved for the treatment of osteoporosis in the United States are alendronate, ibandronate, and risedronate. Alendronate was the first bisphosphonate approved for treatment of osteoporosis in the United States. Risedronate was the second bisphosphonate approved by the Food and Drug Administration (FDA) for the treatment of post-menopausal osteoporosis in the United States *(44)*. Studies have been conducted to test the efficacy of risedronate in cutting the risk of fractures in women aged 80 years and older who have osteoporosis. After 1 year, the rate of new vertebral fractures in the risedronate group was 81% lower when compared to the placebo group ($P < 0.001$). The number of women who needed to be treated to avoid one new vertebral fracture after 1 year was 12. These conclusions from the research provide proof that even in the extreme of age, decreasing bone resorption is an effective tactic to manage osteoporosis *(45)*.

One of the major difficulties with the use of these drugs is the upper gastrointestinal irritation as a result of recurrent and lengthy contact of the drug with the esophageal mucosa. This led to debate about degree of compliance in clinical practice when compared with placebo-controlled trials. Because of market research showing that nearly 90% of physicians and patients preferred a weekly therapy, clinical trials were held to show the efficacy of a weekly dosing regime when compared to daily dosing in terms of increase in BMD and stemming bone turnover. This led to the introduction and endorsement of weekly dosing regimes for alendronate and risedronate. Ibandronate is available as a monthly pill and quarterly intravenous (IV) formulation *(45)*. In addition, Ibandronate (Boniva—Roche) is the first bisphosphonate backed up by the FDA for IV treatment of osteoporosis in post-menopausal women. It can be administered as a bolus injection once every 3 months. Ibandronate is also available as once per month 150-mg pill or 2.5-mg daily tablet. Ibandronate, like other bisphosphonates, inhibits osteoclastic action and diminishes

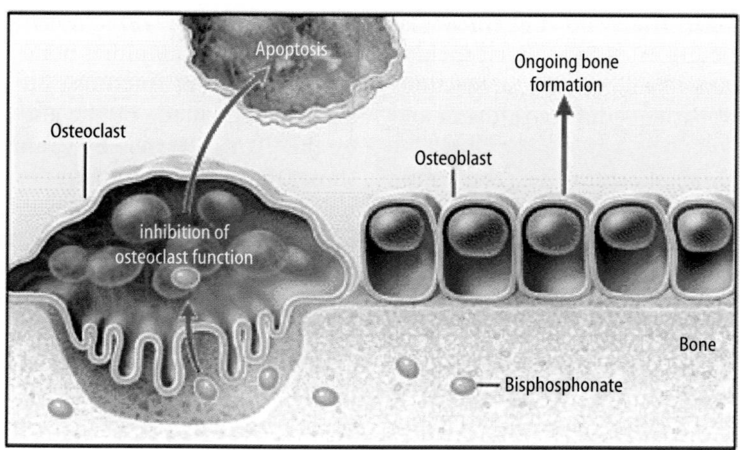

Figure 6.2. For proposed mechanism of action of bisphosphonates (From N Engl J Med 2002;346(9):642).

bone resorption, in turn enhancing bone mass. Approximately 40–50% of IV ibandronate attaches to the bone, and the remaining 40–50% is eliminated unchanged in urine. There are no studies showing that IV ibandronate decreases the fracture rate. FDA endorsement was based on a study showing that IV ibandronate was "not inferior" to the oral form of the drug in increasing BMD. A temporary acute phase reaction including fever, joint pain, and/or myalgias has been reported with IV use of ibandronate, most commonly with the first dose. Zoledronic acid and pamidronate are parenteral bisphosphonates approved by the FDA for the treatment of hypercalcemia of malignancy and multiple myeloma; they have been used off-label for the treatment of postmenopausal osteoporosis *(46)*. Osteonecrosis of the jaw has been linked with the use of high doses of IV bisphosphonates in patients with multiple myeloma and breast carcinoma, and is reported to occur in up to 10% of these patients *(47)*. Osteonecrosis of the jaw occurs less frequently (patient per 100,000 treated) in subjects who use oral bisphosphonates to treat osteoporosis *(48)*.

Pamidronate was developed in the 1980s before the launch of alendronate, ibandronate, and risedronate. It has not been approved for treatment of osteoporosis in the United States. Its current indication for use includes treating hypercalcemia of malignancy and Paget's disease. Pamidronate has been used off-label to treat osteoporosis, especially in patients who cannot swallow, sit upright for 30 minutes, or with other significant gastrointestinal tract problems. There are at present no randomized controlled trials showing efficacy of pamidronate on fracture rates. Side effects include myalgia and influenza-like illness. These reactions occur in 20–25% of patients during infusion and are transient *(49)*.

Of all the available bisphosphonates, zoledronic acid produces the most effective inhibition of the osteoclasts *in vitro*. At high doses, zoledronic acid produces adverse renal effects as confirmed by increase in serum creatinine. Because of the undesirable outcome, the recommended dose was decreased to 4 mg and the time of intravenous infusion was increased from 5 to 15 minutes. A phase II trial evaluated different dosing regimens of IV zoledronic acid (0.25, 0.5, or 1 mg at 3 month intervals, 2 mg biannually, and 4 mg annually) with placebo over the period of 1 year in 351 postmenopausal women with a BMD of T score less than −2.0. All the women in the study were supplemented with calcium 1000 mg/day. After 1 year there was a significant increase in both lumbar spine BMD and femoral neck BMD, P value of less than 0.001 in all regimes versus placebo. At present, a study is underway to evaluate the antifracture efficacy of zoledronic acid in the treatment of osteoporosis. Zoledronic acid should be used with vigilance when administered with other nephrotoxic drugs because of the danger of worsening renal function. Simultaneous use with loop diuretics can increase the risk of hypocalcemia *(50)*.

PTH is the first anabolic therapy for osteoporosis approved by the FDA in the United States. The use of PTH can seem paradoxical given its effect of bone loss in hyperparathyroidism. Experiments in animals have suggested that the method of delivery decides whether the action of the hormone is anabolic or catabolic. The exact mechanism by which once daily dosing of the hormone generates new bone formation is unclear. It has been postulated that the effect is caused by the modulation of IGF-1 and the RANK/RANKL/osteoprotegerin (OPG) system. Clinical trials have been done with both intact PTH (hPTH 1–84) and with 34 amino acid peptide (hPTH 1–34), now called teriparatide *(37)*. Teriparatide is the only FDA-approved treatment for osteoporosis that augments bone mass and decreases risk for fracture by stimulating osteoblastic activity and furthering bone formation, as opposed to bisphosphonates and other therapies, which slow down bone resorption. hPTH I-84 Also amplifies bone bulk and trims the risk of vertebral fractures, but the fracture data has not been made public and it is not endorsed by the FDA. A review by Cranney and associates shows that daily administration of PTH for 12–18 months improves bone mass and, among postmenopausal women, lowers the vertebral and non-spine fracture risk. The review included patients with severe osteoporosis and concluded that PTH increases the BMD of the lumbar spine and femoral neck *(16)*. A recent study using teriparatide in the treatment of post-menopausal osteoporosis demonstrated that the skeletal response of teriparatide is largely independent of age and original BMD *(17)*.

Results from a phase III trial with teriparatide in 1637 post-menopausal women showed a 65% reduction in new vertebral fractures and a 53% reduction in non-vertebral fractures *(2)*. Teriparatide is approved for use at a dose of 20 μg/day subcutaneously for 2 years in women with osteoporosis who are an elevated risk of fracture and who have failed or are not able to endure other therapies. PTH 1–34 is approved for use in men as well for the treatment of osteoporosis caused by primary or secondary hypogonadism. Teriparatide is well tolerated; it can occasionally cause leg cramps and dizziness. The safety of teriparatide has not been probed beyond 2 years. There is "black box" warning for teriparatide because of incidence of osteogenic sarcoma in rats exposed to a lifetime therapy *(15)*.

BMD begins to decline after terminating treatment with teriparatide. This has led to the hypothesis that intermixing two different anti-resorptive agents may result in a synergistic effect. Studies are being conducted at present to test this theory. There is current information on joint effects of PTH and hormone replacement therapy and alendronate with PTH. The use of PTH and hormone replacement therapy has produced noteworthy increase in BMD when compared with a placebo ($P < 0.05$). One study found that a combination of PTH and alendronate diminished both the BMD and the bone marker response when compared to using PTH alone. The assumption was that alendronate being a potent anti-resorptive agent suppressed the osteoblast turnover, thus diminishing the PTH effect *(15)*.

Future/In the Pipeline

Strontium ranelate is a new agent that is approved in the European Union for the treatment of post-menopausal osteoporosis. Its mode of action currently remains unknown. In a phase III trail among 1649 post-menopausal women, strontium ranelate lessened the risk of new vertebral fractures by 49% after 1 year and by 41% over 3 years *(35)*. Strontium ranelate is well tolerated aside from some gastrointestinal effects and unexplained increase in venous thrombosis. This drug is not approved for use in the United States.

Realization of the RANKL mechanism connecting the osteoblasts and osteoclasts has opened a new horizon for the treatment of osteoporosis. Denosumab *(52)* is a fully human monoclonal antibody with a high affinity for RANKL. The joining of this antibody to RANKL inhibits the RANKL from interacting with its receptor, which in turn interferes with osteoclast differentiation. This suppressive effect is long lasting, and in a phase II trial, twice-yearly injections increased the BMD at the hip similar to that seen with alendronate. A phase III trial is now underway *(2)*.

A forthcoming challenge is to recognize risk factors that can give us tools to calculate the fracture risk for the future. This will impact several developing regions of the world where the risk factors can be used to foretell individuals at a higher risk of developing osteoporotic fractures independent of the BMD test. Professor John Kanis and his colleagues are working on such a model in conjunction with the World Health Organization, National Osteoporosis Foundation, and the International Osteoporosis Foundation. Risk factors such as age, prior history of a fracture, family history of osteoporotic fracture, smoking history, steroid use, alcohol use, and rheumatoid arthritis are being taken into consideration in order to develop a set of guidelines that will be able to predict the 10-year fracture risk for men and women worldwide *(53)*.

In summary, osteoporosis in older adults manifests differently than post-menopausal osteoporosis in multiple ways. From its pathophysiology to its therapeutic approach, senile osteoporosis is a geriatric syndrome that, as with all other geriatric syndromes, requires a complete understanding of its particular characteristics and its potential biological, functional, and social consequences in the older population. Only after understanding the particularities of this syndrome will we be able to approach it from a multi-dimensional perspective where the prevention of falls and fractures should be the most important goal of the health professional.

Acknowledgments. Dr. Lyles receives consulting and lecture fees from Novartis, Proctor & Gamble/ Aventis, Merck, Amgen, and Bone Medical LTD. He currently receives grant support from

Novartis, Proctor & Gamble/Aventis, and Amgen. He also is co-inventor with Novartis Pharmaceuticals on a use patent for zoledronic acid (US Provisional Patent Application No. 60/411,067.

Grant Support: The Claude A. Pepper Older American Independence Center AG-11268 and VA Medical Research Services.

References

1. Colon-Emeric CS, Saag KG. Osteoporotic fractures in older adults. Best Prac Res Clin Rheumatol 2006;20:695–706.
2. Sambrook P, Cooper C. Osteoporosis. Lancet 2006;367:2010–2018.
3. Dolan P, Torgerson DJ. The cost of treating osteoporotic fractures in the United Kingdom female population. Osteoporos Int 2000;11:551–552.
4. Lyles KW, Gold DT, Shipp KM, et al. Association of osteoporotic vertebral compression fractures with impaired functional status. Am J Med 1993;94: 595–601.
5. Chan GK, Duque G. Age-related bone loss: old bone, new facts. Gerontology 2002;48:62–71.
6. Tidermark J, Ponzer S, Carlsson P, et al. Effects of protein-rich supplementation and nandrolone in lean elderly women with femoral neck fractures. Clin Nutr 2004;23:587–596.
7. Sambrook PN, Cameron ID, Chen JS, et al. Influence of fall related factors and bone strength on fracture risk in the frail elderly. Osteoporos Int 2007;18)5):603–610.
8. Court-Brown CM, Caesar B. Epidemiology of adult fractures: a review. Injury 2006;37:691–697.
9. Brainsky A, Glick H, Lydick E, et al. The economic cost of hip fractures in community-dwelling older adults: a prospective study. J Am Geriatr Soc 1997;45:281–287.
10. Cooper C, Campion G, Melton LJ. Hip-fractures in the elderly—a worldwide projection. Osteoporos Int 1992;2:285–289.
11. Gullberg B, Johnell O, Kanis JA. World-wide projections for hip fracture. Osteoporos Int 1997;7: 407–413.
12. Rosen CJ. Clinical practice. Postmenopausal osteoporosis. N Engl J Med 2005;353:595–603.
13. Poole KE, Compston JE. Osteoporosis and its management. BMJ 2006;333:1251–1256.
14. Heffernan MP, Saag KG, Robinson JK, et al. Prevention of osteoporosis associated with chronic glucocorticoid therapy. JAMA 2006;295:1300–1303.
15. No authors listed. Prevention and management of osteoporosis. World Health Organ Tech Rep Ser 2003;921:1–164.
16. Prestwood KM, Duque G. Osteoporosis. In: *Textbook of principles of geriatric medicine and gerontology, 5th edition.* Hazzard (ed.) New York: McGraw Hill, 2003, 973–986.
17. Kenny AM, Prestwood KM, Marcello KM, et al. Determinants of bone density in healthy older men with low testosterone levels. J Gerontol A Biol Sci Med Sci 2000;55:M492–M497.
18. Mundy GR, Elefteriou F. Boning up on ephrin signaling. Cell 2006;126:441–443.
19. Nuttall ME, Gimble JM. Is there a therapeutic opportunity to either prevent or treat osteopenic disorders by inhibiting marrow adipogenesis? Bone 2000;27:177–184.
20. Delmas PD, van de Langerijt L, Watts NB, et al. IMPACT Study Group. Underdiagnosis of vertebral fractures is a worldwide problem: the IMPACT study. J Bone Miner Res 2005;20:557–563.
21. Black DM, Steinbuch M, Palermo L, et al. An assessment tool for predicting fracture risk in postmenopausal women. Osteoporos Int 2001;12: 519–528.
22. De Laet CE, van Hout BA, Burger H, et al. Bone density and risk of hip fracture in men and women: cross sectional analysis. BMJ 1997;315:221–225.
23. Guideline for the prevention of falls in older persons. American Geriatrics Society, British Geriatrics Society, and American Academy of Orthopedic Surgeons Panel on Falls Prevention. J Am Geriatr Soc 2001;49:664–672.
24. Hillier TA, Stone KL, Bauer DC, et al. Evaluating the value of repeat bone mineral density measurement and prediction of fractures in older women: the study of osteoporotic fractures. Arch Intern Med 2007;167:155–160.
25. Pieper CF, Colon-Emeric CS, Caminis J, et al. Distribution and correlates of serum 25-hydroxyvitamin D levels in a sample of hip fracture patients. Am J Geriatr Pharmacother [In press].
26. Heaney RP, Dowell MS, Hale CA, et al. Calcium absorption varies within the reference range for serum 25-hydroxyvitamn D. J Amer Coll Nutr 2003;22:142–146.
27. Gallagher JC, Rapuri PB, Smith LM. An age-related decrease in creatinine clearance is associated with an increase in number of falls in untreated women but not in women receiving calcitriol treatment. J Clin Endocrinol Metab 2007;92:51–58.
28. Bischoff-Ferrari HA, Dawson-Hughes B, Willett WC, et al. Effect of vitamin D on falls: a meta-analysis. JAMA 2004;291:1999–2006.

29. Broe KE, Chen TC, Weinberg J, et al. A higher dose of vitamin d reduces the risk of falls in nursing home residents: a randomized, multiple-dose study. J Am Geriatr Soc 2007;55:234–239.
30. Stone LM, Lyles KW. Generations—chronic conditions in later life. Journal of the American Society on Aging. Osteoporos Int 2006;30(3):65–70.
31. Sjosten NM, Salonoja M, Piirtola M, et al. A multifactorial fall prevention programme in home-dwelling elderly people: a randomized-controlled trial. Am J Public Health 2007;12:308–318.
32. Rubin C, Recker R, Cullen D, et al. Prevention of postmenopausal bone loss by a low-magnitude, high-frequency mechanical stimuli: a clinical trial assessing compliance, efficacy, and safety. J Bone Miner Res 2004;19:343–351.
33. Kita K, Hujino K, Nasu T, et al. A simple protocol for preventing falls and fractures in elderly individuals with musculoskeletal disease. Osteoporos Int 2007;18(5):611–619.
34. Neer RM, Arnaud CD, Zanchetta JR, et al. Effect of parathyroid hormone (1–34) on fractures and bone mineral density in postmenopausal women with osteoporosis. N Engl J Med 2001;344:1434–1441.
35. Seeman E, Vellas B, Benhamou C, et al. Strontium ranelate reduces the risk of vertebral and nonvertebral fractures in women eighty years of age and older. J Bone Miner Res 2006;21:1113–1120.
36. Goltzman D. Discoveries, drugs and skeletal disorders. Nat Rev Drug Discov 2002;1:784–796.
37. Marcus R, Wang O, Satterwhite J, et al. The skeletal response to teriparatide is largely independent of age, initial bone mineral density, and prevalent vertebral fractures in postmenopausal with osteoporosis. J Bone Miner Res 2003;18:18–23.
38. Chapuy MC, Arlot ME, Duboeuf F, et al. Vitamin D3 and calcium to prevent hip fractures in the elderly women. N Engl J Med 1992;327:1637–1642.
39. Bischoff-Ferrari HA, Willett WC, Wong JB, et al. Fracture prevention with vitamin D supplementation: a meta-analysis of randomized controlled trials. JAMA 2005;293:2257–2264.
40. Gompel A, Barlow D, Rozenberg S, et al. EMAS Executive Committee. The EMAS 2006/2007 update on clinical recommendations on postmenopausal hormone therapy. Maturitas 2007;56:227–229.
41. Qu Y, Wong M, Thiebaud D, et al. The effect of raloxifene therapy on the risk of new clinical vertebral fractures at three and six months: a secondary analysis of the MORE trial. Curr Med Res Opin 2005;21:1955–1959.
42. Gaudio A, Morabito N. Pharmacological management of severe postmenopausal osteoporosis. Drugs Aging 2005;22:405–417.
43. Wehren LE, Hosking D, Hochberg MC. Putting evidence-based medicine into clinical practice: comparing anti-resorptive agents for the treatment of osteoporosis. Curr Med Res Opin 2004;20:525–531.
44. Mulder JE, Kolatkar NS, LeBoff MS. Drug insight: existing and emerging therapies for osteoporosis. Nat Clin Pract Endocrinol Metab 2006;2:670–680.
45. Boonen S, McClung MR, Eastell R, et al. Safety and efficacy of risedronate in reducing fracture risk in osteoporotic women aged 80 and older: implications for use of the antiresorptive agents in the old and oldest old. J Am Geriatr Soc 2004;52:1832–1839.
46. Croom KF, Scott LJ. Intravenous ibandronate: in the treatment of osteoporosis. Drugs 2006;66:1593–1601.
47. Woo SB, Hellstein JW, Kalmar JR. Narrative review: bisphosphonates and osteonecrosis of the jaws. Ann Intern Med 2006;144:753–761.
48. Bilezikian JP. Osteonecrosis of the jaw—do bisphosphonates pose a risk? N Engl J Med 2006;355:2278–2281.
49. Stokkers PC, Deley M, Van Der Spek M, et al. Intravenous pamidronate in combination with calcium and vitamin D: highly effective in the treatment of low bone mineral density in inflammatory bowel disease. Scand J Gastroenterol 2006;41:200–204.
50. Colon-Emeric CS, Caminis J, Suh TT, et al. HORIZON Recurrent Fracture Trial. The HORIZON Recurrent Fracture Trial: design of a clinical trial in the prevention of subsequent fractures after low trauma hip fracture repair. Curr Med Res Opin 2004;20:903–910.
51. Cranney A, Papaioannou A, Zytaruk N, et al. Parathyroid hormone for the treatment of osteoporosis: a systematic review. CMAJ 2006;175:52–59.
52. Shoback D. Update in osteoporosis and metabolic bone disorders. J Clin Endocrinol Metab 2007;92:747–753.
53. Kanis JA, Black D, Cooper C, et al. A new approach to the development of assessment guidelines for osteoporosis. Osteoporos Int 2002;13:527–536.
54. Green AD, Colon-Emeric CS, Bastian L, et al. Does this woman have osteoporosis? JAMA 2004;292:2890–2900.

7
Genetics of Osteoporosis in Older Age

David Karasik and Douglas P. Kiel

Osteoporosis results from a failure to acquire optimal peak bone mass during growth *(1)* and/or to maintain bone mass in later years. There are two backgrounds for the pathophysiology of involutional osteoporosis: a rapid bone loss after menopause as a result of estrogen withdrawal, and a gradual age-related bone loss thereafter. Women experience a more rapid phase of bone loss after the menopause, caused mainly by estrogen deficiency *(2,3)*, but a less rapid bone loss persists in older persons, in both men and women *(4,5)*. Some authors thus distinguish between two types of pathophysiology of osteoporosis: menopausal and age-related ("senile.").

Bone health in old age depends on a susceptibility to osteoporotic fractures, which seems to be dependent on genetic factors (heritable). The genetic contribution to involutional osteoporosis is substantial and has been extensively studied. With recent advances in the elucidation of the mechanisms involved in osteoporosis, there is a recognition that the two types of syndromes may have different genetic components. Genetic contributions to fractures and fragility in elderly persons in comparison with younger individuals distinguish age-related osteoporosis.

The susceptibility to fractures depends on many factors, including non-skeletal ones such as propensity to fall, diminished soft tissue cushion, and so on. The most reliable predictor of fracture is bone mineral density (BMD). This is also evident in the World Health Organization (WHO) definition of the osteoporosis ("low bone mass leading to structural fragility" *[6]*). In order to identify and quantify the genetic contributions to a complex disease, there is a need to define an "endophenotype". This is especially challenging in the case of osteoporosis, where the phenotype of interest is clinically occult until the "structural fragility" does ultimately manifest as a fracture *(7)*.

In many complex diseases, an "upstream" intermediate measurable phenotype between genotype and disease is chosen as an endophenotype and serves as a target for gene mapping. These are usually well-known risk factors with pathophysiological importance, biological meanings, and measurability before the onset of disease *(8)*. Measurable endophenotypes belonging to simple biological pathways allow complexity reduction. Many traditional biochemical and endocrinologic measures (e.g., serum cholesterol, serotonin, insulin, and so on) fit into this category *(8)*. However, biochemical and endocrinologic markers are not generally used in osteoporosis genetics *(9,10)*, despite advanced understanding of pathophysiologic pathways.

Combining several phenotypes by principal components or factor analysis or simultaneously testing more than one trait (bi- and multivariate analysis *[11]*) may also be considered as productive strategies *(7)*. We proposed a composite clinical phenotypic measure (a principal component score of BMD measures) as an endophenotype for the study of osteoporosis genetics *(12)*. However, genes that contribute to variation in BMD evidently do not always contribute to osteoporotic fractures *(7)*. For these reasons, the "end-point disease" (e.g., osteoporotic fracture *per se*) may still be a valuable phenotype for genetic studies.

In this chapter, we will thus consider at least three domains of phenotypes that play a role in the osteoporosis of old age: fracture *per se*, BMD, and bone loss (measured as BMD change with age). Genetic factors contribute to all of these phenotypes, although genetics may contribute in unique ways to each of the phenotypes.

Heritability of Osteoporotic Fracture

Parental history of fracture (particularly a family history of hip fracture) confers an increased risk of fracture that is notably independent of BMD *(13)*. Deng et al. have reported relatively low heritability of wrist (Colles) fracture in older Caucasian females *(14)*, and a marginal heritability of hip fracture *(15)* in a sample of Caucasian pedigrees. In a cohort of 33,432 Swedish twins born from 1896 to 1944 (data from the Swedish Inpatient Registry), the age-adjusted heritability of any osteoporotic fracture was 0.27 (95% confidence interval [CI], 0.09–0.28) and of hip fracture alone, 0.48 (95% CI, 0.28–0.57) *(16)*. Age-adjusted heritability was considerably greater for first hip fractures before the age of 69 years (0.68; 95% CI, 0.41–0.78) and between 69 and 79 years (0.47; 95% CI, 0.04–0.62) than for hip fractures after 79 years of age (0.03; 95% CI, 0.00–0.26) *(16)*. Notably, a study of concordance of osteoporotic fractures in a large sample of Finnish twin pairs did not find heritability of fractures, apparently owing to an older age of the sample and failure to stratify the twin pairs by age groups *(17)*.

Similarly, the risk of developing fracture for the offspring of patients with osteoporotic fractures was apparently higher at younger ages in a meta-analysis of Kanis et al. *(13)*. Figure 7.1 shows the risk ratios of fractures for the persons with parental history of any fracture, and those with family history of hip fracture in particular, by age (sexes combined). It is clear that risk ratios decline between the ages 65 and 85; thus, for example, the relative risk (RR) for having hip fracture in those with a parental history of hip fracture declines from 2.44 (95% CI, 1.27–4.68) to 1.33 (95% CI, 0.87–2.02) in this period of adult life.

Shorter life expectancy in men compared to women *(18)* and relatively rare occurrence of "andropause" (the age-related hypogonadism affects only approximately 30% of aging males *[19]*) correspond to a lower life-long risk of osteoporotic fractures in men. It has been suggested, but remains to be determined definitively, that the larger skeletal size of men is a critical factor contributing to their lower incidence of age-related fractures than women. Also, it is generally thought that men undergo a pattern of favorable geometric adaptation to a greater extent than women, and that this may contribute to lower fracture rates in elderly men than women *(20–26)*. However, recent data from a cross-sectional study employing 3D-quantitative computed tomography

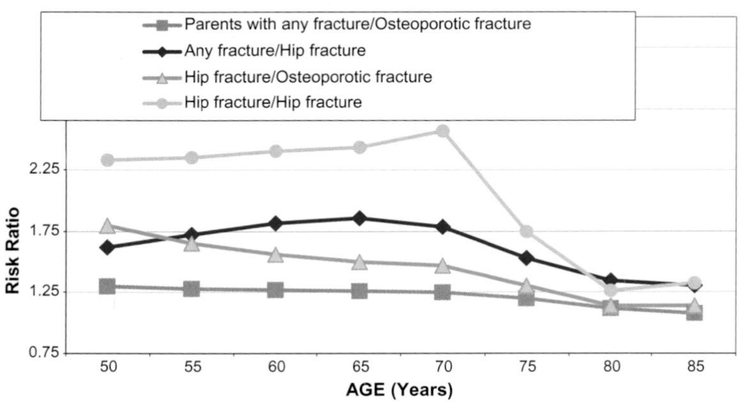

FIGURE 7.1. Risk ratios of fractures with age, for persons with parental history of any fracture and specifically history of hip fracture, by type of fracture they suffered (sexes combined). Data from Kanis et al. *(13)*.

(QCT) challenge this paradigm, demonstrating that the extent to which bone geometry exhibits favorable geometric changes with aging is similar in men and women *(27)*.

In any case, because men do not experience a process analogous to menopausal osteoporosis, they may serve better as a model of senile osteoporosis. However, the ease of recruitment of large cohorts of post-menopausal women such as the Study of Osteoporotic Fractures (SOF) and other samples *(28)*, provides a more realistic chance of successful mapping of osteoporosis genes *(29)*. The majority of studies dealing with genetics of osteoporotic fractures and osteoporosis-related phenotypes to date have been performed in this sex- and age group. Because bone loss is pronounced in women, it is logical that associations with genetic factors are found more often in women *(30)*. However, based on the previous observations, it may be more difficult to identify genes for fracture phenotype in this older age cohort, because the contributions of genes to fractures seem to fade with age *(13,16)*. On the other hand, because the incidence rates of fracture increase at an earlier age in women than men, this earlier age-at-onset of fractures affords an opportunity to recruit large samples of women.

Genetic Contribution to BMD

Although BMD has been commonly used as an endophenotype for fractures caused by osteoporosis, the shared genetic variance between BMD and osteoporotic fractures is modest. Variance component analysis suggested that less than 1% of additive genetic variance is shared between BMD and osteoporotic fractures at the hip *(15)*. Studies of many candidate genes (such as estrogen receptor α *[ESR1] [31]*, collagen 1 α 1 *[Col1A1] [32]*, and insulin-like growth factor-I *[IGF-1] [30,33]*) confirmed this early observation that bone density and fractures have a different genetic milieu. Thus, a *CA* repeat polymorphism in the promoter region of the *IGF-1* gene explained only a minor portion of the variance in BMD (0.2%) and BMD change (0.1%) among females *(30)*, but noncarriers of the *192-bp* allele of this repeat polymorphism had 1.5 (95% CI, 1.1–2.0) times increased risk of having fragility fractures in the same sample *(33)*.

Similarly, the *COL1A1* gene was originally proposed as a candidate gene because it encodes type I collagen, the most abundant protein of bone *(34)*. A meta-analysis of published data found a modest effect of the *s* allele on BMD (equivalent to 0.1–0.2 standard deviation decrease compared to the *S* allele) but a more prominent association with fracture risk (odds ratio [OR] 1.5 and 1.9 in *Ss* and *ss* compared to *SS* genotypes, respectively) *(32)*. Taken together with the functional data mentioned previously, these results indeed suggest that *COL1A1 Sp*1 polymorphisms may affect some "bone quality" component, which is poorly reflected by BMD alone.

However, because BMD at present is among the strongest risk factors for fracture *(35,36)* and thus remains a gold standard for assessment of fracture risk, most of the studies use BMD (in g/cm^2) measured by dual-energy X-ray absorptiometry (DXA) as a preferred phenotype. From the point of view of quantitative analysis, BMD also has a benefit because it is a normally distributed trait. It is highly heritable, with genetic factors contributing up to 60–80% of the total variation in BMD *(37,38)*. Multiple genome-wide linkage screens for genes underlying BMD variability have been conducted in mice *(39–41)* and humans *(42–44)*, including a recent meta-analysis of human linkage studies *(45)*. In our sample of 330 Caucasian pedigrees from the Framingham Study Cohorts, we reported suggestive linkage of BMD at the femur and lumbar spine on chromosomes 6p21.2, 8q24.13, 12q23, 14q31, and 21qter *(44)*. We further postulated that there may be age and gender differences among individuals, as well as differences according to ponderosity. We thus stratified our pedigrees by age ["60 or younger" (age 29–60 years) and "older than 60" (61–96 years)], by sex, and by body mass index (BMI) [into "low" or "high" BMI, by the median cut-off of 27.7 kg/m^2 in males and 25.8 kg/m^2 in females]. Age of 60 years was chosen to create a group of men who were young enough not to have manifested the more significant bone loss that comes with advanced age, while providing sufficient sample size for analyses. Heritability estimates of BMD after adjustment for covariates were comparable in the age-specific subsamples, a finding similar to some previously reported studies *(46)* but not others in which phenotypic resemblance was lower among older subjects *(47)*. We observed a heterogeneity of linkage on 6p21.2 and 21qter, where findings from the total sample *(44)* were not supported by any subsample. Also, age subsample-specific linkage peaks were found, on 9q22–9q31 (in "younger" subsample) and 17p13.3 (in "older"), which were not reflected by the total sample results. Similarly, the loci identified after stratification by gender differed among men and women *(48)*. Our study was the first genome scan in humans that provided evidence for difference in the linked chromosomal regions between younger and older subjects, men and women.

Other studies, such as the FAMilial Osteoporosis Study (FAMOS) *(49)* and Amish osteoporosis study *(50)*, stratified their families at 50 years old. Ralston et al. *(49)* based their choice of an age cutoff of 50 years on the fact that this was the median age of their study sample and is also close to the average age of menopause in women. The large sample size of the FAMOS study (3691 individuals from 715 families) allowed the investigators to conduct age- and gender-specific analyses simultaneously. Thus, in each gender, they were able to distinguish quantitative trait loci (QTL) for peak bone mass (in individuals younger than 50 years) from those that influence bone mass in older people. The linkage peaks were age- and sex-specific; thus, no overlap was found between chromosomal loci for BMD in older men and older women *(49)*. Similarly, in analyses of age-specific subgroups, Streeten et al. *(50)* in the Amish study found suggestive evidence for linkage for those younger than 50 years of age on chromosomes 11q22 and 14q23 (LODs = 2.11 and 2.16, respectively) and for those older than 50 years of age on 3p25.2 (LOD = 2.32); again, no overlap was found between chromosomal loci for BMD in older and younger family members.

Genetic Contribution to Change in BMD

As mentioned, the BMD phenotype in elderly persons is perceived as a mix of bone mass acquired at peak (in young adults) and ensuing loss, caused by either menopause, senescence, or both (reviewed in Yang et al. *[51]*). There is also evidence of a heritable component for age-related bone loss, although less well studied than cross-sectional BMD. It has been proposed that the genes regulating peak bone mass might differ from those regulating bone loss *(52)*, and that genetic factors contributing to change in BMD are those responsible for the bone remodeling ability *(53)*. As originally suggested back in 1993, at a median follow-up of approximately 3 years, BMD change of both hip and spine was heritable in twins aged 24–75 years *(54)*. A number of ensuing studies have attempted to dissect the genetic basis for the rate of bone loss, with various levels of success, in humans (55–58) and mice *(53)*.

Yang et al. *(51)* warn that caution should be exercised while interpreting results of these studies, particularly in light of the presumption that the rate of bone loss can be treated as a phenotype independent of BMD. By re-analyzing the data from a 9.5-years longitudinal study *(59)*, Yang and colleagues *(51)* found that approximately 67% of post-menopausal BMD variation is attributable to the pre-menopausal BMD ("peak BMD"), and approximately 29% to the bone loss rate. The contribution of the rate of bone loss to low BMD is thus fairly small, but not negligible. The estimated pre- and post-menopausal bone loss rates are generally approximately 0.3–1.5% per year, varying at different skeletal sites; even during the peri-menopausal period when "rapid" bone loss occurs, the annual rate of bone loss is between 0.6–2% (reviewed by Yang et al. *[51]*). Bone loss is a relatively slow process, but once triggered, it tends to steadily progress with age. Hannan et al. found an average 4-year BMD loss ranging from 3.4–4.8% in women and 0.2–3.6% in men at all skeletal sites *(4)*. The mean rate of BMD change from baseline to follow-up (~2 years) was 1.2% and 1.1% for women and men, respectively, in the Rotterdam study *(30)*. Recently, Khosla et al. *(60)* used high-resolution 3D pQCT imaging at the wrist to describe age-related patterns of bone change in a cross-sectional study design. Relative to young women (age 20–49 years), whose cortical volumetric BMD decreased with age, young men actually had an apparent increase in vBMD. Both men and women had decreased vBMD with advanced age in the 50–90 years age group (−22% in women and −18% in men). Thus, despite significantly higher bone loss in women than men ($p = 0.01$) after age 50, Khosla et al. *(60)* could not specifically show an effect of menopause on the BMD change (alternatively, this finding can be interpreted as an effect of andropause *[61]* in men!). Cross-sectional studies such as these *(4,60)* are not totally free from secular trend and survival bias. Notable is a finding of Parsons et al. *(62)* that the major predictors of bone loss in post-menopausal women were menopausal status, hormone replacement therapy (HRT) use, and BMI, but not the genetic polymorphisms associated with BMD.

Changes in BMD may obviously depend on errors in bone density measurement, technology changes from old to new densitometric devices, as well as changes in anthropometric measures of the patient (such as advanced kyphosis and weight loss). The baseline and follow-up scan comparability needs to be rigorously assessed before using such data for genetic analyses; further adjustment needs to be done for change in weight and BMI, as well as for the type of device used at each measurement occasion, in order to avoid or control measurement errors.

Candidate Genes for Fractures and Bone Mass in Aging

There are indications that genotype-phenotype associations with regard to osteoporosis and BMD in older-age individuals differ from those in younger ages. There are several examples, focusing on the most widely studied biological candidate genes for osteoporosis.

Interleukin (IL)-6 Gene Promoter Polymorphisms

Estrogen deficiency is involved in bone loss via the direct action of estrogen on bone cells, as well as mediation of cytokines in bone marrow. The decline in estrogen production after menopause leads to increased production of pro-inflammatory cytokines, such as IL-6, which are normally suppressed by estrogen *(63)*. Increased levels of IL-6, in turn, promote the differentiation of osteoclast precursor cells into mature osteoclasts, which increase resorption within the bones *(64)*.

Several studies have identified the IL-6 gene locus (7p21) to be linked to BMD in post-menopausal women *(65,66)* and in families of osteoporotic probands *(67,68)*, whereas no linkage was found in young, healthy sister pairs *(69)*. These observations suggest that IL-6 genetic variation might specifically contribute to the population variance in bone mass *primarily in older women (64,70)*. Dinucleotide repeat polymorphisms at the IL-6 locus have been associated with or linked to BMD in post-menopausal, but not pre-menopausal, women *(64,70)*.

In order to elucidate the contribution of the IL-6 gene to BMD in women, we studied an interaction between IL-6 promoter polymorphisms and factors known to affect bone turnover, namely years since menopause, estrogen status, dietary calcium and vitamin D intake, physical activity, smoking, and alcohol in the Offspring Cohort of the Framingham Heart Study *(71)*. We found that BMD was significantly lower in women with genotype −174 *GG* compared to *CC*, and intermediate with *GC*, who were more than 15 years past menopause, estrogen-deficient, or who had insufficient calcium intake (<940 mg/day). No associations were observed in pre-menopausal women. (Of note, in the Belfast Elderly Longitudinal Ageing Study, a reduction in frequency of GG homozygotes was associated with higher serum levels of IL-6 in the oldest [octo/nonagenarian] age group *[72]*). In women with both estrogen-deficiency and poor calcium intake, BMD differences at the hip between *IL-6* −174 *CC* and *GG* were as high as 16.8% *(71)*. Results of this study may be interpreted not only as an age-specific, but also syndrome-specific genetic influence. Thus, a phenotype in women more than 15 years post-menopause may be an indication of the "senile" rather than "menopausal" osteoporosis.

Most recently, the IL-6 −174 *G* allele was confirmed to also be associated with lower bone ultrasound properties and an increased risk of fracture (OR 1.5, 95% CI 1.1–2.0) in a large cohort of 964 post-menopausal women aged 75 years *(73)*. Together, these data indicate that the influence of *IL-6* gene variants on bone mass may depend on gender, age, estrogen status, and dietary calcium.

Another group specifically studied the rate of decline in hip BMD *(64)*. Compared with women having the *GG* phenotype, women having the *CC* genotype also had slower rates of bone loss in the total hip and femoral neck in approximately 3.5 years of follow-up and 33% lower risk of wrist fractures over an average of 10.8 years *(64)*. Also important was the observation that the association between the −174*GC* polymorphism and hip bone loss was independent of weight loss during follow-up *(74)*, which conforms to a primary action of IL-6 on bone rather than indirectly via age-related weight loss.

Vitamin D Receptor (VDR) Gene Polymorphisms

The VDR mediates the effects of calcitriol [1,25(OH)$_2$D$_3$] on the intestinal absorption of calcium and phosphate, and on bone mineralization. Morrison et al. first reported that VDR 3′-UTR *Bsm*I alleles were associated with BMD in adult women and post-menopausal bone loss *(75)*. The association between the *VDR* gene and osteoporosis-related traits has been extensively studied. The frequently studied markers include *Bsm*I, *Apa*I, *Taq*I, and *Fok*I, which currently have unknown functional effects *(76)*. Numerous population-based studies including hundreds to thousands of subjects, mostly pre- and post-menopausal women, looked at the association between VDR alleles, BMD, and bone loss, with discordant results *(77–88)*. In addition, some investigators noted a *vanishing* influence of VDR genotypes on bone mass with advancing age *(84,89)*.

Morita et al. *(90)* analyzed BMD change over 3 years in Japanese women (15–79 years old) for *Apa*I, *Taq*I, and *Fok*I polymorphisms of the 5-year age-stratified groups. The annual percent changes in lumbar spine BMD were different in the *Taq*I *tt* subjects from other genotypes in women who were pre-menopausal at the follow-up, and in the women who already had been post-menopausal at the baseline. Interestingly, the effect of the *tt* genotype on BMD change was opposite in the two groups of Japanese women; bone loss at the lumbar spine in the pre-menopausal subjects with tt genotype was significantly greater than that of *tt* homozygous post-menopausal women, who actually showed a tendency toward bone gain *(90)*. This finding suggests an interaction between the menopausal status and the *Taq*I alleles. The meta-analysis of Thakkinstian et al. *(91)* focused on the relationship between VDR *Bsm*I and BMD/osteoporosis at the femoral neck or spine in adult women. They also studied the association between *Bsm*I and mean percent BMD change over time and revealed a significant effect of *Bsm*I, with BB and Bb genotypes having greater bone loss per year than the bb genotype *(91)*.

It remains uncertain whether VDR genotypes contribute significantly to fracture risk in the elderly *(18)*. However, because VDR is also involved in the aging of muscles *(92)*, it might contribute to non-BMD risk factors of the osteoporotic fractures (frailty and fall-related).

Estrogen Receptor α (ESR1) and Estrogen Receptor β (ESR2) Genes

Estradiol plays a major role in the acquisition and maintenance of peak bone mass in both females *(93,94)* and males *(30,95,96)*. Genotypes identified by *Pvu*II and *Xba*I restriction enzymes in the first intron of the gene *ESR1* are in strong linkage disequilibrium with one another and only 46 base pairs apart. *ESR1* gene polymorphisms, including *Pvu*II, *Xba*I and a TA repeat polymorphism in the promoter region, were subsequently analyzed with bone mass, bone loss, and/or fractures in women, with contrasting results *(58,83,85,88,97–102)*.

A meta-analysis of the association between *ESR1* genotypes and BMD, including more than five thousand women from 22 eligible studies (n = 11 in Caucasians and n = 11 in Asians), concluded that homozygotes for the *Xba*I *XX* genotype have a modestly but significantly higher BMD (+1–2%) at lumbar spine or hip compared to *xx* *(31)*. No differences were found between *PvuII* genotypes, despite the fact that *XbaI* and *PvuII* sites are in strong linkage disequilibrium. In this meta-analysis, differences between genotypes tended to be up to five time greater in pre- menopausal compared to post-menopausal women, suggesting that ESR1 genotypes might influence peak bone mass acquisition, although only three studies included pre-menopausal women. Most interestingly, differences in fracture risk were disproportionately high compared to the small differences in bone mass observed between genotypes (OR 0.66 [95% CI 0.47–0.93] in *XX* vs *xx*) *(31)*, suggesting that *ESR1* genotypes might influence bone "quality" above and beyond BMD.

Indeed, a recent study of these polymorphisms in 18,917 individuals from 8 European centers found evidence of association with fracture risk but not BMD *(103)*, which again points out the dissimilar genetic composition of these two phenotypes. Some authors reported an interaction between *ESR1* polymorphisms and HRT *(58,104)*, as well as a gene-by-gene interaction between *ESR1* and *VDR* alleles on BMD *(85,97)*.

Low-Density Lipoprotein (LDL)-Receptor Related Protein 5 (LRP5) Gene

LRP5 is a member of the LDL-receptor related family coding for a transmembrane co-receptor for Wnt signaling *(105)*. Mutations of this gene were shown to be associated with osteoporosis-pseudoglioma syndrome (loss-of-function mutations) *(106)* and a high bone mass phenotype (gain-of-function mutations) *(107–109)*. *LRP5* polymorphisms were also associated with idiopathic osteoporosis in 78 European-Caucasian men (mean age ~50 years) *(110)*. Moreover, 1-year changes in lumbar spine bone mass and size in pre-pubertal boys were also significantly associated with these *LRP5* variants *(111)*, suggesting that *LRP5* polymorphisms could contribute to the risk of spine osteoporosis in men by influencing vertebral bone growth during childhood *(111)*.

In a large-scale population-based genetic association study performed in the Framingham Study Offspring Cohort and including a subset of 1797 unrelated individuals, 10 single-nucleotide polymorphisms (SNPs) spanning the *LRP5* gene were genotyped and used for association and interaction analyses with BMD by regression methods. After adjustment for co-variates, in men no older than 60 years, three SNPs were significantly associated with BMD: rs2306862 on Exon 10 with femoral neck BMD (p = 0.01) and Ward's BMD (p = 0.01); rs4988321/p. V667M with Ward's BMD (p = 0.02); and intronic rs901825 with trochanter BMD (p = 0.03). In women, 3 SNPs in intron 2 were significantly associated with BMD: rs4988330 for trochanter (p = 0.01) and spine BMD (p = 0.003); rs312778 with femoral neck BMD (p = 0.05); and rs4988331 with spine BMD (p = 0.04). For each additional rare allele, BMD changed by 3–5% in males and 2–4% in females. Moreover, there was a significant interaction between physical activity and rs2306862 in exon 10 (p for interaction = 0.02) and rs3736228/p. A1330V in exon 18 (p for interaction = 0.05) on spine BMD in men. In both cases, the *TT* genotype was associated with lower spine BMD in men with higher physical activity scores, conversely with higher BMD in men with lower physical activity scores (Figure 7.2) (112). Therefore, in addition to the differ-

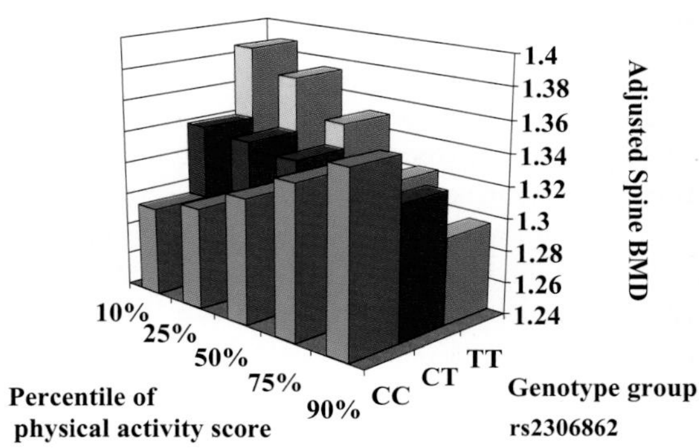

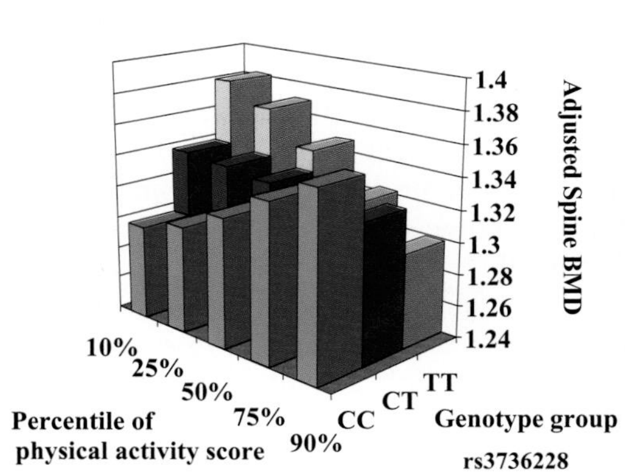

FIGURE 7.2. Significant interaction between two SNPs (rs2306862 and rs3736228) and physical activity on BMD of the spine in men. The *x*-axis provides continuously measured PASE scores divided into percentiles, the *y*-axis provides adjusted BMD of the lumbar spine, and the *z*-axis provides the three genotype groups for each SNP. For rs2306862 there were 535 men with CC, 192 men with CT, and 18 men with TT genotypes. For rs3736228 there were 529 men with CC, 187 men with CT, and 16 men with TT genotypes. Modified from Kiel et al. *(112)*.

ences by age and gender, analyses of *LRP5* polymorphisms in the Framingham Osteoporosis Study suggested an interaction with physical activity in men.

As shown previously using *IL-6, ESR1,* and *LRP5* as examples, the effect of genes on osteoporosis-related traits is gender- and age-related. Thus Pluijm et al. *(113)* found that only among the younger men and women (65–69 years) was the presence of *ApoE* ε4 allele associated with lower hip BMD values. In older men, no associations between *ApoE* status and BMD were found. Also, variation in SNPs in the *TNSALP (ALPL)* gene has been shown to be associated with BMD in *older post-menopausal women*, and the effects on age-related bone loss seemed to accumulate with aging *(114)*. Other genes association studies have found the opposite effects of age. Similarly, polymorphisms in the sclerostin (*SOST*) gene were found to be associated with BMD, and the effect became more pronounced with increasing age in the Rotterdam study *(115)*. In another case-control study, *SOST* polymorphisms were not found to be associated with BMD, probably in part because of the younger age of the participants than those in the Rotterdam study *(116)* (For more information on *SOST* gene, see *[117]*).

Biological Processes That Exert Age-Related Genetic Effects

To study a complex age-related process such as osteoporosis, investigators in the field have to reach some basic consensus on characterizing the major change occurring in bone with aging. For example, the changes could include hydroxyapatite crystallite size *(118)*, hydration, osteoclastic proliferation or other processes influencing bone mineral content, the extent of secondary mineralization, or bone tissue spatial arrangement, which in turn impacts the tissue mechanical properties. In genetic epidemiological terms, this task is intertwined with the definition of the "endophenotype" for bone aging, as explained previously. The susceptibility to fractures depends on many non-skeletal factors; conditions such as sarcopenia, which itself may have genetic components. Yet sarcopenia may result in reduced muscular input on the skeleton *(119)* and thus contribute to the etiology of osteopenia *(120)* along with the effect on propensity to fall. These conditions, although important contributors to the osteoporotic fracture risk in the elderly, probably have their own genetic predispositions, which may make it difficult to detect specific genetic effect on bone aging *per se*. Defining the pathophysiologically or biologically sound endophenotypes is key in the successful study into the mechanisms and genetic contributions to the aging of the skeleton.

Bone aging is a model of general aging. Some general processes of senescence/aging are present within the bone microenvironment and may be well represented by bone phenotypes *(121)*, ultimately contributing to degeneration of the skeleton. Combined bone scoring systems (osseographic score) have been proposed as integrative measures of bone aging *(122,123)*. These integrative phenotypes have been shown to contribute to the prediction of mortality in most age groups of both sexes. Also, the heritability of such phenotypes adjusted for sex, height, BMI, alcohol intake, smoking status, physical activity, and in women, menopausal status and estrogen use, was quite substantial (heritability = 57%). Genome-wide linkage analysis of the score suggested the presence of quantitative trait loci with logarithm of the odds (LOD) scores higher than 1.8 on chromosomes 3p, 7q, 11p, 16q, and 21q *(122,124)*.

As shown previously, inflammation is linked to bone turnover both directly *(71,125)* and via estrogen pathways *(126,127)*. Prostaglandins and cytokines have long been reported to both stimulate and inhibit bone formation and resorption *(128)*. Circulating concentrations of inflammatory markers *(74)* and polymorphisms *(129–131)* have been related to variation in BMD and fracture risk. The expression levels of many of the inflammatory genes have recently been shown to be up-regulated with muscle aging *(132,133)*, which indicates their involvement also in the sarcopenia phenotype and in aging in general.

One of the intriguing mechanisms of aging is adipogenesis. Osteoblasts and adipocytes share a common precursor cell in the bone marrow stroma, termed a marrow stromal cell (MSC). Cultures of MSCs were established from young donors (age 18–42 years), elderly healthy donors (age

66–78), and patients with osteoporosis (age 58–76) by Justesen et al. *(134)*. They found no age-related changes in the osteoblastic or adipocytic colony formation or the steady-state levels of mRNA of the adipogenic or osteogenic gene markers. In another study, changes in gene expression in fracture healing were expected to differ at differing ages. To explore this, 6-, 26-, and 52-week-old female Sprague-Dawley rats were subjected to mid-diaphyseal femoral fracture *(135)*. Nearly all genes presently associated with bone metabolism showed the same response to fracture healing regardless of the age of the animal, thus there was no difference in the healing anabolic response with age.

Conclusions

Much of the variability of osteoporosis and related fractures has a genetic basis. A full picture of the complex genetic architecture of osteoporosis has been elusive in the absence of an optimal endophenotype for osteoporosis, especially for bone loss in elderly persons. Osteoporotic phenotypes, such as fracture, BMD, and bone loss are all heritable. The question is, to what extent do the same genetic factors contribute to all these phenotypes, and how do genetics regulate these traits at different periods of adult life? Much can be learned by studying the disconnect between BMD and fragility fracture phenotypes in genetic epidemiologic studies of osteoporosis. On one hand, this poses challenges in the study of genetic variants regulating both bone mass and fragility; on the other, the genetic variants that are independent of BMD could be combined with BMD measurements to improve risk assessment for complications of osteoporosis *(117)*. The research efforts need to focus on these important questions.

Ferrari *(18)* urges physicians to start evaluating whether candidate gene polymorphisms so far identified in association studies could be translated into clinical practice (i.e., evaluate the positive and negative predictive values of gene markers with respect to osteoporosis and fracture risk, and response to therapy). Rather than looking disdainfully at the "genetic revolution of medicine" *(136)*, we should make an effort to bring this increasing knowledge from the bench to the bed-side *(18)*.

Guidelines for population screening as applied to genetic susceptibility to disease have recently been published *(137)*. Investigators should be aware that the strength of the association between the gene and osteoporosis-related phenotypes may depend on gender, age, ethnicity, and interactions with a number of life style and environmental risk factors for osteoporosis *(18)*.

Translational research in the field of osteoporosis requires that clinicians recognize the important contribution of aging *per se* to the osteoporosis syndrome and bone loss. Tailoring of medicines will require a better understanding of pathogenesis, especially the genetic mechanisms underlying age-related bone loss.

References

1. Bonjour JP, Theintz G, Law F, Slosman D, Rizzoli R. Peak bone mass. Osteoporos Int 1994;4(Suppl 1):7–13.
2. Riggs BL, Khosla S, Melton LJ. A unitary model for involutional osteoporosis: estrogen deficiency causes both type I and type II osteoporosis in postmenopausal women and contributes to bone loss in aging men. J Bone Miner Res 1998;13: 763–773.
3. Melton LJ III, Atkinson EJ, O'Connor MK, O'Fallon WM, Riggs BL. Determinants of bone loss from the femoral neck in women of different ages. J Bone Miner Res 2000;15(1):24–31.
4. Hannan MT, Felson DT, Dawson-Hughes B, et al. Risk factors for longitudinal bone loss in elderly men and women: the Framingham Osteoporosis Study. J Bone Miner Res 200;15(4): 710–720.
5. Burger H, de Laet CE, van Daele PL, et al. Risk factors for increased bone loss in an elderly population: the Rotterdam Study. Am J Epidemiol 1998;147(9):871–879.
6. Bone health and osteoporosis: a report of the surgeon general. U.S. Department of Health and Human Services, Office of the Surgeon General, Rockville, MD, 2004.
7. Schulze TG, McMahon FJ. Defining the phenotype in human genetic studies: forward genetics and reverse phenotyping. Hum Hered 2004;58(3–4): 131–138.
8. Pan WH, Lynn KS, Chen CH, Wu YL, Lin CY, Chang HY. Using endophenotypes for pathway

clusters to map complex disease genes. Genet Epidemiol 2006;30(2):143–154.
9. Havill LM, Bredbenner TL, Mahaney MC, Nicolella DP. Normal variation in cross-sectional geometry of the femoral midshaft in baboons is heritable and is associated with ANKH expression. J Bone Min Res 2006;21(Suppl 1):S239.
10. Livshits G, Yakovenko C, Kobyliansky E. Quantitative genetic analysis of circulating levels of biochemical markers of bone formation. Am J Med Genet 2000;94(4):324–331.
11. Otremski I, Karasik D, Livshits, G. Genetic variation and covariation of parathyroid hormone levels and bone density in human population. Calcif Tissue Int 2000;66:168–175.
12. Karasik D, Cupples LA, Hannan MT, Kiel DP. Genome screen for a combined bone phenotype using principal component analysis: the Framingham study. Bone 2004;34(3):547–556.
13. Kanis JA, Oden A, Johnell O, De Laet C, Jonsson B. Excess mortality after hospitalisation for vertebral fracture. Osteoporos Int 2004;15(2):108–112.
14. Deng HW, Chen WM, Recker S, et al. Genetic determination of Colles' fracture and differential bone mass in women with and without Colles' fracture. J Bone Miner Res 2000;15(7):1243–1252.
15. Deng HW, Mahaney MC, Williams JT, et al. Relevance of the genes for bone mass variation to susceptibility to osteoporotic fractures and its implications to gene search for complex human diseases. Genet Epidemiol 2002;22(1):12–25.
16. Michaelsson K, Melhus H, Ferm H, Ahlbom A, Pedersen NL. Genetic liability to fractures in the elderly. Arch Intern Med 2005;165(16):1825–1830.
17. Kannus P, Palvanen M, Kaprio J, Parkkari J, Koskenvuo M. Genetic factors and osteoporotic fractures in elderly people: prospective 25 year follow up of a nationwide cohort of elderly Finnish twins. BMJ 1999;319(7221):1334–1337.
18. Ferrari S. Osteoporosis: A Complex Disorder of Aging with Multiple Genetic and Environmental Determinants. In: *Nutrition and Fitness: Mental Health, Aging, and the Implementation of a Healthy Diet and Physical Activity Lifestyle, vol. 95*. Basel: Karger, 2005, pp 35–51.
19. Orwoll ES, Klein RF. Osteoporosis in men. Endocr Rev 1995;16(1):87–116.
20. Smith R, Walker R. Femoral expansion in aging women: implications for osteoporosis and fractures. Science 1994;145:156–157.
21. Ruff CB, Hayes WC. Subperiosteal expansion and cortical remodeling of the human femur and tibia with aging. Science 1982;217(4563):945–948.
22. Ruff CB, Hayes WC. Sex differences in age-related remodeling of the femur and tibia. J Orthop Res 1988;6:886–896.
23. Beck TJ, Ruff CB, Bissessur K. Age-related changes in female femoral neck geometry: implications for bone strength. Calcif Tissue Int 1993;53(Suppl 1): S41–S46.
24. Seeman E. From density to structure: growing up and growing old on the surfaces of bone. J Bone Miner Res 1997;12(4):509–521.
25. Duan Y, Turner CH, Kim BT, Seeman E. Sexual dimorphism in vertebral fragility is more the result of gender differences in age-related bone gain than bone loss. J Bone Miner Res 2001; 16(12):2267–2275.
26. Kaptoge S, Dalzell N, Loveridge N, Beck TJ, Khaw KT, Reeve J. Effects of gender, anthropometric variables, and aging on the evolution of hip strength in men and women aged over 65. Bone 2003;32(5):561–570.
27. Riggs BL, Melton LJ III, Robb RA, et al. Population-based study of age and sex differences in bone volumetric density, size, geometry, and structure at different skeletal sites. J Bone Miner Res 2004;19(12):1945–1954.
28. Deng HW, Chen WM, Conway T, et al. Determination of bone mineral density of the hip and spine in human pedigrees by genetic and life-style factors. Genet Epidemiol 2002;19(2):160–177.
29. Brown MA. Genetic studies of osteoporosis–a rethink required. Calcif Tissue Int 2005;76(5): 319–325.
30. Rivadeneira F, Houwing-Duistermaat JJ, Vaessen N, et al. Association between an insulin-like growth factor I gene promoter polymorphism and bone mineral density in the elderly: the Rotterdam Study. J Clin Endocrinol Metab 2003;88(8): 3878–84.
31. Ioannidis JP, Stavrou I, Trikalinos TA, et al. Association of polymorphisms of the estrogen receptor alpha gene with bone mineral density and fracture risk in women: a meta-analysis. J Bone Miner Res 2002;17(11):2048–2060.
32. Mann V, Hobson EE, Li B, et al. A COL1A1 Sp1 binding site polymorphism predisposes to osteoporotic fracture by affecting bone density and quality. J Clin Invest 2001;107(7):899–907.
33. Rivadeneira F, Houwing-Duistermaat JJ, Beck TJ, et al. The influence of an insulin-like growth factor I gene promoter polymorphism on hip bone geometry and the risk of nonvertebral fracture in the elderly: the Rotterdam Study. J Bone Miner Res 2004;19(8):1280–1290.

34. Grant SF, Reid DM, Blake G, Herd R, Fogelman I, Ralston SH. Reduced bone density and osteoporosis associated with a polymorphic Sp1 binding site in the collagen type I alpha 1 gene. Nat Genet 1996;14(2):203–205.
35. Marshall D, Johnell O, Wedel H. Meta-analysis of how well measures of bone mineral density predict occurrence of osteoporotic fractures [see comments]. BMJ 1996;312(7041):1254–1259.
36. Cummings SR, Melton LJ. Epidemiology and outcomes of osteoporotic fractures. Lancet 2002; 359(9319):1761–1767.
37. Zmuda JM, Cauley JA, Ferrell RE. Recent progress in understanding the genetic susceptibility to osteoporosis. Genet Epidemiol 1999;16(4):356–367.
38. Nguyen TV, Blangero J, Eisman JA. Genetic epidemiological approaches to the search for osteoporosis genes. J Bone Miner Res 2000;15: 392–401.
39. Klein R, Mitchell S, Phillips T, Belknap J, Orwoll E. Quantitative trait loci affecting peak bone mineral density in mice. J Bone Miner Res 1998;13:1648–1656.
40. Beamer WG, Shultz KL, Donahue LR, et al. Quantitative trait loci for femoral and lumbar vertebral bone mineral density in C57BL/6J and C3H/HeJ inbred strains of mice. J Bone Miner Res 2001; 16(7):1195–206.
41. Benes H, Weinstein R, Zheng W, et al. Chromosomal mapping of osteopenia-associated quantitative trait loci using closely related mouse strains. J Bone Miner Res 2000;15:626–633.
42. Devoto M, Shimoya K, Caminis J, et al. First-stage autosomal genome screen in extended pedigrees suggests genes predisposing to low bone mineral density on chromosomes 1p, 2p and 4q. Eur J Hum Genet 1998;6:151–157.
43. Koller DL, Econs MJ, Morin PA, et al. Genome screen for QTLs contributing to normal variation in bone mineral density and osteoporosis. J Clin Endocrinol Metab 2000;85(9):3116–3120.
44. Karasik D, Myers RH, Cupples LA, et al. Genome screen for quantitative trait loci contributing to normal variation in bone mineral density: the Framingham Study. J Bone Miner Res 2002; 17(9):1718–1727.
45. Ioannidis J, Ng MY, Sham PC, et al. Meta-analysis of genome wide scans provides evidence for gender and site specific regulation of bone mass. J Bone Min Res 2007;22(2):173–183.
46. Mitchell BD, Kammerer CM, Schneider JL, Perez R, Bauer RL. Genetic and environmental determinants of bone mineral density in Mexican Americans: results from the San Antonio Family Osteoporosis Study. Bone 2003;33(5):839–846.
47. Baudoin C, Cohen-Solal ME, Beaudreuil J, De Vernejoul MC. Genetic and environmental factors affect bone density variances of families of men and women with osteoporosis. J Clin Endocrinol Metab 2002;87(5):2053–2059.
48. Karasik D, Cupples LA, Hannan MT, Kiel DP. Age, gender, and body mass effects on quantitative trait loci for bone mineral density: the Framingham study. Bone 2003;33(3):308–316.
49. Ralston SH, Galwey N, MacKay I, et al. Loci for regulation of bone mineral density in men and women identified by genome wide linkage scan: the FAMOS study. Hum Mol Genet 2005;14(7): 943–951.
50. Streeten EA, McBride DJ, Pollin TI, et al. Quantitative trait loci for BMD identified by autosome-wide linkage scan to chromosomes 7q and 21q in men from the Amish Family Osteoporosis Study. J Bone Miner Res 2006;21(9):1433–1442.
51. Yang TL, Zhao LJ, Liu YJ, Liu JF, Recker RR, Deng HW. Genetic and environmental correlations of bone mineral density at different skeletal sites in females and males. Calcif Tissue Int 2006;78(4):212–217.
52. Harris M, Nguyen TV, Howard GM, Kelly PJ, Eisman JA. Genetic and environmental correlations between bone formation and bone mineral density: a twin study. Bone 1998;22(2):141–145.
53. Szumska D, Benes H, Kang P, et al. A novel locus on the X chromosome regulates post-maturity bone density changes in mice. Bone 2007;40(3): 758–766.
54. Kelly PJ, Nguyen T, Hopper J, Pocock N, Sambrook P, Eisman J. Changes in axial bone density with age: a twin study. J Bone Miner Res 1993;8(1):11–17.
55. Christian JC, Yu PL, Slemenda CW, Johnston CC Jr. Heritability of bone mass: a longitudinal study in aging male twins. Am J Hum Genet 1989;44(3): 429–433.
56. Wynne F, Drummond FJ, Daly M, et al. Suggestive linkage of 2p22–25 and 11q12–13 with low bone mineral density at the lumbar spine in the Irish population. Calcif Tissue Int 2003;72(6): 651–658.
57. Khosla S, Riggs BL, Atkinson EJ, et al. Relationship of estrogen receptor genotypes to bone mineral density and to rates of bone loss in men. J Clin Endocrinol Metab 2004;89(4):1808–1816.
58. Salmen T, Heikkinen AM, Mahonen A, et al. Early postmenopausal bone loss is associated with PvuII estrogen receptor gene polymorphism in Finnish

women: effect of hormone replacement therapy. J Bone Miner Res 2000;15(2):315–321.
59. Recker R, Lappe J, Davies K, Heaney R. Characterization of perimenopausal bone loss: a prospective study. J Bone Miner Res 2000;15(10): 1965–1973.
60. Khosla S, Riggs BL, Atkinson EJ, et al. Effects of sex and age on bone microstructure at the ultradistal radius: a population-based noninvasive in vivo assessment. J Bone Miner Res 2006;21(1): 124–131.
61. Khosla S, Melton LJ III, Atkinson EJ, O'Fallon WM. Relationship of serum sex steroid levels to longitudinal changes in bone density in young versus elderly men. J Clin Endocrinol Metab 2001;86(8):3555–3561.
62. Parsons CA, Mroczkowski HJ, McGuigan FE, et al. Interspecies synteny mapping identifies a quantitative trait locus for bone mineral density on human chromosome Xp22. Hum Mol Genet 2005;14(21):3141–3148.
63. Manolagas SC, Jilka RL. Bone marrow, cytokines, and bone remodeling. Emerging insights into the pathophysiology of osteoporosis. N Engl J Med 1995;332(5):305–311.
64. Moffett SP, Zmuda JM, Oakley JI, et al. Tumor necrosis factor-alpha polymorphism, bone strength phenotypes, and the risk of fracture in older women. J Clin Endocrinol Metab 2005; 90(6):3491–3497.
65. Murray RE, McGuigan F, Grant SF, Reid DM, Ralston SH. Polymorphisms of the interleukin-6 gene are associated with bone mineral density. Bone 1997;21(1):89–92.
66. Tsukamoto K, Yoshida H, Watanabe S, et al. Association of radial bone mineral density with CA repeat polymorphism at the interleukin 6 locus in postmenopausal Japanese women. J Hum Genet 1999;44(3):148–151.
67. Duncan EL, Brown MA, Sinsheimer J, et al. Suggestive linkage of the parathyroid receptor type 1 to osteoporosis [see comments]. J Bone Miner Res 1999;14(12):1993–1999.
68. Hamanaka Y, Yamamoto I, Takada M, et al. Comparison of bone mineral density at various skeletal sites with quantitative ultrasound parameters of the calcaneus for assessment of vertebral fractures. J Bone Miner Metab 1999;17(3):195–200.
69. Lakatos P, Foldes J, Nagy Z, et al. Serum insulin-like growth factor-I, insulin-like growth factor binding proteins, and bone mineral content in hyperthyroidism. Thyroid 2000;10:417–423.
70. Takacs I, Koller DL, Peacock M, et al. Sibling pair linkage and association studies between bone mineral density and the insulin-like growth factor I gene locus. J Clin Endocrinol Metab 1999; 84(12):4467–4471.
71. Ferrari SL, Karasik D, Liu J, et al. Interactions of interleukin-6 promoter polymorphisms with dietary and lifestyle factors and their association with bone mass in men and women from the framingham osteoporosis study. J Bone Miner Res 2004;19(4):552–559.
72. Rea IM, Ross OA, Armstrong M, et al. Interleukin-6-gene C/G 174 polymorphism in nonagenarian and octogenarian subjects in the BELFAST study. Reciprocal effects on IL-6, soluble IL-6 receptor and for IL-10 in serum and monocyte supernatants. Mech Ageing Dev 2003;124(4):555–561.
73. Nordstrom A, Gerdhem P, Brandstrom H, et al. Interleukin-6 promoter polymorphism is associated with bone quality assessed by calcaneus ultrasound and previous fractures in a cohort of 75-year-old women. Osteoporos Int 2004;15(10): 820–826.
74. Scheidt-Nave CE, Bismar H, Leidug-Bruckner G, Seibel MJ, Ziegler R, Pfeilschifter J. Serum interleukin-6 is a major predictor of bone loss in women specific to the first decade past menopause. J Bone Min Res 1999;14 (Suppl 1):S147.
75. Morrison NA, Qi JC, Tokita A, et al. Prediction of bone density from vitamin D receptor alleles [see comments] [published erratum appears in Nature 1997 May 1;387(6628):106]. Nature 1994;367(6460): 284–287.
76. Gross C, Eccleshall TR, Malloy PJ, Villa ML, Marcus R, Feldman D. The presence of a polymorphism at the translation initiation site of the vitamin D receptor gene is associated with low bone mineral density in postmenopausal Mexican-American women [see comments]. J Bone Miner Res 1996;11(12):1850–1855.
77. Hustmyer FG, Peacock M, Hui S, Johnston CC, Christian J. Bone mineral density in relation to polymorphism at the vitamin D receptor gene locus. J Clin Invest 1994;94(5):2130–2134.
78. Eccleshall TR, Garnero P, Gross C, Delmas PD, Feldman D. Lack of correlation between start codon polymorphism of the vitamin D receptor gene and bone mineral density in premenopausal French women: the OFELY study. J Bone Miner Res 1998;13(1):31–35.
79. Garnero P, Borel O, Sornay-Rendu E, Delmas PD. Vitamin D receptor gene polymorphisms do not predict bone turnover and bone mass in healthy premenopausal women. J Bone Miner Res 1995; 10(9):1283–1288.

80. Garnero P, Borel O, Sornay-Rendu E, Arlot ME, Delmas PD. Vitamin D receptor gene polymorphisms are not related to bone turnover, rate of bone loss, and bone mass in postmenopausal women: the OFELY Study. J Bone Miner Res 1996;11(6):827–834.
81. Houston LA, Grant SF, Reid DM, Ralston SH. Vitamin D receptor polymorphism, bone mineral density, and osteoporotic vertebral fracture: studies in a UK population. Bone 1996;18(3): 249–252.
82. Jorgensen HL, Scholler J, Sand JC, Bjuring M, Hassager C, Christiansen C. Relation of common allelic variation at vitamin D receptor locus to bone mineral density and postmenopausal bone loss: cross sectional and longitudinal population study. BMJ 1996;313(7057):586–590.
83. Vandevyver C, Vanhoof J, Declerck K, et al. Lack of association between estrogen receptor genotypes and bone mineral density, fracture history, or muscle strength in elderly women. J Bone Miner Res 1999;14(9):1576–1582.
84. Ferrari S, Rizzoli R, Slosman D, Bonjour JP. Familial resemblance for bone mineral mass is expressed before puberty. J Clin Endocrinol Metab 1998;83(2):358–361.
85. Gennari L, Becherini L, Masi L, et al. Vitamin D and estrogen receptor allelic variants in Italian postmenopausal women: evidence of multiple gene contribution to bone mineral density. J Clin Endocrinol Metab 1998;83(3):939–944.
86. Salamone LM, Ferrell R, Black DM, et al. The association between vitamin D receptor gene polymorphisms and bone mineral density at the spine, hip and whole-body in premenopausal women [published erratum appears in Osteoporos Int 1996;6(3):187–8]. Osteoporos Int 1996;6(1):63–68.
87. Uitterlinden AG, Pols HA, Burger H, et al. A large-scale population-based study of the association of vitamin D receptor gene polymorphisms with bone mineral density. J Bone Miner Res 1996; 11(9):1241–1248.
88. Langdahl BL, Lokke E, Carstens M, Stenkjaer LL, Eriksen EF. A TA repeat polymorphism in the estrogen receptor gene is associated with osteoporotic fractures but polymorphisms in the first exon and intron are not. J Bone Miner Res 2000;15(11):2222–2230.
89. Riggs BL, Nguyen TV, Melton LJ III, et al. The contribution of vitamin D receptor gene alleles to the determination of bone mineral density in normal and osteoporotic women. J Bone Miner Res 1995;10(6):991–996.
90. Morita A, Iki M, Dohi Y, et al. Prediction of bone mineral density from vitamin D receptor polymorphisms is uncertain in representative samples of Japanese Women. The Japanese Population-based Osteoporosis (JPOS) Study. Int J Epidemiol 2004;33(5):979–988.
91. Thakkinstian A, D'Este C, Eisman J, Nguyen T, Attia J. Meta-analysis of molecular association studies: vitamin D receptor gene polymorphisms and BMD as a case study. J Bone Miner Res 2004;19(3):419–428.
92. Bischoff-Ferrari HA, Borchers M, Gudat F, Durmuller U, Stahelin HB, Dick W. Vitamin D receptor expression in human muscle tissue decreases with age. J Bone Miner Res 2004;19(2):265–269.
93. Cummings SR, Browner WS, Bauer D, et al. Endogenous hormones and the risk of hip and vertebral fractures among older women. Study of Osteoporotic Fractures Research Group [see comments]. N Engl J Med 1998;339(11):733–738.
94. Rizzoli R, Bonjour JP. Hormones and bones. Lancet 1997;349 (Suppl 1):SI20–S123.
95. Carani C, Qin K, Simoni M, et al. Effect of testosterone and estradiol in a man with aromatase deficiency. N Engl J Med 1997;337(2):91–95.
96. Amin S, Zhang Y, Sawin CT, et al. Association of hypogonadism and estradiol levels with bone mineral density in elderly men from the Framingham study. Ann Intern Med 2000;133(12):951–963.
97. Willing M, Sowers M, Aron D, et al. Bone mineral density and its change in white women: estrogen and vitamin D receptor genotypes and their interaction. J Bone Miner Res 1998;13(4):695–705.
98. Deng HW, Li J, Li JL, Johnson M, Gong G, Recker RR. Association of VDR and estrogen receptor genotypes with bone mass in postmenopausal Caucasian women: different conclusions with different analyses and the implications. Osteoporos Int 1999;9(6):499–507.
99. Becherini L, Gennari L, Masi L, et al. Evidence of a linkage disequilibrium between polymorphisms in the human estrogen receptor alpha gene and their relationship to bone mass variation in postmenopausal Italian women. Hum Mol Genet 2000;9(13):2043–2050.
100. Albagha OM, McGuigan FE, Reid DM, Ralston SH. Estrogen receptor alpha gene polymorphisms and bone mineral density: haplotype analysis in women from the United Kingdom. J Bone Miner Res 2001;16(1):128–134.
101. Bagger YZ, Jorgensen HL, Heegaard AM, Bayer L, Hansen L, Hassager C. No major effect of estrogen receptor gene polymorphisms on bone mineral

density or bone loss in postmenopausal Danish women. Bone 2000;26(2):111–116.
102. van Meurs JB, Schuit SC, Weel AE, et al. Association of 5′ estrogen receptor alpha gene polymorphisms with bone mineral density, vertebral bone area and fracture risk. Hum Mol Genet 2003; 12(14):1745–1754.
103. Ioannidis JP, Ralston SH, Bennett ST, et al. Differential genetic effects of ESR1 gene polymorphisms on osteoporosis outcomes. JAMA 2004; 292(17):2105–2114.
104. Han KO, Moon IG, Kang YS, Chung HY, Min HK, Han IK. Nonassociation of estrogen receptor genotypes with bone mineral density and estrogen responsiveness to hormone replacement therapy in Korean postmenopausal women [see comments]. J Clin Endocrinol Metab 1997;82(4): 991–995.
105. Hey PJ, Twells RC, Phillips MS, et al. Cloning of a novel member of the low-density lipoprotein receptor family. Gene 1998;216(1):103–111.
106. Gong Y, Slee RB, Fukai N, et al. LDL receptor-related protein 5 (LRP5) affects bone accrual and eye development. Cell 2001;107(4):513–523.
107. Little RD, Carulli JP, Del Mastro RG, et al. A mutation in the LDL receptor-related protein 5 gene results in the autosomal dominant high-bone-mass trait. Am J Hum Genet 2002;70(1):11–19.
108. Boyden LM, Mao J, Belsky J, et al. High bone density due to a mutation in LDL-receptor-related protein 5. N Engl J Med 2002;346(20):1513–1521.
109. Van Wesenbeeck L, Cleiren E, Gram J, et al. Six novel missense mutations in the LDL receptor-related protein 5 (LRP5) gene in different conditions with an increased bone density. Am J Hum Genet 2003;72(3):763–771.
110. Ferrari SL, Deutsch S, Baudoin C, et al. LRP5 gene polymorphisms and idiopathic osteoporosis in men. Bone 2005;37(6):770–775.
111. Ferrari SL, Deutsch S, Choudhury U, et al. Polymorphisms in the low-density lipoprotein receptor-related protein 5 (LRP5) gene are associated with variation in vertebral bone mass, vertebral bone size, and stature in whites. Am J Hum Genet 2004;74(5):866–875.
112. Kiel D, Ferrari S, Cupples LA, et al. Genetic variation at the low density lipoprotein receptor-related protein 5 (LRP5) locus modulates Wnt signaling and the relationship of physical activity with bone mineral density in men. Bone 2007;40(3):587–596.
113. Pluijm SM, Dik MG, Jonker C, Deeg DJ, van Kamp GJ, Lips P. Effects of gender and age on the association of apolipoprotein E epsilon4 with bone mineral density, bone turnover and the risk of fractures in older people. Osteoporos Int 2002; 13(9):701–709.
114. Goseki-Sone M, Sogabe N, Fukushi-Irie M, et al. Functional analysis of the single nucleotide polymorphism (787T>C) in the tissue-nonspecific alkaline phosphatase gene associated with BMD. J Bone Miner Res 2005;20(5):773–782.
115. Uitterlinden AG, Arp PP, Paeper BW, et al. Polymorphisms in the sclerosteosis/van Buchem disease gene (SOST) region are associated with bone-mineral density in elderly whites. Am J Hum Genet 2004;75(6):1032–1045.
116. Balemans W, Foernzler D, Parsons C, et al. Lack of association between the SOST gene and bone mineral density in perimenopausal women: analysis of five polymorphisms. Bone 2002;31 (4):515–519.
117. Ralston SH, de Crombrugghe B. Genetic regulation of bone mass and susceptibility to osteoporosis. Genes Dev 2006;20(18):2492–2506.
118. Boskey AL, DiCarlo E, Paschalis E, West P, Mendelsohn R. Comparison of mineral quality and quantity in iliac crest biopsies from high- and low-turnover osteoporosis: an FT-IR microspectroscopic investigation. Osteoporos Int 2005;16(12): 2031–2038.
119. Melton LJ III, Riggs BL, Achenbach SJ, et al. Does reduced skeletal loading account for age-related bone loss? J Bone Miner Res 2006;21(12):1847–1855.
120. Gilsanz V, Wren TA, Sanchez M, Dorey F, Judex S, Rubin C. Low-level, high-frequency mechanical signals enhance musculoskeletal development of young women with low BMD. J Bone Miner Res 2006;21(9):1464–1474.
121. Kuro-o M, Matsumura Y, Aizawa H, et al. Mutation of the mouse klotho gene leads to a syndrome resembling ageing. Nature 1997;390(6655):45–51.
122. Karasik D, Hannan MT, Cupples LA, Felson DT, Kiel DP. Genetic contribution to biological aging: the Framingham Study. J Gerontol A Biol Sci Med Sci 2004;59(3):218–226.
123. Karasik D, Yakovenko K, Barakh I, et al. Comparative analysis of age prediction by markers of bone change in the hand as assessed by roentgenography. Am J Hum Biol 1999;11:31–44.
124. Karasik D, Demissie S, Cupples LA, Kiel DP. Disentangling the genetic determinants of human aging: biological age as an alternative to the use of survival measures. J Gerontol A Biol Sci Med Sci 2005;60(5):574–587.
125. Ferrari SL, Ahn-Luong L, Garnero P, Humphries SE, Greenspan SL. Two promoter polymorphisms

regulating interleukin-6 gene expression are associated with circulating levels of C-reactive protein and markers of bone resorption in postmenopausal women. J Clin Endocrinol Metab 2003;88(1):255–259.
126. Baldini V, Mastropasqua M, Francucci CM, D'Erasmo E. Cardiovascular disease and osteoporosis. J Endocrinol Invest 2005;28(10 Suppl):69–72.
127. Weitzmann MN, Pacifici R. Estrogen deficiency and bone loss: an inflammatory tale. J Clin Invest 2006;116(5):1186–1194.
128. Raisz LG. Pathogenesis of osteoporosis: concepts, conflicts, and prospects. J Clin Invest 2005; 115(12):3318–3325.
129. Urano T, Shiraki M, Fujita M, et al. Association of a single nucleotide polymorphism in the lipoxygenase ALOX15 5′-flanking region (-5229G/A) with bone mineral density. J Bone Miner Metab 2005;23(3):226–230.
130. Yamada Y. Association of polymorphisms of the transforming growth factor-beta1 gene with genetic susceptibility to osteoporosis. Pharmacogenetics 2001;11(9):765–771.
131. Yamada Y, Miyauchi A, Takagi Y, Tanaka M, Mizuno M, Harada A. Association of the C-509–T polymorphism, alone of in combination with the T869->C polymorphism, of the transforming growth factor-beta1 gene with bone mineral density and genetic susceptibility to osteoporosis in Japanese women. J Mol Med 2001;79(2–3):149–156.
132. Giresi PG, Stevenson EJ, Theilhaber J, et al. Identification of a molecular signature of sarcopenia. Physiol Genomics 2005;21(2):253–263.
133. Zahn JM, Sonu R, Vogel H, et al. Transcriptional profiling of aging in human muscle reveals a common aging signature. PLoS Genet 2006;2(7):e115.
134. Justesen J, Stenderup K, Eriksen EF, Kassem M. Maintenance of osteoblastic and adipocytic differentiation potential with age and osteoporosis in human marrow stromal cell cultures. Calcif Tissue Int 2002;71(1):36–44.
135. Meyer RA Jr, Desai BR, Heiner DE, Fiechtl J, Porter S, Meyer MH. Young, adult, and old rats have similar changes in mRNA expression of many skeletal genes after fracture despite delayed healing with age. J Orthop Res 2006;24(10):1933–1944.
136. Holtzman NA, Marteau TM. Will genetics revolutionize medicine? N Engl J Med 2000;343(2):141–144.
137. Khoury MJ, McCabe LL, McCabe ER. Population screening in the age of genomic medicine. N Engl J Med 2003;348(1):50–58.

8
Fracture Epidemiology Among Individuals 75+

Heike A. Bischoff-Ferrari

Introduction

Fractures contribute significantly to morbidity and mortality in older individuals. Among individuals age 60 years and older, the mortality-adjusted residual lifetime risk of fracture has been estimated to be 44–65% for women and 25–42% for men *(1)*.

After age 75, hip fractures are the most frequent fractures, and up to 50% of older individuals suffering a hip fracture will have permanent functional disability, 15–25% will require long-term nursing home care, and up to 20% will die within the first year after the event *(2–4)*. The exponential increase in hip fractures after age 75 translates into an estimated 1 in 3 women, and 1 in 6 men, who will have sustained a hip fracture by their 90th decade *(5)*. Consequently, hip fractures account for substantial and increasing health care expenses with annual costs in the United States projected to increase from 7.2 billion in 1990 to 16 billion in 2020 *(6)*.

This chapter reviews epidemiologic data on the rates of hip and other common fractures among older individuals. In addition, future projections, geographic, and seasonal patterns of hip and other common fractures will be summarized.

Critical for the understanding of fractures at later age is their close relationship with muscle weakness *(7)* and falling *(8)*. Thus, at the beginning of this chapter, the epidemiology of falls, and their importance in regard to fracture risk among older individuals, will be reviewed.

Falls and Why They Need to Be Addressed for Optimal Fracture Prevention in Older Individuals

With the focus of this chapter being on fractures in older individuals, it is essential to take falling into consideration. More than 90% of fractures occur after a fall. In addition, falls are common. Fall rates increase 10% per decade, and more than 30% of all community-dwelling and 50% of all institutionalized men and women aged 65 fall once per year *(9)*. Serious injuries occur with 10–15% of falls *(8)*, resulting in fractures in 5% and hip fracture in 1–2%. As an independent determinant of functional decline *(10)*, falls lead to 40% of all nursing home admissions *(3)*.

Because of the increasing proportion of older individuals, annual costs from all fall-related injuries in the United States in persons 65 years or older are projected to increase from $20.3 billion in 1994 to $32.4 billion in 2020 *(11)*. Thus, interventions that reduce the risk and thereby consequences of falls, such as fractures, may have substantial public health value.

Mechanistically, the circumstances and the direction *(12,13)* of a fall determine the type of fracture, whereas bone density and factors that attenuate a fall, such as better strength or better padding, critically determine whether a fracture will take place when the faller lands on a certain bone *(14)*. Thus, for optimal fracture prevention, both falls and bone health need attention.

However, in the history of osteoporosis treatment, the focus has been on bone. Only recently has the prevention of falls gained significant attention *(15–17)*.

Consistent with the understanding that factors unrelated to bone are at play in fracture epidemiology, the circumstances of different fractures are strikingly different. Hip fractures tend to occur in less-active individuals falling indoors from a standing height with little forward momentum, and they tend to fall sideways or straight down on their hip *(18–20)*. On the other hand, other nonvertebral fractures, such as distal forearm or humerus fractures, tend to occur among more-active older individuals who are correspondingly more likely to be outdoors and have a greater forward momentum when they fall *(21–23)*.

Even if bone is the primary target, falling may indirectly affect bone density through increased immobility from self-restriction of activities *(24)*. It is well known that falls may lead to a psychological trauma known as fear of falling *(25)*. In a recent survey among community-dwelling older persons, 13% of men and 21% of women aged 66–70 years old are reported to be moderately or very fearful of falling *(25)*. After their first fall, approximately 30% of individuals develop fear of falling *(24)*, resulting in self-restriction of activities *(24)*, increasing immobility, and decreased quality of life *(25)*. What makes the assessment of falls challenging is the fact that falls tend to be forgotten if not associated with significant injury *(26)*, requiring short periods of follow-up.

Site-Specific Fracture Epidemiology Among Older Individuals

Hip Fractures

Hip fractures are the most common fractures among white and black individuals age 75 and older *(27,28)*. Future projections indicate that hip fractures will increase in many countries *(29)*. This is in part explained by increased life expectancy plus the expected demographic changes, with a significant rise of the oldest and frailest segment of the population. Based on a world-wide projection, the total number of hip fractures in 1990 was estimated to be 338,000 in men and 917,000 in women *(29)*. Assuming no change in the age- and sex-specific incidence, the number of hip fractures are estimated to double by the year of 2025, and more than triple by the year 2050. Most pronounced increases are expected for Asia, where in 1990 26% of all hip fractures occurred. In 2025 it has been predicted that 37% of all hip fractures will occur in Asia, with a further increase in 2050 of 45%. The 10-year hip fracture probability varies world-wide and is shown in Figure 8.1 *(30)*.

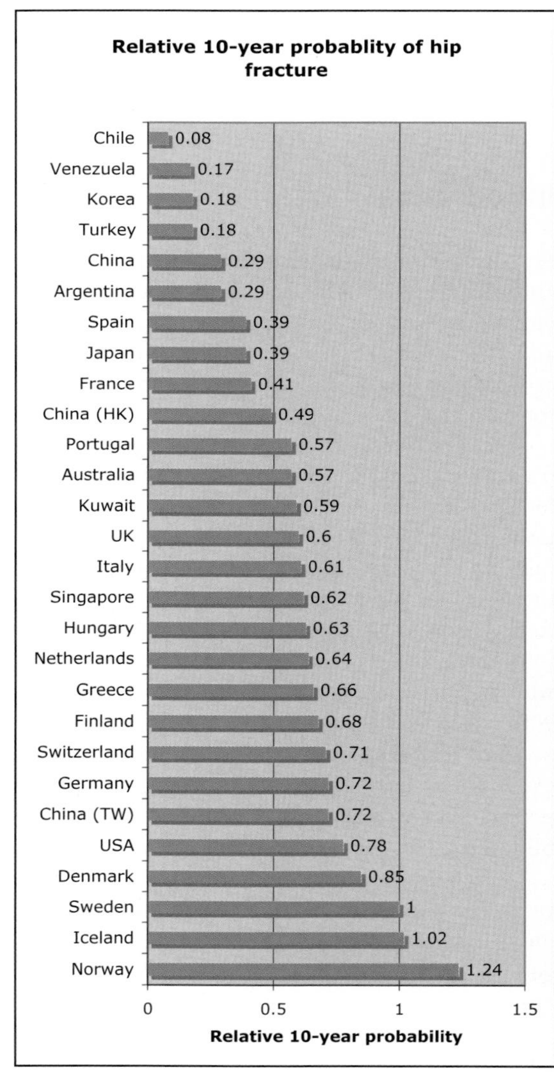

FIGURE 8.1. **World-wide comparison of hip fracture probability standardized to Sweden.** Standardized to Swedish hip fracture data. Within Europe the highest 10-year hip fracture probability is observed in Norway, followed by Iceland. (Adapted from Kanis JA. et al. *[30]*.)

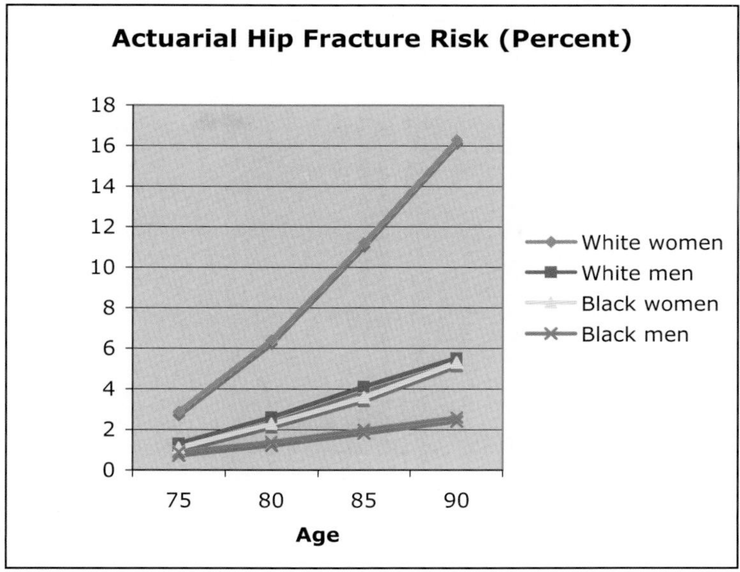

FIGURE 8.2. Actuarial risk of hip fracture (in percentages) of a 65-year-old individual. More than 16% of 65-year-old white women and 5.5% of white men, as well as 5.3% of black women and 2.6% of black men, can expect to sustain a hip fracture by age 90. The actuarial risk takes into consideration that after age 75, death rates become substantial and reduce the number of individuals at risk for a fracture. (Data is adapted from Barrett JA et al. *[27]*.)

Within different countries and race/ethnicity groups, hip fracture risk increases exponentially with age. Figure 8.2 gives US population-based data on the actuarial risk of hip fracture among individuals with age 65 (Medicare recipients), according to Barrett et al. *(27)*. In addition, hip fracture rates vary considerably by type of dwelling and based on selection criteria from randomized controlled trials. The highest hip fracture rates were observed in the placebo group of vitamin D trials among nursing home residents. Table 8.1 shows calculated hip fracture rates among older individuals per 10,000 person-years based on different cohort studies, as well as the placebo groups from several large bisphosphonate and vitamin D trials. Table 8.2 shows risk factors for hip fracture among women age 65 and older. Risk factors for hip fractures among older men include falls *(15)*, low estradiol and low testosterone levels *(31)*, prior fracture, and low hip bone density *(13)*.

Other Non-Vertebral Fractures

The actuarial risk of fracture in a person 65 years of age is shown for three common non-vertebral fractures in Figures 8.3–8.5: distal forearm, proximal humerus, and ankle fractures *(27)*. Similar to hip fractures, distal forearm and proximal humerus fractures show a steep increase with age, which is most pronounced in white women. Ankle fractures only show a small increase with age.

Vertebral Fractures

Vertebral fractures cause disability, back pain *(32)*, and decreased quality of life among older individuals *(33)*. Women with a first vertebral fracture, have a more than 19% risk of developing a second vertebral fracture in the subsequent year *(34)*, a 2.5-fold increased risk for any subsequent fracture *(35)*, and a 2.8-fold increased mortality rate within the following 10 years *(36)*.

Compared to hip fractures, the epidemiology of vertebral fractures is challenging, with less than 30% of vertebral fractures coming to clinical attention *(28)*. Based on data from Cooper and colleagues, vertebral fractures increase exponentially after age 65 among men and women, and incidence rates for vertebral fractures project between hip and radius fractures for both genders after age 75 *(28)*. Figure 8.6 illustrates data from

Table 8.1. Hip Fracture Rates From Different Settings

Data source	Age	Hip fracture rates per 10,000 person-years
Cohort data		
NHANES I—men *(71)*	70+	37
NHANES I—women		
Framingham—men *(72)*	70+	87
	75–79	3.2
	80–84	6.6
	85–89	18.8
	90–94	30.6
Framingham—women	95+	45.5
	75–79	7.8
	80–84	15
	85–89	28.4
	90–94	43.5
Dubbo—men *(73)*	95+	70.2
Dubbo—women	85+	119
	85+	260
Trial data		
FIT trial for alendronate (low bone density, no fracture) *(74)*	68 (SD ± 6)	26
HORIZON trial with zolendronate; 18-month data as published in abstract form 2006 *(75)* (T score ≤ −2.5 or ≤ −1.5 with prevalent vertebral fracture)	73 (55–89)	62
HIP trial for residronate (T score of < −4.0 or T score < −3.0 plus a non-skeletal risk factor for hip fracture) *(76)*	74 (SD ± 3)	101
HIP trial for residronate (at least one non-skeletal risk factor for hip fracture or low bone density) *(76)*	83 (SD ± 3)	124
Vitamin D trial Lips et al. *(77)*	80 (SD ± 6)	107
Assisted living Decalyos I Vitamin D trial *(63)*	84 (SD ± 6)	523
Nursing home Decalyos II Vitamin D trial *(78)*	86 (SD ± 8)	553
Nursing home		

Table 8.2. Risk Factors for First Incident Hip and Radiographic Vertebral Fracture in Women Age 65 and Older

Hip fracture	Radiographic vertebral fracture
Older age	Older age
Any previous fracture	Previous non-spine fracture
Low calcaneal bone density	Low bone density at all sites
No increase in weight since age 25	Low body mass index
Current smoking was not associated with risk of hip fracture	Current smoking
	Low milk consumption during pregnancy (<1 glass/day)
Low calcium intake was not associated with risk of hip fracture	
On feet <4 hours per day	Low levels of daily physical activity (walks <1 block/day or <1 hour/day household chores)
(falls not considered in this model)	Having a fall
(antacid use not considered in this model)	Regular use of aluminum-containing antacids
History of maternal hip fracture	**Maternal hip fracture was not associated with risk of vertebral fracture**
Tall at age 25	(Tall at age 25 not considered in this model)
Low self-rated health	**Self-rated health was not associated with risk of vertebral fracture**
Previous hyperparathyroidism	**Previous hyperparathyroidism was not associated with risk of vertebral fracture**
Current use of long-acting benzodiacepins	(Long-acting benzodiacepin use not considered in this model)
Current use of anticonvulsant drugs	(Anticonvulsant drug use not considered in this model)
Current caffeine intake	**Caffeine intake was not associated with risk of vertebral fracture**
Inability to rise from a chair	**Inability to rise from a chair was not associated with risk of vertebral fracture**
Resting pulse >80 beats/minute	(resting pulse use not considered in this model)
Vitamin D deficiency/latitude	
Previous fall	

Table 8.2 summarizes and compares risk factors for hip and radiographic incident vertebral fractures assessed from the Study of Osteoporotic Fractures (SOF) among white women age 65 and older. Risk factors for both outcomes are based on multivariate analyses.

Risk factors for hip fracture are adapted from Cummings SR et al. *(7)*. Hip fracture rates were 11 per 10,000 person-years among women with no more than two risk factors and normal calcaneal bone density. Hip fracture rates were 270 per 10,000 person-years among women with five or more risk factors plus a calcaneal bone density in the lowest one-third for their age. Added to the table in dark red are two established risk factors for hip fracture not assessed in the model within the SOF cohort (falls *[8,13,15]*, vitamin D deficiency *[59,62,64]*, and latitude away from the equator *[65]*).

Risk factors for radiographic incident fractures are adapted from Nevitt MC et al. *(37)*. For radiographic vertebral fractures, women in the lowest third of wrist bone density plus five or more risk factors had a 12-fold greater risk than women in the highest third of wrist bone density with no additional risk factors. Radiographic vertebral fracture was defined as a 20% and at least 4-mm decrease in vertebral height.

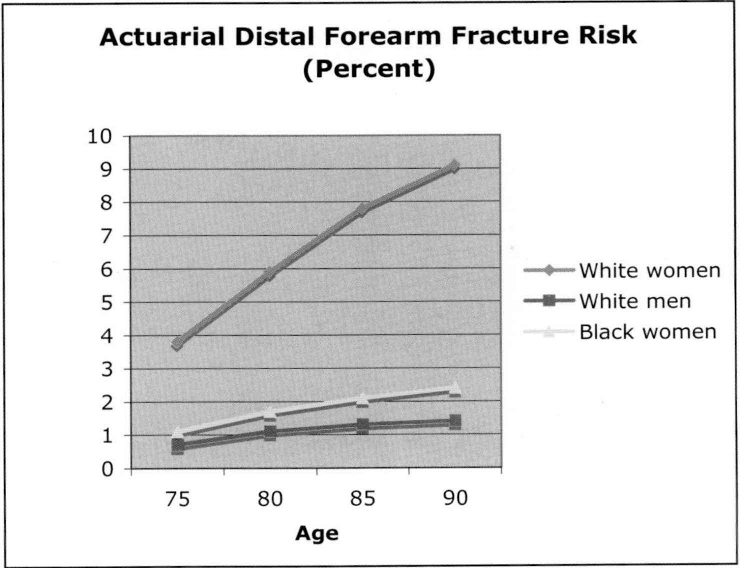

FIGURE 8.3. Actuarial risk of distal forearm fracture (in percentages) of a 65-year-old individual. More than 9% of 65-year-old white women and 1.4% of white men, as well as 2.4% of black women, can expect to sustain a distal forearm fracture by age 90. Cases in black men were too small to explore. The actuarial risk takes into consideration that after age 75, death rates become substantial and reduce the number of individuals at risk for a fracture. (Data is adapted from Barrett JA et al. *[27]*.)

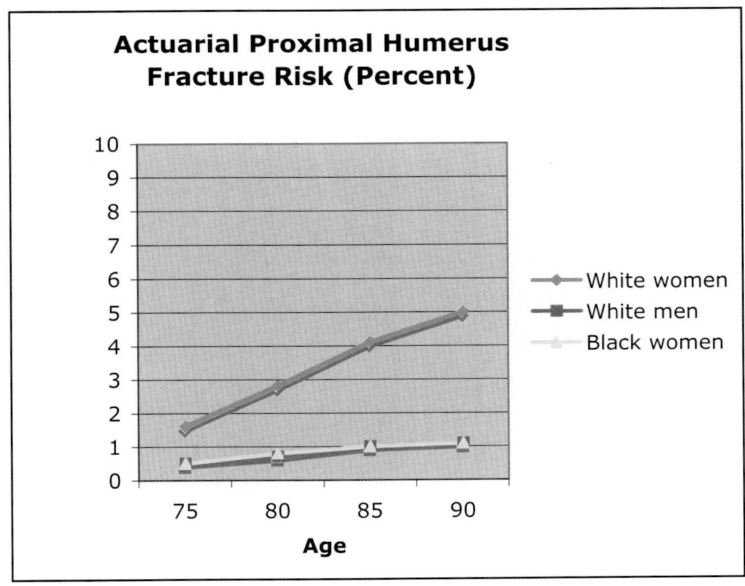

FIGURE 8.4. Actuarial risk of proximal humerus fracture (in percentages) of a 65-year-old individual. More than 5% of 65-year-old white women and 1.1% of white men, as well as 1.1% of black women, can expect to sustain a distal forearm fracture by age 90. Cases in black men were too small to explore. The actuarial risk takes into consideration that after age 75, death rates become substantial and reduce the number of individuals at risk for a fracture. (Data is adapted from Barrett JA et al. *[27]*.)

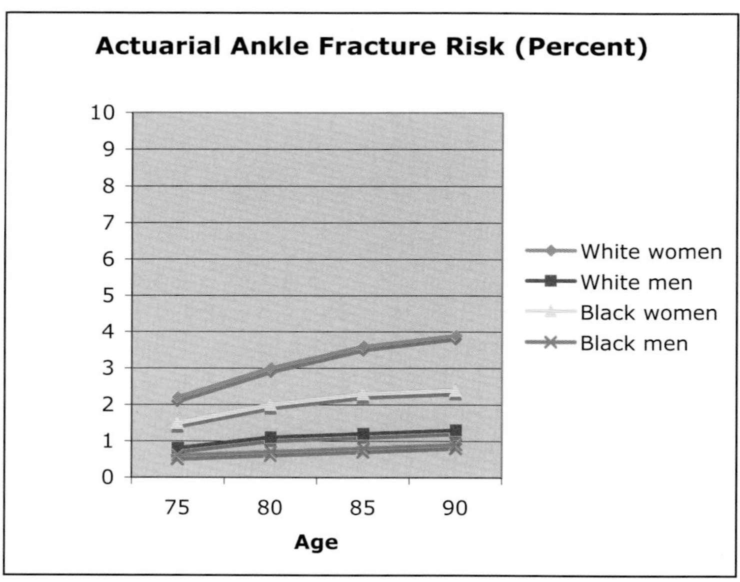

FIGURE 8.5. Actuarial risk of ankle fracture (in percentages) of a 65-year-old individual. 3.9% of 65-year-old white women and 1.3% of white men, as well as 2.4% of black women, can expect to sustain a distal forearm fracture by age 90. Cases in black men were too small to explore. The actuarial risk takes into consideration that after age 75, death rates become substantial and reduce the number of individuals at risk for a fracture. (Data is adapted from Barrett JA et al. *[27]*.)

the SOF study on prevalence of vertebral fractures among women by age, suggesting that one in three women will have a prevalent fracture at age 80 *(37)*. In regards to men, after age 80, vertebral fracture rates have been reported to be similar to those in women *(38)*. In fact, based on radiological deformities, data from a multi-center European study found equal sex incidence between the ages

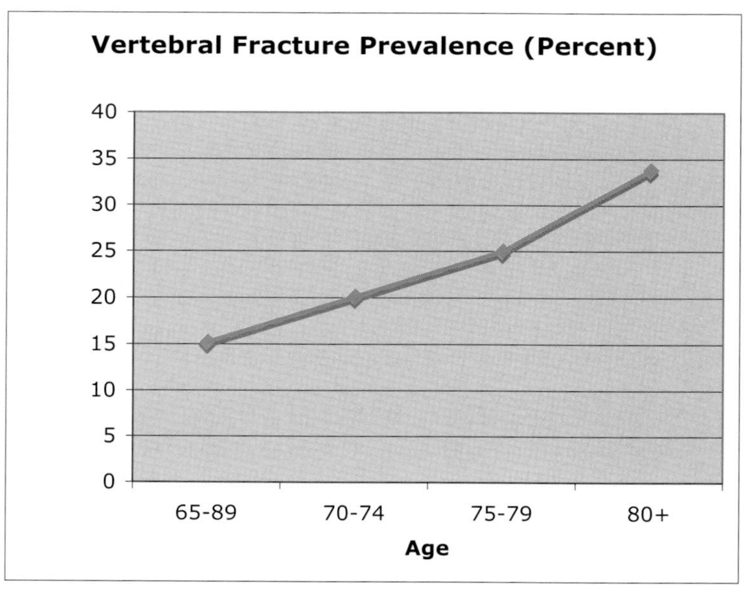

FIGURE 8.6. Vertebral fracture prevalence by age among women. Based on data from women of the Study of Osteoporotic Fractures (SOF), 1 in 3 will have a prevalent vertebral fracture at age 80+. (Adapted from Nevitt MC et al. *[37]*.)

50 and 79. The latter study further suggested a geographical variation of vertebral fractures within Europe, with higher rates in Skandinavia *(39)*.

More than 90% of vertebral fractures in women result from mild to moderate trauma, whereas this proportion is only 55% among men *(40)*. Severe vertebral deformities appear to have a predilection between T10 and L1 *(40)*. Risk factors for a first radiographic vertebral fracture among women age 65 and older are shown in Table 8.2 *(37)*.

Geographic and Seasonal Variations in Hip and Other Non-Vertebral Fractures

Excess winter morbidity and mortality continue to be important public health problems, especially among older persons *(41–43)*. In addition to clear seasonal variations in respiratory *(42–45)* and cardiovascular diseases *(46)*, fractures of the hip *(47–53)* and distal forearm *(54)* contribute to high winter morbidity rates in older persons.

Some studies indicate that falls caused by snow and ice may play an important role in seasonality of fractures *(48,49)*. One cause of the increased fracture risk in winter compared to summer may be that older persons are more likely to slip and fall during periods of snow and ice *(55)*. On the other hand, hip fractures, which mostly occur indoors *(18–20)*, may be less affected by snow and ice.

In a large population-based study from the United States, fracture rates for hip, distal forearm, proximal humerus, and ankle were higher in winter than in other seasons, although the winter peak was small for hip fractures (*see* Figure 8.7) *(56)*. This seasonal pattern was most evident in "warm" states that are only minimally affected by ice and snow. Furthermore, in the same study, hip fractures had strikingly different associations with weather than fractures of the distal forearm, proximal humerus, and ankle. In winter, total snowfall was associated with a reduced risk of hip fracture (−5% per 20 inches) but an increased risk of non-hip fractures (6–12%; $p < 0.05$ at all sites). In summer, hip fracture risk tended to be lower during sunny weather (−3% per 2 weeks of sunny days; $p = 0.13$), although there was an increased

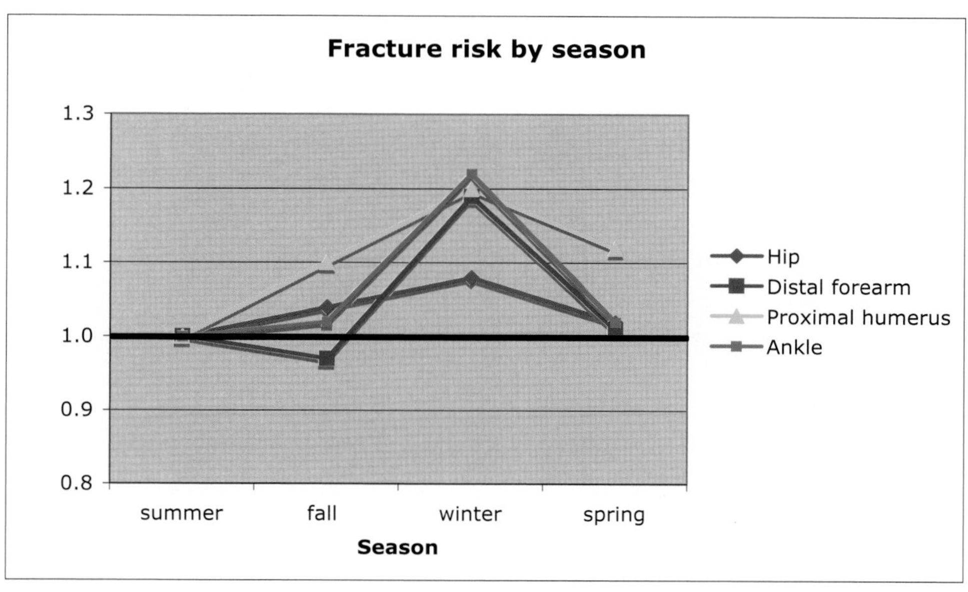

FIGURE 8.7. Relative risks of fractures, by season. Relative risks are adjusted for gender, age, and race/ethnicity. For all sites, fracture risk in winter was significantly higher than in each of the other seasons (95% CI excluded 1 for the comparison of each season with winter). (Adapted from Bischoff-Ferrari HA et al. *[56]*.)

risk of the other fractures (15–20%; $p < 0.05$) in sunny weather *(56)*.

One plausible explanation for the strikingly different seasonal and weather patterns between hip and non-hip fractures may be found in the circumstances surrounding these fractures. Hip fractures tend to occur indoors among relatively frail individuals *(18–20)*, whereas the others tend to occur among more active individuals who are correspondingly more likely to be outdoors *(21–23)*. Clearly, weather would affect the latter group differently than the former *(18)*. It is likely, for example, that active individuals would expose themselves to adverse weather conditions more readily than their more frail counterparts, thus increasing their risks of ice- and snow-related falls and fractures. A possible support of this hypothesis is suggested by the subgroup analyses, in which individuals who are more likely to be frail and less active (women and individuals aged 80 years and older), had a smaller winter/summer difference in hip fracture risk than the more robust population groups (men and individuals younger than 80; *see* Table 8.3).

The protective association of sunshine with risk of hip fracture in the summer and fall may be due to the higher serum concentrations of 25-hydroxyvitamin D associated with sun exposure *(57,58)*. Improved vitamin D status through supplementation with vitamin D may reduce the risk of falls *(59)*, improve bone mineral density (BMD) *(60,61)*, and reduce risk of fractures *(60,62–64)* in older individuals. The benefit of sun exposure is supported by a recent review suggesting that for each 10° change in latitude from the equator (e.g., from Paris to Stockholm), fracture probability increased by 0.3% in men, by 0.8% in women, and by 0.6% in men and women combined *(65)*. On the other hand, for the fractures outside the hip, an incremental gain in vitamin D from sunlight exposure may be outweighed by the increased risk associated with outdoor activities in more-active older persons in sunny weather.

Corroborating the findings on snowfall in winter being protective against hip fractures on a geographic level are studies indicating a distinct North-South gradient in hip fracture risk, with lower rates in the northern United States, where colder weather is more common *(66)*. At the same time, there is no indication of a North-South gradient for non-hip fractures. Rather, lower rates for non-hip fractures (distal forearm and proximal humerus) are found in the Western states and higher rates in the Eastern states *(66)*. Ankle fractures appear to have a somewhat similar pattern as distal forearm and proximal humerus, but not consistently so. All patterns appear to be similar in men and in women.

Geographic variations of hip fractures have been investigated for Europe, where rates appear to be higher in the north compared to the south (Figure 8.1). This apparent inconsistency with the US pattern for hip fractures may be explained by additional genetic influences within Europe, or lower sunshine exposure with a greater distance from the equator *(64)*.

Table 8.3. Winter/Summer Relative Fracture Risks, by Fracture Type in Subgroups of the Population

Fracture site	Winter/summer RR by gender		Winter/summer RR by age		Winter/summer RR by race	
	RR (95% CI) men	RR (95% CI) women	RR (95% CI) younger (65–80)	RR (95% CI) older (>80)	RR (95% CI) white individuals	RR (95% CI) black individuals
Hip	1.15 [1.08–1.23]	1.07 [1.03–1.10]*	1.10 [1.05–1.15]	1.08 [1.04–1.12]	1.08 [1.05–1.12]	1.21 [1.03–1.42]
Distal forearm	1.51 [1.33–1.71]	1.15 [1.11–1.21]***	1.25 [1.19–1.32])	1.08 [1.00–1.16]**	1.20 [1.15–1.25]	1.05 [0.81–1.37]
Proximal humerus	1.23 [1.07–1.42]	1.19 [1.12–1.27]	1.28 [1.19–1.38]	1.10 [1.01–1.20]**	1.19 [1.12–1.26]	1.50 [1.02–2.20]
Ankle	1.25 [1.10–1.42]	1.21 [1.13–1.29]	1.23 [1.15–1.31]	1.18 [1.04–1. 34]	1.22 [1.14–1.29]	1.30 [1.01–1.68]

Adapted from Bischoff-Ferrari HA et al. (56).

RR, relative risk; CI, confidence interval.

RRs are based on Poisson Regression Models. The models by gender included age and race, the models by age included gender and race, and the model by race included gender and age. Stars indicate level of significance of difference by gender, age, and race in regard to winter/summer relative fracture risk:

$^{*}p < 0.05$; $^{**}p < 0.01$; $^{***}p < 0.$

Gender-Specific Mortality From Hip Fracture

Mortality from hip fractures is significant and has been estimated between 12–20% among women in the first year after the event *(4)*. Men, despite their lower incidence of hip fractures, have a twofold higher risk of death after hip fracture compared to women *(67)*. The increased risk among men is still unclear. One explanation, however, has been suggested by the Baltimore Hip studies *(68)*, where mortality rates after hip fracture were similar between men and women if deaths caused by infections were excluded. Deaths related to infections (pneumonia, influenza, and septicemia) explained the gender difference in the Baltimore cohort, and the gender difference appeared to be maintained throughout the second year after hip fracture. Independent of gender, pre-existing morbidity and poor functional status have been identified as risk factors for mortality after hip fracture *(69,70)*.

Repeat Fractures

Based on a 16-year follow-up of the Dubbo Osteoporosis Study *(35)*, the absolute risk for a repeat fracture increases steeply and equally in men and women with age (*see* Figure 8.8) despite a lower absolute risk for a first fracture among men. The relative risk for a repeat fracture among women age 60–69, 70–79, and 80+ is 1.65 (95% confidence interval [CI] 1.18–2.32), 2.36 (1.91–2.92), and 1.80 (1.45–2.25), respectively. The relative risk for a repeat fracture among men age 60–69, 70–79, and 80+ is 3.75 (2.19–6.43), 4.32 (3.00–6.21), and 2.77 (1.69–4.54), respectively. Among women, the incident fracture associated with the highest repeat fracture risk is hip fracture, with a 2.79-fold increased risk for a repeat fracture (95% CI 2.06–3.77). Among men, the incident fracture associated with the highest repeat fracture risk is vertebral fracture, with a 6.18-fold increased risk (95% CI 4.17–9.14). Absolute repeat fracture rates according to initial fracture site are illustrated in Figure 8.9 *(35)*.

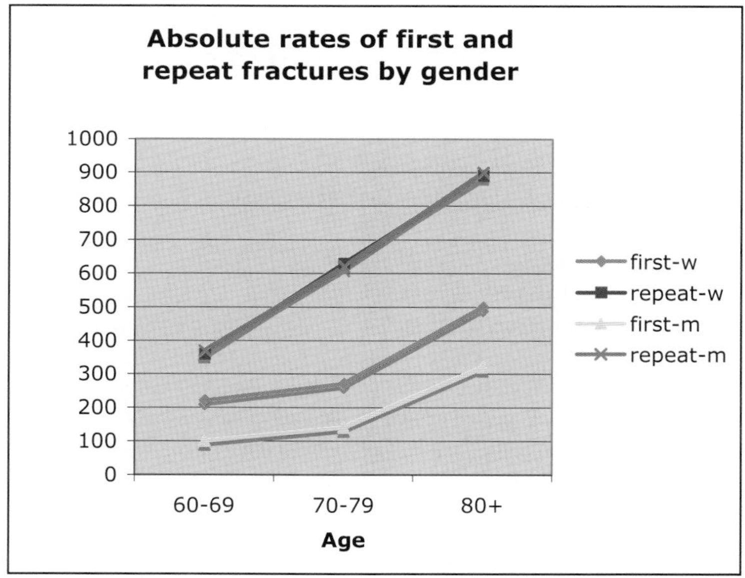

FIGURE 8.8. **Absolute rates of first and repeat fractures according to gender and age.** "W" stands for women and "M" stands for men. The absolute risk for a first fracture increases with age in both genders, with higher rates among women at all ages. Repeat fracture rates increase more steeply and are similar between men and women. Women age 80 or older have an 80% increased risk for a repeat fracture (RR 1.80; 95% CI 1.45–2.25). Men age 80 or older have a 2.77-fold increased risk for a repeat fracture (RR 2.77; 95% CI 1.69–4.54). (Adapted from Center JR et al. *[35]*.)

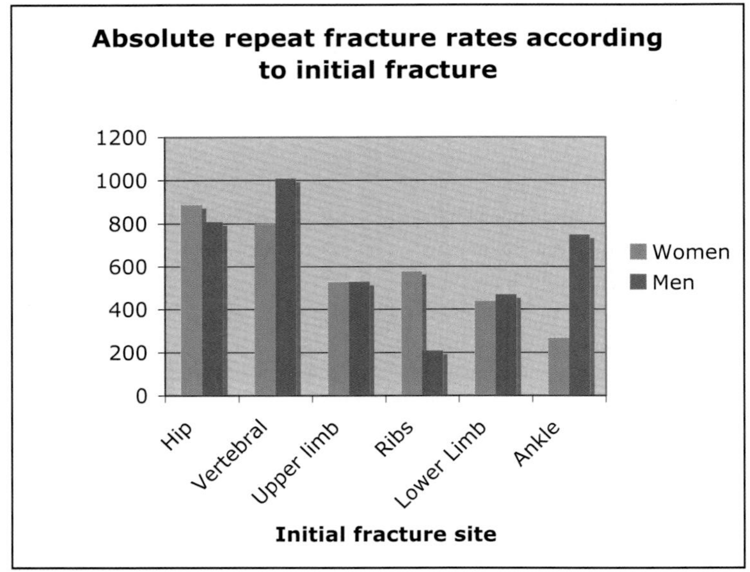

FIGURE 8.9. **Absolute repeat fracture rates by initial fracture site and gender.** Hip fractures among women and vertebral fractures among men age 60 years and older carry the highest gender-specific absolute risk for a repeat fracture. (Adapted from Center JR et al. *[35]*.)

Summary

Fractures among older individuals are frequent, contribute significantly to morbidity and mortality, and are closely linked to falls. Among all fractures, hip fractures result in the greatest personal and societal burden, and are the most frequent fractures among individuals age 75 and older. Future projections indicate a world-wide increase of hip fractures, which is in part explained by prolonged life expectancy and the absolute increase of the oldest segment of the population in many countries.

A significant part of age-related fracture morbidity is explained by the high risk of a repeat fracture, which rises steeply with age, and is similar in men and women despite lower incident fracture rates among men. Thus, fractures among older individuals are an indicator of frailty, which is also reflected by markedly higher hip fracture rates among nursing homes residents if compared to the general older population.

Furthermore, fractures among older individuals vary by season; with a marked winter peak for distal forearm, proximal humerus, and ankle fractures. The winter peak for hip fractures is relatively small, which may be explained by strikingly different associations with weather. For example, regional snowfall and summer sunshine are inversely related to hip fracture risk, but associated with higher rates of the other fractures.

References

1. Nguyen ND, Ahlborg HG, Center JR, Eisman JA, Nguyen TV. Residual Lifetime Risk of Fractures in Women and Men. J Bone Miner Res 2007;12:12.
2. Magaziner J, Hawkes W, Hebel JR, et al. Recovery from hip fracture in eight areas of function. J Gerontol A Biol Sci Med Sci 2000;55(9):M498–M507.
3. Tinetti ME, Williams CS. Falls, injuries due to falls, and the risk of admission to a nursing home. N Engl J Med 1997;337(18):1279–1284.
4. Cummings SR, Kelsey JL, Nevitt MC, O'Dowd KJ. Epidemiology of osteoporosis and osteoporotic fractures. Epidemiol Rev 1985;7:178–208.
5. Birge SJ, Morrow-Howell N, Proctor EK. Hip fracture. Clin Geriatr Med 1994;10(4):589–609.
6. Cummings SR, Rubin SM, Black D. The future of hip fractures in the United States. Numbers, costs, and potential effects of postmenopausal estrogen. Clin Orthop 1990;(252):163–166.

7. Cummings SR, Nevitt MC, Browner WS, et al. Risk factors for hip fracture in white women. Study of Osteoporotic Fractures Research Group. N Engl J Med 1995;332(12):767–773.
8. Fatalities and injuries from falls among older adults—United States, 1993–2003 and 2001–2005. MMWR Morb Mortal Wkly Rep 2006;55(45):1221–1224.
9. Tinetti ME. Risk factors for falls among elderly persons living in the community. N Engl J Med 1988;319:1701–1707.
10. Tinetti ME, Williams CS. The effect of falls and fall injuries on functioning in community-dwelling older persons. J Gerontol A Biol Sci Med Sci 1998;53(2):M112–M119.
11. Englander F, Hodson TJ, Terregrossa RA. Economic dimensions of slip and fall injuries. J Forensic Sci 1996;41(5):733–746.
12. Cummings SR, Nevitt MC. Non-skeletal determinants of fractures: the potential importance of the mechanics of falls. Study of Osteoporotic Fractures Research Group. Osteoporos Int 1994;4 Suppl 1:67–70.
13. Nguyen ND, Frost SA, Center JR, Eisman JA, Nguyen TV. Development of a nomogram for individualizing hip fracture risk in men and women. Osteoporos Int 2007;17:17.
14. Nevitt MC, Cummings SR. Type of fall and risk of hip and wrist fractures: the study of osteoporotic fractures. The Study of Osteoporotic Fractures Research Group. J Am Geriatr Soc 1993;41(11): 1226–1234.
15. Lewis CE, Ewing SK, Taylor BC, et al. Predictors of non-spine fracture in elderly men: the MrOS study. J Bone Miner Res 2007;22(2):211–219.
16. Nevitt MC, Cummings SR. Type of fall and risk of hip and wrist fractures: the study of osteoporotic fractures. The Study of Osteoporotic Fractures Research Group. J Am Geriatr Soc 1993;41(11): 1226–1234.
17. Stone KL, Ewing SK, Lui LY, et al. Self-reported sleep and nap habits and risk of falls and fractures in older women: the study of osteoporotic fractures. J Am Geriatr Soc 2006;54(8):1177–1183.
18. Nevitt MC, Cummings SR. Type of fall and risk of hip and wrist fractures: the study of osteoporotic fractures. J Am Geriatr Soc 1994;42(8):909.
19. Carter SE, Campbell EM, Sanson-Fisher RW, Gillespie WJ. Accidents in older people living at home: a community-based study assessing prevalence, type, location and injuries. Aust N Z J Public Health 2000;24(6):633–636.
20. Campbell AJ, Borrie MJ, Spears GF, Jackson SL, Brown JS, Fitzgerald JL. Circumstances and consequences of falls experienced by a community population 70 years and over during a prospective study. Age Ageing 1990;19(2):136–141.
21. O'Neill TW, Marsden D, Adams JE, Silman AJ. Risk factors, falls, and fracture of the distal forearm in Manchester, UK. J Epidemiol Community Health 1996;50(3):288–292.
22. Graafmans WC, Ooms ME, Bezemer PD, Bouter LM, Lips P. Different risk profiles for hip fractures and distal forearm fractures: a prospective study. Osteoporos Int 1996;6(6):427–431.
23. Keegan TH, Kelsey JL, King AC, Quesenberry CP Jr, Sidney S. Characteristics of fallers who fracture at the foot, distal forearm, proximal humerus, pelvis, and shaft of the tibia/fibula compared with fallers who do not fracture. Am J Epidemiol 2004;159(2):192–203.
24. Vellas BJ, Wayne SJ, Romero LJ, Baumgartner RN, Garry PJ. Fear of falling and restriction of mobility in elderly fallers. Age Ageing 1997;26(3):189–193.
25. Arfken CL, Lach HW, Birge SJ, et al. The prevalence and correlates of fear of falling in elderly persons living in the community. Am J Public Health 1994;84(4):565–570.
26. Cummings SR, Nevitt MC, Kidd S. Forgetting falls. The limited accuracy of recall of falls in the elderly. J Am Geriatr Soc 1988;36(7):613–616.
27. Barrett JA, Baron JA, Karagas MR, Beach ML. Fracture risk in the U.S. Medicare population. J Clin Epidemiol 1999;52(3):243–249.
28. Cooper C, Melton LJ III. Epidemiology of osteoporosis. Trends Endokrin Metab 1992;314:224–229.
29. Gullberg B, Johnell O, Kanis JA. World-wide projections for hip fracture. Osteoporos Int 1997;7(5): 407–413.
30. Kanis JA, Johnell O, De Laet C, Jonsson B, Oden A, Ogelsby AK. International variations in hip fracture probabilities: implications for risk assessment. J Bone Miner Res 2002;17(7):1237–1244.
31. Amin S, Zhang Y, Felson DT, et al. Estradiol, testosterone, and the risk for hip fractures in elderly men from the Framingham Study. Am J Med 2006;119(5):426–433.
32. Nevitt MC, Ettinger B, Black DM, et al. The association of radiographically detected vertebral fractures with back pain and function: a prospective study. Ann Intern Med 1998;128(10):793–800.
33. Silverman SL, Minshall ME, Shen W, Harper KD, Xie S. The relationship of health-related quality of life to prevalent and incident vertebral fractures in postmenopausal women with osteoporosis: results from the Multiple Outcomes of Raloxifene Evaluation Study. Arthritis Rheum 2001;44(11):2611–2619.

34. Lindsay R, Silverman SL, Cooper C, et al. Risk of new vertebral fracture in the year following a fracture. JAMA 2001;285(3):320–323.
35. Center JR, Bliuc D, Nguyen TV, Eisman JA. Risk of subsequent fracture after low-trauma fracture in men and women. JAMA 2007;297(4):387–394.
36. Hasserius R, Karlsson MK, Jonsson B, Redlund-Johnell I, Johnell O. Long-term morbidity and mortality after a clinically diagnosed vertebral fracture in the elderly—a 12- and 22-year follow-up of 257 patients. Calcif Tissue Int 2005;76(4):235–242.
37. Nevitt MC, Cummings SR, Stone KL, et al. Risk factors for a first-incident radiographic vertebral fracture in women > or = 65 years of age: the study of osteoporotic fractures. J Bone Miner Res 2005;20(1):131–140.
38. Praemer A, Furner S, Rice DP. Musculoskeletal conditions in the United States. Rosemont: American Academy of Orthopedic Surgeons, 1992, pp. 145–170.
39. O'Neill TW, Felsenberg D, Varlow J, Cooper C, Kanis JA, Silman AJ. The prevalence of vertebral deformity in european men and women: the European Vertebral Osteoporosis Study. J Bone Miner Res 1996;11(7):1010–1018.
40. Melton LJ III, Lane AW, Cooper C, Eastell R, O'Fallon WM, Riggs BL. Prevalence and incidence of vertebral deformities. Osteoporos Int 1993;3(3): 113–119.
41. Douglas AS, Allan TM, Rawles JM. Composition of seasonality of disease. Scott Med J 1991;36(3): 76–82.
42. Wilkinson P, Pattenden S, Armstrong B, et al. Vulnerability to winter mortality in elderly people in Britain: population based study. BMJ 2004;17:17.
43. Wilkinson P, Pattenden S, Armstrong B, et al. Vulnerability to winter mortality in elderly people in Britain: population based study. BMJ 2004; 329(7467):647.
44. Lieberman D, Friger MD. Seasonal variation in hospital admissions for community-acquired pneumonia: a 5-year study. J Infect 1999;39(2):134–140.
45. Vilkman S, Keistinen T, Tuuponen T, Kivela SL. Seasonal variation in hospital admissions for chronic obstructive pulmonary disease in Finland. Arctic Med Res 1996;55(4):182–186.
46. Spencer FA, Goldberg RJ, Becker RC, Gore JM. Seasonal distribution of acute myocardial infarction in the second National Registry of Myocardial Infarction. J Am Coll Cardiol 1998;31(6):1226–1233.
47. Jacobsen SJ, Sargent DJ, Atkinson EJ, O'Fallon WM, Melton LJ III. Population-based study of the contribution of weather to hip fracture seasonality. Am J Epidemiol 1995;141(1):79–83.
48. Bulajic-Kopjar M. Seasonal variations in incidence of fractures among elderly people. Inj Prev 2000; 6(1):16–19.
49. Hemenway D, Colditz GA. The effect of climate on fractures and deaths due to falls among white women. Accid Anal Prev 1990;22(1):59–65.
50. Jacobsen SJ, Goldberg J, Miles TP, Brody JA, Stiers W, Rimm AA. Seasonal variation in the incidence of hip fracture among white persons aged 65 years and older in the United States, 1984–1987. Am J Epidemiol 1991;133(10):996–1004.
51. Lau EM, Gillespie BG, Valenti L, O'Connell D. The seasonality of hip fracture and its relationship with weather conditions in New South Wales. Aust J Public Health 1995;19(1):76–80.
52. Mannius S, Mellstrom D, Oden A, Rundgren A, Zetterberg C. Incidence of hip fracture in western Sweden 1974–1982. Comparison of rural and urban populations. Acta Orthop Scand 1987;58(1): 38–42.
53. Zetterberg C, Andersson GB. Fractures of the proximal end of the femur in Goteborg, Sweden, 1940–1979. Acta Orthop Scand 1982;53(3):419–426.
54. Jacobsen SJ, Sargent DJ, Atkinson EJ, O'Fallon WM, Melton LJ III. Contribution of weather to the seasonality of distal forearm fractures: a population-based study in Rochester, Minnesota. Osteoporos Int 1999;9(3):254–259.
55. Ralis ZA. Epidemic of fractures during period of snow and ice. Br Med J (Clin Res Ed) 1981; 282(6264):603–605.
56. Bischoff-Ferrari HA, Orav JE, Barrett JA, Baron JA. Effect of seasonality and weather on fracture risk in individuals 65 years and older. Osteoporos Int 2007;24:24.
57. Holick MF. The photobiology of vitamin D and its consequences for humans. Ann N Y Acad Sci 1985;453:1–13.
58. Harris SS, Dawson-Hughes B. Seasonal changes in plasma 25-hydroxyvitamin D concentrations of young American black and white women. Am J Clin Nutr 1998;67(6):1232–1236.
59. Bischoff-Ferrari HA, Dawson-Hughes B, Willett CW, et al. Effect of vitamin D on falls: a meta-analysis. JAMA 2004;291(16):1999–2006.
60. Dawson-Hughes B, Harris SS, Krall EA, Dallal GE. Effect of calcium and vitamin D supplementation on bone density in men and women 65 years of age or older. N Engl J Med 1997;337(10):670–676.
61. Bischoff-Ferrari HA, Zhang Y, Kiel DP, Felson DT. Positive association between serum 25-hydroxyvitamin D level and bone density in osteoarthritis. Arthritis Rheum 2005;53(6):821–826.

62. Trivedi DP, Doll R, Khaw KT. Effect of four monthly oral vitamin D3 (cholecalciferol) supplementation on fractures and mortality in men and women living in the community: randomised double blind controlled trial. BMJ 2003;326(7387):469.
63. Chapuy MC, Arlot ME, Duboeuf F, et al. Vitamin D3 and calcium to prevent hip fractures in the elderly women. N Engl J Med 1992;327(23):1637–1642.
64. Bischoff-Ferrari HA, Willett WC, Wong JB, Giovannucci E, Dietrich T, Dawson-Hughes B. Fracture prevention with vitamin D supplementation: a meta-analysis of randomized controlled trials. JAMA 2005;293(18):2257–2264.
65. Johnell O, Borgstrom F, Jonsson B, Kanis J. Latitude, socioeconomic prosperity, mobile phones and hip fracture risk. Osteoporos Int 2007;18(3): 333–337.
66. Karagas MR, Baron JA, Barrett JA, Jacobsen SJ. Patterns of fracture among the United States elderly: geographic and fluoride effects. Ann Epidemiol 1996;6(3):209–216.
67. Myers AH, Robinson EG, Van Natta ML, Michelson JD, Collins K, Baker SP. Hip fractures among the elderly: factors associated with in-hospital mortality. Am J Epidemiol 1991;134(10):1128–1137.
68. Wehren LE, Hawkes WG, Orwig DL, Hebel JR, Zimmerman SI, Magaziner J. Gender differences in mortality after hip fracture: the role of infection. J Bone Miner Res 2003;18(12):2231–2237.
69. Lyons AR. Clinical outcomes and treatment of hip fractures. Am J Med 1997;103(2A):51S–63S; discussion 63S–64S.
70. Browner WS, Pressman AR, Nevitt MC, Cummings SR. Mortality following fractures in older women. The study of osteoporotic fractures. Arch Intern Med 1996;156(14):1521–1525.
71. Looker AC, Harris TB, Madans JH, Sempos CT. Dietary calcium and hip fracture risk: the NHANES I Epidemiologic Follow-Up Study. Osteoporos Int 1993;3(4):177–184.
72. Samelson EJ, Zhang Y, Kiel DP, Hannan MT, Felson DT. Effect of birth cohort on risk of hip fracture: age-specific incidence rates in the Framingham Study. Am J Public Health 2002;92(5): 858–862.
73. Chang KP, Center JR, Nguyen TV, Eisman JA. Incidence of hip and other osteoporotic fractures in elderly men and women: Dubbo Osteoporosis Epidemiology Study. J Bone Miner Res 2004;19(4): 532–536.
74. Cummings SR, Black DM, Thompson DE, et al. Effect of alendronate on risk of fracture in women with low bone density but without vertebral fractures: results from the Fracture Intervention Trial. JAMA 1998;280(24):2077–2082.
75. Black DM, Boonen S, Cauley J, Delmas PD, Eastell R, Reid IR. Effects of once-yearly infusion of zolendronic acid 5 mg on spine and hip fracture reduction in postmenopausal women with osteoporosis: The HORIZON Pivotal Fracture Trial. JBMR 2006;21 Suppl 1;Abstract 1054(September 2006):S16.
76. McClung MR, Geusens P, Miller PD, et al. Effect of risedronate on the risk of hip fracture in elderly women. Hip Intervention Program Study Group. N Engl J Med 2001;344(5):333–340.
77. Lips P, Graafmans WC, Ooms ME, Bezemer PD, Bouter LM. Vitamin D supplementation and fracture incidence in elderly persons. A randomized, placebo-controlled clinical trial. Ann Intern Med 1996;124(4):400–406.
78. Chapuy MC, Pamphile R, Paris E, et al. Combined calcium and vitamin D3 supplementation in elderly women: confirmation of reversal of secondary hyperparathyroidism and hip fracture risk: the Decalyos II study. Osteoporos Int 2002;13(3): 257–264.

9
Falls as a Geriatric Syndrome: How to Prevent Them? How to Treat Them?

Manuel Montero-Odasso

"It takes a child 1 year to acquire independent movement and 10 years to acquire independent mobility. An old person can lose both in a day."

Bernard Isaacs *(1)*

Introduction

This quotation from the late Bernard Isaacs still portrays, four decades after being written, the crude consequence that an older adult may experience after a single fall *(1)*. Despite the enormous efforts of researchers and clinicians to understand the falls syndrome, there is still a significant gap between the knowledge gained about this challenging syndrome and the clinical application of the proven interventions available. The aim of this chapter is to reduce this gap and to provide a rationale for the integration of a risk assessment for falls and fractures into research on the emerging problem of senile osteoporosis in older population.

Falls and fall-induced injuries in older people are worldwide problems with substantial clinical and public health implications. They are both associated with advancing age and an increased risk of disability, dependency, premature nursing home admission, and mortality *(2)*. First described almost 40 years ago as the geriatric syndrome "Instability," falls have become increasingly important in recent years *(3)*. A fall is defined as "an unintentional change in position resulting in coming to rest at a lower level or on the ground" *(4)*. Loss of consciousness owing to seizures or acute stroke are not included in the fall definition, although they can also present as an episode of instability and a change of position to a lower level *(5,6)*. Although falls can have multiple and diverse etiologies, they generally share similar risk factors, as they frequently result from the accumulated effect of impairments in multiple systems. Therefore, an intelligent approach to address such a complex problem must first take into consideration the most likely causes, contributing factors, and associated comorbidities. Because falls and fractures in older adults have an entangled relationship, a characterization of the risk factors for fractures caused by falls must be also considered in this joint approach.

Historical Perspectives: Falls as a Geriatric Syndrome

Falls, as a geriatric syndrome, have always been with us. They have been described for millennia as natural accidents that occur with old people. For instance, the ancient Egyptians represented older persons in their hieroglyphs as a man bend over and using a cane, indicating an understanding of an older individual's tendency to experience falls. This begs the question: if falls have been a known problem in the elderly for so long, why the increased interest in the topic today? One possible reason might relate to the number of scientific discoveries and social improvements that have been made in recent decades. Advances in medicine, nutrition, and better social and working conditions have caused the proportion of elderly people in the population to increase

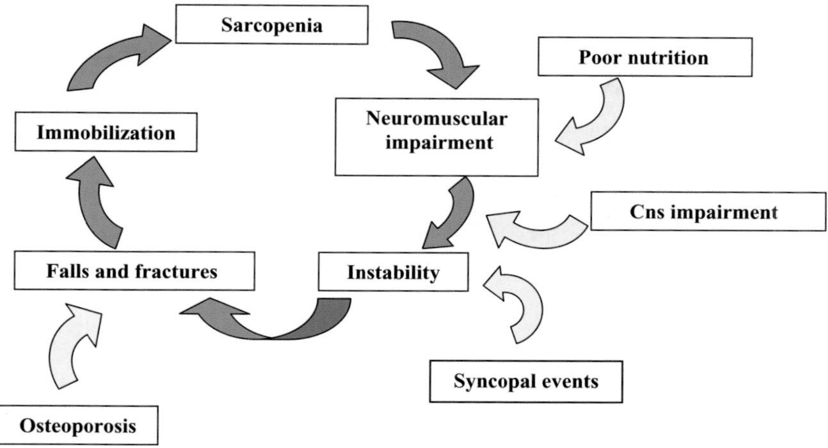

FIGURE 9.1. Vicious cycle in falls and fractures and principal contributors.

dramatically, a pattern that is seen in most of the Western world. This increased longevity, has also been accompanied by increasing levels of disability including an increased incidence of falls and fractures, which are now being studied and are frequently appearing in the medical literature. In the beginning, the primary focus of falls research was on the mechanical consequences of the fall, namely physical injury and fractures, both of which were assumed to be an expected result of the normal aging process. However, to consider falls as an inevitable or even normal phenomenon associated with aging has significantly delayed the creation of a systematic approach to this syndrome. As a result, the initial approach was based exclusively on treating the consequences of falls, which generated a kind of therapeutic nihilism to the syndrome itself. With the creation of geriatrics as a distinct medical specialty, this view has changed and falls have started to be considered as a syndrome with concomitant risk factors and etiologies. Falls and fractures are major components of the geriatric giants of "Instability" and "Immobility" *(1)*, and both are principal components in the vicious circle involving fall and fracture in older adults. As shown in Figure 9.1, once immobilization owing to falls or muscle weakness starts, it exacerbates the neuromuscular impairment leading to deconditioning, increasing muscle weakness and potentially sarcopenia, and increasing the risk of future falls and fractures.

Cohort and retrospective observational studies conducted during the early 1980s described the epidemiology, consequences, and underlying factors responsible for the falls syndrome *(3,4, 6–10)*. Clinical trials conducted in the late 1980s demonstrated that interventions based on multi-factorial and multi-disciplinary approaches may prevent falls and their associated consequences *(3,11–15)*. Despite the myriad of successful clinical trials in preventing falls, however, important gaps still exist in the current clinical knowledge of the area. This gap is even more evident when we look at the applicability of falls prevention and fractures treatment to everyday clinical scenarios.

Epidemiology of Falls

The incidence and severity of the falls consequences rises steadily entering the sixth decade and tends to be higher among persons age 80 years old and over. The high incidence of falls in this population is not the actual problem, because other populations such as children and professional athletes have an even higher frequency of falls. Rather, the problem for the elderly is the increased morbidity associated with falls. Because of the number of co-morbidities associated with the aging process, in particular osteoporosis and the loss of the adaptive and defensive mechanisms related to falling, older people are much more susceptible to sustain serious injury after even a minor fall. Accidents are generally ranked as the

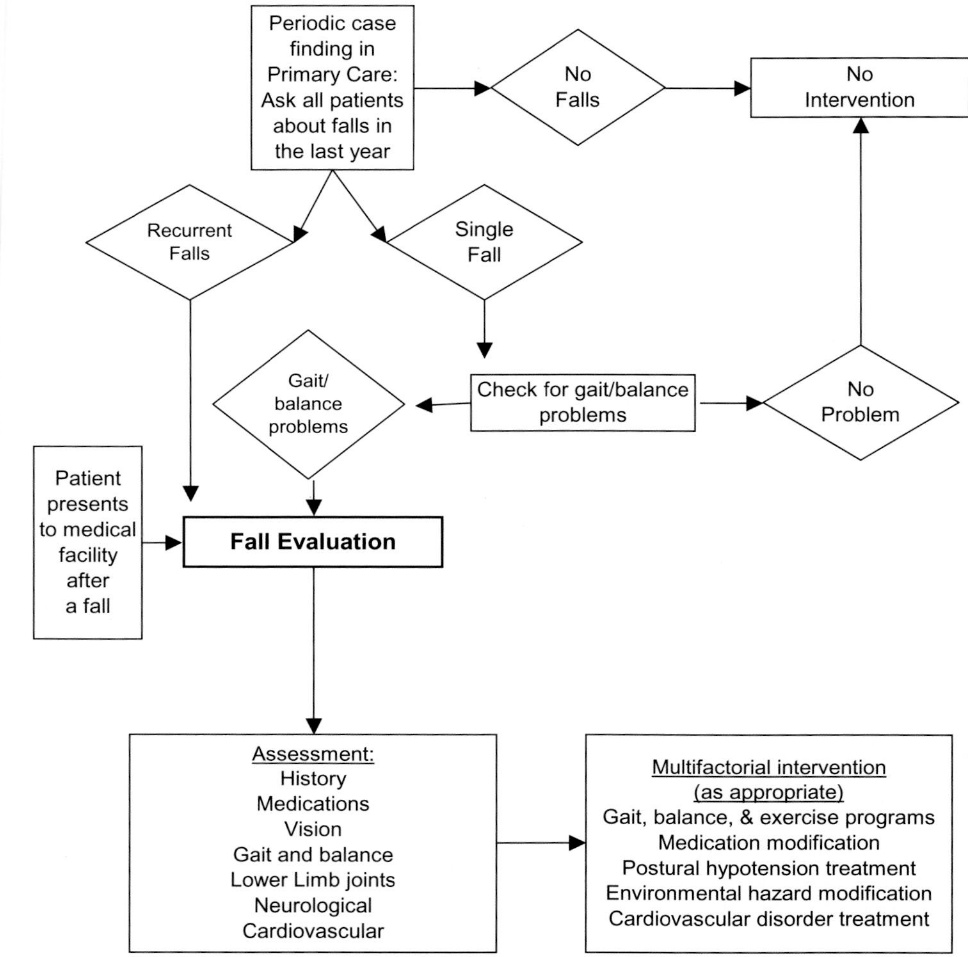

FIGURE 9.2. American Geriatrics Society, British Geriatrics Society, and American Academy of Orthopaedic Surgeons approach to falls *(2)*. (Guideline for the prevention of falls in older persons. American Geriatrics Society, British Geriatrics Society, and American Academy of Orthopaedic Surgeons Panel on Falls Prevention[16]. Used with permission of Blackwell Publishers.)

fourth or fifth leading cause of death in the developed world (after cardiovascular disorders, cancer, stroke, and pulmonary diseases), with falls being the leading cause of accidental death in older adults, accounting for two-thirds of these deaths *(16)* (Figure 9.2).

The prevalence and incidence of falls vary according the population and setting being analyzed. Clinical trials conducted by Tinetti and colleagues have reported that the incidence of falls in community-dwelling older people is approximately 30% per year for those aged 65 and older, and between 40–50% for those aged 80 and older *(14)*. Among individuals who have a history of falls in the previous year, the annual incidence is closer to 60%. In older hospitalized patients the prevalence of falls rises to 40%, whereas older adults living in long-term care facilities have a prevalence of falls ranging from 45–50% *(16–18)*. As was stated earlier, falls constitute the largest single cause of injury-related mortality in elderly individuals; moreover, falls are an independent determinant of functional decline, leading to 40% of all nursing home admissions. This increased prevalence in institutional settings may be caused by a variety of factors including the intrinsic characteristics of the residents with the majority being frail, and the more accurate reporting of falls which generally occurs in these settings *(17)*.

Complications of Falling

Falls can have a number of serious medical, physiological, and social consequences, which are sometimes underreported or underestimated in the literature (*see* Table 9.1).

Morbidity and Mortality

Complications and consequences resulting from falls are the leading cause of death from injury in men and women aged 65 and older. One rule of thumb used to describe the frequency of various outcomes of sustaining an unexpected fall by older adults: 20% of the individuals develop "fear of falling;" 15% sustain sufficient injury that they frequently visit the Emergency Department because of the pain, bruises, or dizziness; 10% sustain a severe injury but not a fracture (e.g., head injury, brain hematomas, or chest trauma); and 5% sustain a fracture with 1% of these being a hip fracture *(17,19)*. These percentages can be more than doubled for women aged 75 and older *(20)*.

It has long been understood that the way a person falls can determine the type of injury that follows. For example, wrist fractures often result from forward falls onto a hand, hip fractures typically happen from falls on the side, and falling backwards tends to have the lowest rate of fracture. Older adults between the ages of 65 and 75 tend to have more wrist fractures, whereas those over age 75 suffer more hip fractures. Several hypotheses have been postulated in an attempt to explain this apparent shift from wrist to hip fractures, with one of the most accepted being that the shift is a result of a slowing of defensive reflexes in individuals over 75 years of age *(21)*.

Table 9.1. Frequent Consequences of the Fall Syndrome in Older People

Cause	Consequence
Medical	Hematoma
	Fracture
	Chronic pain
	Death
Psychological	Fear of falling
	Anxiety
	Loss of confidence
	Depression
Social	Dependency
	Isolation
	Placement in long-term care
Functional	Immobility
	Deconditioning
	Disability and dependence

Psychological and Social Consequences

No less important, and in some cases even more frequent, are the social and psychological consequences of the falls and how they may impact on functional domains. Fear of falling has been described as a serious problem, with prevalence rates ranging from 25 to 55% of community-dwelling elderly *(17,22–24)*. Fear of falling can strongly influence an elderly individual's quality of life as it can lead to isolation and poor satisfaction with life. Moreover, fear of falling itself has been shown to be a predictor of actual falling. The consensus is that individuals develop a fear of falling and depression secondary to recurrent falls. Fear of experiencing another fall (known as "post-fall anxiety") may trigger something of a downward spiral for the individual in terms of their social and psychological life. It can lead the individual to restrict their social activities, possibly owing to a decrease in confidence about their abilities. This in turn can gradually lead to isolation, feelings of loneliness, hopelessness, and potentially even depression. What makes this pattern particularly unfortunate is that the social isolation stage may be the easiest point at which to intervene; however, it is frequently not reported or identified, which leads to much needless suffering for the individual.

Causes of Falling and Risk Factors

Although it may be possible to determine the precipitating factor for a given fall, the actual underlying causes tend to be varied and complex. Multiple risk factors have been identified as contributors to the fall syndrome and accordingly, the list is highly heterogeneous, including such factors as age-associated changes, sensory impairments, muscular weakness, co-morbidities, cardiovascular-mediated problems, polypharmacy, and environmental hazards, among others *(8,25,26)*. The most accepted classification of falls is based on whether risk factors are related to an extrinsic hazard or owing to an intrinsic disorder *(16,27)*. Extrinsic falls are usually related to environmental hazards that cause the individual to slip, trip, or sustain an externally induced displacement, whereas intrinsic falls are generally related to mobility or balance disorders, muscle weakness, orthopedic problems, sensory impairment, or a neurally-mediated cardiovascular disorder such as postural hypotension or post-prandial hypotension *(28)*. However, for almost 80% of fallers, this classification is of limited clinical applicability, as their falls were caused by a combination of intrinsic and extrinsic factors *(29)*.

Through studies conducted by Tinetti and her colleagues, it is now known that the risk of falling increases consistently as the number of risk factors increases. Although modifying only one of these risk factors may reduce incidence of falls, the risk reduction is likely to be greater when multiple risk factors are modified *(15)*. From a clinical point of view, it is more efficient to select interventions that simultaneously address several risk factors; this chapter proposes an aggregation of risk factors into four categories related to potential interventions. These categories are the following: neuromuscular problems, medical problems, cardiovascular problems, and environmental problems. Table 9.2 lists these domains as well as their proposed risk factors, assessment measures and tests, and some potential interventions appropriate for each giving disorder. One important precipitator of falls is medication, which is included under medical problems. Although there

TABLE 9.2. Cause of Falls According to Risk Factor Identification and Grouped Regarding Potential Interventions

Domain assessed	Risk factor/disease:	Assessment	Potential intervention
Neuromuscular	Parkinsonism syndrome Balance and gait problems Lower extremity weakness	Gait velocity test Get Up and Go POMA	1—Supervised home-based exercise programs (structural gait retraining, balance, and lower transfer interventions, limb strengthening and flexibility exercises) 2—Provision of appropriate walking aids 3—Vitamin D and calcium supplementation
Medical	Dizziness or vertigo Visual impairment Peripheral neuropathy Hip problems or deformity Cognitive problems or depression	History and examination, including review of drugs, visual acuity assessment, echocardiograph, short Geriatric Depression Scale	1—Appropriate investigation and management of untreated medical problems 2—Review and modification of psychotropic drugs, other culprit drugs, and polypharmacy 3—Optical correction by an optician or referral to an ophthalmologist 4—Formal psychogeriatric assessment
Environmental	Environmental fall hazards	Occupational therapy: assessment of environmental fall hazards using a standard checklist	1—Home hazard modification using standard protocol
Cardiovascular	Orthostatic hypotension Post-prandial hypotension Vasovagal syndrome Carotid sinus hypersensitivity	Measurement of morning orthostatic blood pressure, carotid sinus massage supine and tilted upright, prolonged head-up tilt	1—Advice on avoiding precipitants and modification of drugs 2—Postural hypotension: compression socks, fludrocortisone, or midodrine 3—Cardioinhibitory carotid sinus hypersensitivity: permanent pacemaker 4—Symptomatic vasodepressor carotid sinus hypersensitivity or vasovagal syncope: fludrocortisone or midodrine

POMA, performed oriented mobility assessment; MMSE, mini-mental status exam; GDS, gereatric depression exam.

are inherent difficulties in studying the role of medication as a risk factor for falls, there already exists strong evidence that both the type and class of medication, in particular psychotropics, sedatives, and vasodilators, and the sheer number of medications taken can be an important cause of falls in older adults *(22,30–32)*.

Classification of Falls: The Value of the Gait Assessment

Falls can be classified in a number of diverse ways, including by their number (single fall versus multiple falls); whether or not an injury was sustained (injurious falls versus non-injurious falls); and what risk factors may have been involved (intrinsic versus extrinsic factors). The traditional classification, based on the presence of intrinsic and extrinsic factors, has been validated and is accepted worldwide *(27)*; however, to attribute a fall to an extrinsic factor can be difficult as the majority of environmentally related falls result from an interaction with the intrinsic factors of that individual. Although the intrinsic-extrinsic categorization was originally intended to separate and identify multiple contributors to the fall, older people who experience an extrinsic fall often have an underlying intrinsic condition that decreases their ability to compensate for the hazardous situation. In other words, there may be an intrinsic incapacity to avoid the external factors. As explained earlier, falls are often related to a complex interaction among these factors that can challenge postural control and the ability of the individual to maintain an upright position.

Problems in balance and gait performance are common in older people, having a profound impact on health and quality of life *(22,33–35)*. A number of the disorders associated with the aging process affect mobility and gait in older persons: loss of muscle mass (sarcopenia), decreased visual acuity, impairment in proprioception and nerve conduction, and loss of the defence reflexes, to list just a few. In addition to these age-related changes, many chronic diseases, including arthritis, neurological problems, and cardiac and respiratory conditions, have marked effects on gait and balance *(36,37)*. The more frequent factors which can affect gait performance in older persons include muscle weakness, chronic pain, reduced joint mobility, and impaired central nervous system (CNS) processing *(33)*.

Gait performance is a complex task that depends on the normal functioning of multiple systems working in a highly coordinated and integrated manner *(33,38)*. As impairments in different domains can alter this delicate system, it has been hypothesized that different chronic conditions such as visual or hearing problems, muscular weakness, osteoarthritis, or peripheral neuropathy could be evidenced through gait performance *(38)*. In addition, certain psychotropic medications such as benzodiazepines and neuroleptics, which have CNS action, may also affect gait performance. Because gait is affected by several different conditions, gait performance reflects different factors that can cause the fall syndrome. This fact may explain why gait problems *per se* are among the highest predictive risk factor for fall in older adults *(6,33,38,39)*. Rather than looking for a single, rare disease that causes gait problems in older people, such as myelopathy or normal pressure hydrocephalus, more prevalent causes should be sought. The identification of these major contributors will allow the formulating of an operational diagnosis for the individual's gait problem and, in turn, provide further information on which to base a therapeutic plan.

Clinical observation can detect the main gait problems in the majority of the older adults, so formal testing in a gait laboratory is not necessary for everyone. However, this kind of high-tech analysis might be useful in particular cases, or for developing specific rehabilitation strategies, and for research purposes. A focused and careful observation of the gait performance can detect subtle abnormalities, underlying impairments, and the pathologic process involved. Table 9.3 describes some of the common causes of falls and gait problems in older adults, and their relation to performance-based evaluation. Operationally, underlying impairments on gait can be grouped into three major hierarchical categories based on the sensorimotor level involved, as outlined in Table 9.4. Nutt and Alexander have proposed this classification of gait disorder in the elderly based on sensorimotor levels coining the term "lower-level gait disorders" to refer to an altered gait that is a

Table 9.3. Common Causes of Falls and Abnormal Mobility and Gait in Older Adults in Relation to Performance-Based Evaluation

Symptom	Potential cause
Difficulty rising from a chair	Weakness Osteoarthritis
Instability on first standing	Hypotension Weakness
Instability with eyes closed	Problems related to proprioception
Decreased step height/ length	Parkinsonism Frontal lobe disease Fear of falling

result of lower extremity problem or peripheral dysfunction *(33,40)*. This impairment can be attributed to joint and/or muscular problem as well as to a peripheral nervous disease. Lower extremity motor problems are prevalent in older adults and can lead to compensatory changes in gait as a result of chronic pain, joint and foot deformities, or focal muscle weakness. Using this approach, Hough and colleagues have found that at least 50% of ambulatory elderly seeking a consultation for gait impairment have joint or muscle problems in the lower limbs *(41)*. A systematic review of the literature found that lower limb muscle weakness is significantly associated with falls and subsequent disability in older adults *(42)*.

At the middle sensorimotor level, the problem is based on the modulation of sensory and motor control of gait without affecting the ignition of the walking problem. Typical examples are the gait problems caused by Parkinson's disease or those caused by spasticity secondary to hemiplegia. However, at the high sensorimotor level, gait characteristic become less specific while cognitive dysfunction, attentional problems, and fear of falling become more prominent features. In this category are "frontal gait" problems, "ignition gait" disturbances, and the "cautious gait" caused by fear of falling. Finally, combinations of these levels are frequently found as older adults may have deficits at more than one level.

Among those older adults who do have a gait disturbance, the cause may be easily identifiable (e.g., Parkinson's disease or previous stroke with hemiparesis); however, there are many older adults with an impaired gait for whom there does not appear to be a well-defined disease. Sudarsky and colleagues found that in patients attending a neurology clinic, the cause of the gait problem was frequently "unknown," even after neuroimaging, in approximately 10–20% of older adults with a disturbed gait *(35)*. In a study of the "oldest old," whose age ranged from 87–97 years, Bloem and colleagues observed that approximately 20% of those studied had a normal gait, 69% had a gait

Table 9.4. Common Cause of Gait Disorder in Older People According the Hierarchic Sensorimotor Level

Level	Deficit/Condition	Gait characteristic
Low	Peripheral sensory ataxia: posterior column, peripheral nerves, vestibular and visual ataxia	Unsteady, uncoordinated (especially without visual input)
	Peripheral motor deficit owing to hip problems	Avoids weight-bearing on affected side Painful knee flexed
	Arthritis (antalgic gait, joint deformity)	Painful spine produces short slow steps and decreased lumbar lordosis, kyphosis and ankylosing spondylosis produce stooped posture
	Peripheral motor deficit owing to myopathic and neuropathic conditions (weakness)	Proximal motor neuropathy produces waddling and foot slap; Distal motor neuropathy produces distal weakness
Middle	Spasticity from hemiplgia, hemiparsis	Leg swings outward and in a semi-circle from hip (circumduction)
	Spasticity from paraplegia, paresis	Circumduction of both legs; steps are short, shuffling, and scraping
	Parkinsonism	Small shuffling steps, hesitation, acceleration (festination), falling forward (propulsion)
	Cerebellar ataxia	Wide-based gait with increased trunk sway, irregular stepping
High	Cautious gait	Fear of falling with appropriate postural responses, normal to widened gait base, shortened stride, slower turning en bloc. Performance improve with assistance or evaluator walking on the side
	Ignition failure	Frontal gait disorder: difficulty initiating gait; short, shuffling gait, like Parkinsonian, but with a wider base, upright posture, and arm swing presence

Adapted with permission from Nutt, et al. *(40)* and Alexander *(33)*.

disorder caused by known disease, and approximately 11% of the subjects had an idiopathic "senile gait disorder," that is to say a gait disorder of unknown origin *(43)*. Interestingly, those subjects with a gait disorder of unknown origin had a higher risk of falls, fractures, hospitalizations and mortality after a 2–3 year follow up period, compared with age-matched subjects with a normal gait *(39,44)*.

An additional value of gait assessment is to help in ruling out cardiovascular contributors to falls. It has been postulated that falls secondary to neurally mediated cardiovascular causes may be expressed by a different mechanism, without necessarily chronically affecting gait performance *(39,45)*. Although the exact mechanism by which a neurally mediated cardiovascular problem causes a fall remains unclear, there is growing clinical evidence for its association with unexplained falls *(46)*. Therefore, the absence of gait problems in older adults with recurrent falls should be an indicator of cardiovascular cause of falls in those individuals *(47)*.

Falls and Fracture Risk Assessment: Who to Assess? How to Assess?

Falls are highly prevalent across the older population; consequently, screening strategies have been developed and a systematic approach has been recommended *(16)*.

The first approach should include taking a history of previous falls, because this is the most important predictor for future falls. For patients who present with a positive history of falls, a complete fall evaluation should include an assessment of balance and gait, vision acuity, and documentation of the individual's medication history. This triad is considered to have a high predictive value for detecting older adults at higher risk for falls in the community *(16)*.

Additionally, because 10 and 20% of falls are related to a hemodynamic episode such as postural hypotension and vasovagal symptoms, these entities should also be considered *(45)*. Information regarding the circumstances of the falls is necessary in order to detect if there is a "medical or environmental pattern" to the falls. For instance, falls after taking certain medications or in an specific place of the house may lead to the identification of drugs associated to falls (e.g., diuretics, vasodilators, and benzodiazepines) or environmental factors that may have contributed to the fall (e.g., a loose carpet, poor lighting, or a displaced piece of furniture).

However, particularly when there is a negative history of falls, gait and balance evaluation is considered to be the more important part of the assessment *(16,25,33,38,48)*. Gait can be assessed from either a quantitative or qualitative perspective. Several tests have been validated that assess gait performance in older adults; however, as is common with most tests, each has its own set of advantages and disadvantages. The majority of the tests in use today have evolved from a test described first by Mathis and Isaacs, namely the Get Up and Go Test *(49)*. Briefly, the Get Up and Go consists of rising from a chair, walking 3 m, turning around, walking back to the start point, and sitting down again. A later modification by Podsialo and Richardson incorporated a timed component to the performance measure of the test, thus providing extra information for analysis and clinical interpretation *(50)*. Because this test was initially created to evaluate frail elderly with disability, a problem faced when evaluating older persons in the community is a ceiling effect, because high-functioning older adults generally perform well on the task. Therefore, for these individuals a cut-off time of 12 seconds has been proposed in order to detect those vulnerable to suffer future falls *(51)*. More complex tests such as the Performed Oriented Mobility Assessment (POMA) test and the Berg Balance Scale has been described and validated for assessing risk of falling in different scenarios *(52–54)*.

A final, powerful test that can be used in different settings is the gait velocity test. It has been demonstrated to be very sensitive test for detecting mobility problems and to predict falls, even in high-functioning older people. Gait velocity is measured as the time taken to walk a known and predetermined distance (e.g., the middle 8 m of 10 m) and it is usually timed by a chronometer *(38)*, with the participants being instructed to "walk at a comfortable and secure pace." The only limitation of the gait velocity test appears when it is used in people using assistive devices. In this situation, changes in the functionality may show less effect on gait velocity *(55)*.

The proper gait and balance test needs to be selected regarding the population assessed. For instance, in long-term care facilities or when evaluating frail older adults with poor functionality, the Get Up and Go test may provide a good discrimination for detecting those at risk. For better-functioning older adults, such as older persons without disability, a more continuous measurement without ceiling effects, such as the gait velocity test may be more appropriate. Once a gait problem has been detected with a quantitative test, it can be categorized with clinical observation using a hierarchical classification (Table 9.4) or using an established quantitative protocol such as that of the POMA test.

In summary, the gait velocity test may serve as an initial step in the approach, and different cut-off points for detecting individuals at high risk of falls can be established according to the population evaluated. For example, it has been suggested to use a gait velocity cut off of 1 m/second in community elderly without disability, 0.8 m/second in older persons with disabilities, and 0.6 m/second in older persons living in nursing homes *(33,38,39)*.

A second step is based on the assessment of the risk of injuries caused by falls. Specifically, the identification of those at risk of falls in the first step should prompt the assessment of risk of fracture. The more important factors for fracture risk are the history of previous osteoporosis fracture, the use of psychotropic medication, and the presence of sarcopenia and impaired mobility *(56)*. This stepped approach is summarized in Figure 9.3. Once assessment is completed and risk categorization determined, appropriate and focused strategies and interventions can be instituted.

Medical Strategies to Reduce Risk of Falls and Fall-Related Injuries: Who to Treat and How to Treat Them?

Interventions to reduce the risk of falls and the subsequent injuries are essential. Two kinds of strategies have been used: single intervention

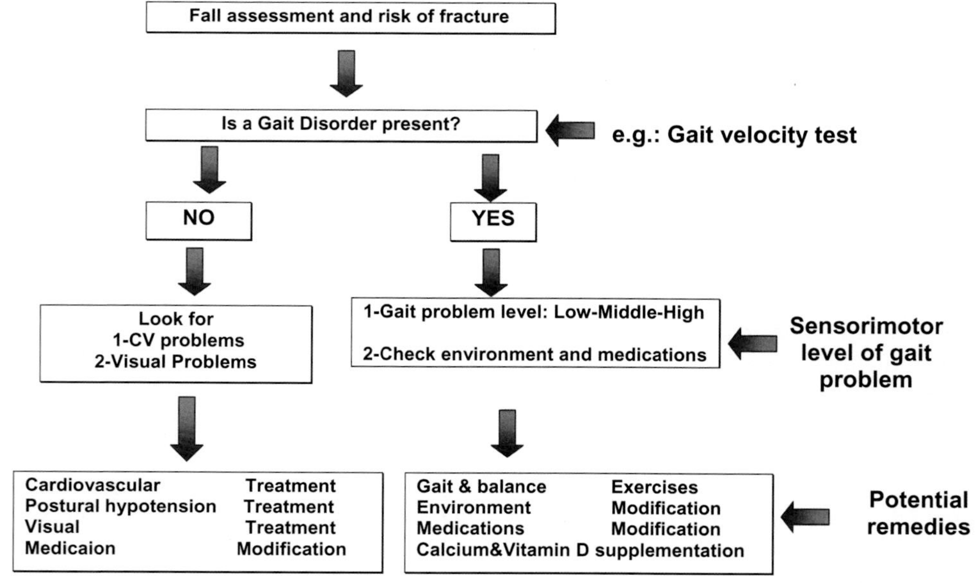

FIGURE 9.3. Proposed approach to analyze falls in person with unexplained falls. (Adapted with permission from Montero-Odasso M, et al. *[38]*.)

strategies and multiple intervention strategies. A recent systematic review demonstrated that multifactorial risk assessments and treatment are among the most effective interventions for reducing falls; however, a single intervention that acts on several levels can provide an effective treatment approach in specific cases *(20,57)*. Two single interventions, which can be included in this area are exercises programs and vitamin D supplementation. Exercise has been shown to have an important affect on muscle strength and balance and is currently the best single intervention available. A detailed description of existing strategies and the impact of this intervention are addressed in Chapter 10.

Vitamin D supplementation is a promising intervention in older persons with high risk of falls. Vitamin D is not merely a vitamin but also a pro-hormone and was, until recently, considered as one of the calciotropic hormones without a major significance to other metabolic processes. Several recent findings have demonstrated that vitamin D also plays a role as a factor for cell differentiation, function, and survival *(60)*. Bone and muscle have also been shown to be significantly affected by the presence or absence of vitamin D. In bone, vitamin D stimulates bone turnover while protecting osteoblasts from dying via apoptosis, whereas in muscle, vitamin D maintains the function of type II fibers, which helps to preserve muscle strength and prevent falls. Two major changes associated with aging, osteoporosis and sarcopenia, have been also linked to the development of frailty in elderly patients. In both cases vitamin D plays an important role, because the low levels of this vitamin seen in the elderly may be associated with a deficit in bone formation and muscle function.

Giving Vitamin D in Older Adults at High Risk of Falls: Does It Work?

Role of Vitamin D on Muscle and Neuromuscular Function

As stated earlier, gait and balance problems are principal contributors of falls in elderly people. Although several mechanisms are implicated in the balance control, muscular function is a main component of the balance system. Previously, the moderate protective effect of vitamin D on fracture risk has been attributed primarily to bone mineral density changes. However, vitamin D may also directly improve muscle strength, thereby reducing fracture risk through fall prevention. Two landmark randomized controlled trials have found that vitamin D reduced fractures within 8–12 weeks, a finding consistent with muscle strength benefits more than improvement in the bone density or bone strength, because treatment for a greater period of time is needed to achieve an improvement in bone mass *(24,56)*. The term osteomalacic myopathy describes the effect that the deficit in vitamin D has on muscular function and strength *(58)*. Clinical findings in osteomalacic myopathy include proximal muscle weakness, diffuse muscle pain, and gait impairments such as a waddling gait *(59)*. The fast and strong type II muscle fibers are the first to be recruited to avoid falling, and because of the fact that primarily these fibers are affected by vitamin D deficiency, it has been hypothesized that vitamin D deficiency may increase the risk of falls in elderly people. Indeed, the histopathological changes of vitamin D-deficit myopathy are quite similar to the changes seen in the age-related muscle loss *(60)*. This process, recently given the name sarcopenia, is attributed to the reduction of the numbers of both type I and type II fibers with marked type II fiber atrophy *(61)*. Although several physiological mechanisms have been implicated in the development of sarcopenia, the role of vitamin D metabolism is still not well understood *(62)*. The cellular effect on muscle after vitamin D supplementation was demonstrated in one study where treatment with vitamin D increased the relative number and size of type II muscle fibers of elderly women within 3 months of treatment *(62)*.

Few studies have been conducted that answer questions about the effects of vitamin D on balance and gait performance, and those few have generally looked for these improvements only in terms of secondary outcomes. Specifically, vitamin D plus calcium compared with calcium alone decreased body sway by 9% within 2 months of treatment in elderly ambulatory women. And similarly, vitamin D plus calcium compared with calcium alone increased musculoskeletal function by 4–11% in institutionalized elderly women *(63)*. Although there is evidence that vitamin D supplementation improves the muscle strength, mass, and function in older adults with a vitamin D deficiency; to extrapolate these findings to the general population is still premature because of the shortage of studies, and it is still an area for further clinical research.

The Fragility Fracture and Vitamin D

This concept is associated to those fractures that are not related to a significant trauma and are associated with a lack of bone strength *(64)*. The presence of fragility fracture in a patient is the strongest known risk factor of future fractures *(65,66)*. There are several studies that suggest that the lack of vitamin D action is an important pre-disposing factor for fragility fractures. In fact, bone strength is the consequence of a coordinated and well-regulated bone turnover with a certain level of coordination among bone cells. The absence of vitamin D will determine an initial reduction in bone turnover owing to the lack of activity followed afterward by a compensatory response induced by parathyroid hormone (PTH). Indeed, the typical feature of senile osteoporosis is a marked deficit in bone turnover, which could be explained by a reduction in the activity of vitamin D as one of the main factors *(67)*.

The Effect of Vitamin D Supplementation and Falls

During the last 10 years, several trials have included among their primary or secondary outcomes variables for addressing the question of whether supplementation with vitamin D improves muscle function and prevents mobility decline, falls, and fractures (Table 9.5). Pfeifer and colleagues compared the effect of 8 weeks of treatment with a daily dose of vitamin D (800 IU) and calcium (1200 mg) versus calcium 1200 mg alone in 148 healthy elderly women *(63)*. After a 1-year follow-up, they found a reduction in both the total number falls and the number of fallers. This study also demonstrated an improvement in balance as measured by body sway in the vitamin D group, suggesting that vitamin D may improve postural stability in people who received the combined treatment. Bischoff and colleagues studied 122 elderly women in a long-term geriatric facility and compared the rate of falls before and after the intervention. The subjects were randomized to either 1200 mg calcium and 800 IU vitamin D or 1200 mg calcium alone. Women treated with vitamin D plus calcium experienced a 49% relative reduction in falls when compared to the group that received calcium alone *(68)*. In both of these studies, the participants had an existing severe vitamin D deficiency. By contrast, study conducted in 445 healthy participants aged 65 years and older that had high serum levels of 25(OH)D did not find differences in the rate of falls after supplementation with vitamin D and calcium. The participants were randomized for taking a daily dose of 700 IU vitamin D and 500 mg calcium or placebo over 3 years. The main outcome evaluated in this particular study was the number of non-vertebral fractures, which was significantly lower in the treatment group, and falls were a secondary outcome *(36)*. Lips and colleagues investigated the effect of vitamin D on falls as a sub-study of a larger trial. This trial involved participants living in apartments for older people who were given 400 IU of vitamin D3 or placebo for an average of 2 years *(69)*. After prospective monitoring of falls over a 28-week period, no difference was found in the risk of falls between the intervention and control groups.

The Frailty Intervention Trial in Elderly Subjects investigated the effect of a single dose of 300,000 IU vitamin D2 supplementation or placebo on muscle strength, walking velocity, and new falls in 243 hospitalized frail older patients *(70)*. The outcomes were evaluated for a period of 6 months. Despite a significant increase in 25(OH)D levels in the treatment group, no differences were found between the vitamin D and control group across any of the outcomes.

The effect of vitamin D on the prevention of fractures shows variable results. A large

TABLE 9.5. Clinical Trials of Treatment With Vitamin D and Effect in Mobility, Falls, and Fractures

Trial/Design	Intervention	Participants	Muscle outcomes	Falls outcomes	Fractures outcomes
Pfeifer et al. *(63)*, 2000 RCT Double blind	800 IU/day and 1200 mg calcium for 8 weeks 1-year follow-up	$N = 148$. Healthy women Baseline levels: 25(OH)D: 10 μg/L	↓ sway in 2/3 measures on balance platform at 8 weeks.	Intervention group had ↓ number of falls (30 vs. 17) and ↓ number of people who fell (19 vs. 11)	Not evaluated
Bischoff et al. (68), 2001 RCT Double blind	800 IU/day and 1200 calcium for 12 weeks	$N = 122$. Older women in long-term stay geriatric institutions Baseline levels: Not reported	Improved muscle performance ($P = 0.0094$)	Intervention group had ↓ number of falls (250 vs. 55), 49% reduction in falls (95% CI 14–71%)	Not evaluated
Dawson-Hughes et al. *(36)*, 1997 RCT Double blind	700 IU/day and 500 mg calcium for 3 years	$N = 445$. Healthy, ambulatory men and women Baseline levels: 25(OH)D: Men = 33.0 ± 16 μg/L Women = 28.7 ± 13.3 μg/L	Not evaluated	No difference in percentage of people who fell, number of falls per person slightly higher in intervention group	Reduced non-vertebral fractures (26 vs. 11)
Graafmans et al. *(77)*, 1996 RCT Double blind	400 IU/day for mean 2 years; falls monitored for 28 weeks	$N = 354$. Men and women living residences Baseline levels: 25(OH)D: Median 10.8	Not evaluated	No difference between groups in the odds of having a fall, OR 1.0 (95% CI 0.6–1.5)	Not evaluated
Latham et al. *(70)*, 2002 RCT Double blind	300,000 IU/single dose	$N = 243$. Frail older people Baseline levels: 25(OH)D: Median 16 μg/L	Manual muscle strength; balance test and timed walk: no difference between groups	Falls over 6 months: no difference between groups	Not evaluated
Chapuy et al *(72)*, 2002 RCT Double blind	Vitamin D 800 IU/day and 1200 mg of calcium for 2 years	$N = 610$. Women residents of apartments for the elderly Baseline levels: 25(OH)D: 8.5 ± 5.3 μg/L	Not evaluated	No significant difference in falls (63.9% in active vs. 62.1% in placebo)	Relative risk of hip fracture in placebo group RR = 1.69 (95% CI 0.96–3.0)
Trivedi et al. *(73)*, 2003 RCT Double blind	100,000 IU/single dose every 4 month	$N = 2686$. Community elderly Baseline levels: not reported	Not evaluated	Not evaluated	Relative risk of hip fracture in placebo group RR = 1.69 (95% CI 0.96–3.0)

RCT, randomized controlled trial; 25(OH)D, 25 hydroxyvitamin D; IU, international units; RR, relative risk; CI, confidence interval.

study conducted by Chapuy and colleagues showed a reduction in fractures in women with a severe vitamin D deficit (serum 25OHD 14 ng/mL) after a supplementation with vitamin D *(71)*. The same author in a study conducted in older women in France found significant increases in 25(OH)D levels and a decreased risk of hip fracture, but no difference in the number of fallers between the experimental and control groups during 2 years of follow-up *(72)*. The study from Dawson-Hughes and colleagues, which failed to detect a reduction in the number and rate of falls, did show a significant reduction in non-vertebral fractures *(36)*. In addition, a recent study by Trivedi, involving 2686 subjects receiving 100,000 IU of vitamin D3 every 4 months, showed a reduced rate of fractures by 22% *(73)*.

Rationale of Giving Vitamin D

The variability of the results assessing the effect of vitamin D on fractures and falls prevention has led the researchers to postulate several different hypothesis. First, as both muscle and brain contain vitamin D receptors (VDR), it has been postulated that vitamin D3 (calcitriol) improves both muscle and CNS function, affecting balance (74). Second, a direct effect on muscle without a significant effect on bone has also been postulated. In a recent meta-analysis combining five randomized controlled trials, there was a 13% reduction in falls after treatment with vitamin D without documented changes on bone mass *(75)*. On the other hand, a systematic review of controlled trials undertaken to assess the effectiveness of vitamin D supplementation on muscle strength, physical function, and falls in older people did not find enough evidence to determine the roll of vitamin D in these issues *(76)*.

All of the studies that found a positive effect on the rate of falls have utilized a vitamin D supplementation regimen of at least 800 IU or equivalent per day and calcium. These findings provide a rationale to use this combined supplementation approach. Although the precise optimal dose of vitamin D has yet to be established, recent studies seem to indicate that dosages higher than the currently recommended 800 IU/day may be required in order to achieve neuromuscular improvement. It has been suggested by some that doses approaching 3000 IU/day may be necessary to achieve the neuromuscular outcomes described.

It has been recommended that serum 25(OH)D concentration be measured after vitamin D supplementation has begun so as to ensure a level higher than 50 nmol/L, and preferably between 50–80 nmol/L, is maintained in those with a high risk of falls and fractures, especially older individuals. Finally, it has been postulated that patients who experience falls may have a deficiency of vitamin D. For instance, studies evaluating patients who attended fall clinics have shown that hypovitaminosis D is very common, affecting roughly 72% of this population *(78)*. Since the benefits of vitamin D supplementation in older people are well recognized and without toxic effects, a pragmatic approach may be to supplement all older adults who are at risk of falls and fracture.

Conclusion

Falls and fractures represent an important and sometimes neglected feature in older adults. A systematic approach based on clinical assessment and performed-based measurements with a simple gait assessment can detect those at higher risk. During the evaluation of the risk of injuries, special attention should be paid to frail older adults with clinical signs of vitamin D deficiency. Interventional strategies based on multi-factorial or single interventions such as medication modification, resistance and balance exercises, as well as vitamin D supplementation may be implemented based on the deficits and impairments detected on evaluation.

An integrated treatment should emerge that involves a combination of medical, rehabilitative, environmental, and psychosocial interventions.

Acknowledgment. I am indebted to Kevin Hansen, MA, Research Associate at the Division of Geriatric Medicine at St. Joseph's Health Care—London, ON, Canada, for his assistance in the preparation of the manuscript.

References

1. Isaacs B. The Giants of Geriatrics. *The Challenge of Geriatric Medicine.* New York: Oxford University Press, 1992, pp. 1–7.
2. Rubenstein LZ, Robbins AS, Josephson KR, Schulman BL, Osterweil D. The value of assessing falls in an elderly population. A randomized clinical trial. Ann Intern Med 1990;113:308–316.
3. Tinetti ME. Where is the vision for fall prevention? J Am Geriatr Soc 2001;49:676–677.
4. Wild D, Nayak US, Isaacs B. Description, classification and prevention of falls in old people at home. Rheumatol Rehabil 1981;20:153–159.
5. King MB, Tinetti ME. A multifactorial approach to reducing injurious falls. Clin Geriatr Med 1996; 12:745–759.
6. Tinetti ME, Speechley M. Prevention of falls among the elderly. N Engl J Med 1989;320:1055–1059.
7. Campbell AJ, Spears GF, Borrie MJ, et al. Falls, elderly women and the cold. Gerontology 1988;34: 205–208.
8. Campbell AJ, Borrie MJ, Spears GF. Risk factors for falls in a community-based prospective study

of people 70 years and older. J Gerontol 1989;44: M112–M117.
9. Campbell AJ, Borrie MJ, Spears GF, et al. Circumstances and consequences of falls experienced by a community population 70 years and over during a prospective study. Age Ageing 1990;19:136–141.
10. Young SW, Abedzadeh CB, White MW. A fall-prevention program for nursing homes. Nurs Manage 1989;20:80Y–80AA, 80DD, 80FF.
11. Kerse N, Butler M, Robinson E, Todd M. Fall prevention in residential care: a cluster, randomized, controlled trial. J Am Geriatr Soc 2004;52:524–531.
12. Shaw FE, Bond J, Richardson DA, et al. Multifactorial intervention after a fall in older people with cognitive impairment and dementia presenting to the accident and emergency department: randomised controlled trial. BMJ 2003;326:73.
13. Theodos P. Fall prevention in frail elderly nursing home residents: a challenge to case management: part II. Lippincotts Case Manag 2004;9:32–44.
14. Tinetti ME, Baker DI, McAvay G, et al. A multifactorial intervention to reduce the risk of falling among elderly people living in the community. N Engl J Med 1994;331:821–827.
15. Tinetti ME, McAvay G, Claus E. Does multiple risk factor reduction explain the reduction in fall rate in the Yale FICSIT Trial? Frailty and Injuries Cooperative Studies of Intervention Techniques. Am J Epidemiol 1996;144:389–399.
16. Guideline for the prevention of falls in older persons. American Geriatrics Society, British Geriatrics Society, and American Academy of Orthopaedic Surgeons Panel on Falls Prevention. J Am Geriatr Soc 2001;49:664–672.
17. Rubenstein LZ, Josephson KR, Osterweil D. Falls and fall prevention in the nursing home. Clin Geriatr Med 1996;12:881–902.
18. Vu MQ, Weintraub N, Rubenstein LZ. Falls in the nursing home: are they preventable? J Am Med Dir Assoc 2004;5:401–406.
19. Tinetti ME. Clinical practice. Preventing falls in elderly persons. N Engl J Med 2003;348:42–49.
20. Kannus P, Sievanen H, Palvanen M et al. Prevention of falls and consequent injuries in elderly people. Lancet 2005;366:1885–1893.
21. Kannus P, Leiponen P, Parkkari J, et al. A sideways fall and hip fracture. Bone 2006;39:383–384.
22. Isaacs B. Clinical and laboratory studies of falls in old people. Prospects for prevention. Clin Geriatr Med 1985;1:513–524.
23. Lach HW. Incidence and risk factors for developing fear of falling in older adults. Public Health Nurs 2005;22:45–52.
24. Lach HW. Self-efficacy and fear of falling: in search of complete theory. J Am Geriatr Soc 2006;54: 381–382.
25. Bloem BR, Boers I, Cramer M, et al. Falls in the elderly. I. Identification of risk factors. Wien Klin Wochenschr 2001;113:352–362.
26. Tinetti ME, Doucette J, Claus E, et al. Risk factors for serious injury during falls by older persons in the community. J Am Geriatr Soc 1995;43:1214–1221.
27. Lach HW, Reed AT, Arfken CL, et al. Falls in the elderly: reliability of a classification system. J Am Geriatr Soc 1991;39:197–202.
28. Lach HW, Reed AT, Arfken CL, et al. Falls in the elderly: reliability of a classification system. J Am Geriatr Soc 1991;39:197–202.
29. Tinetti ME, Speechley M, Ginter SF. Risk factors for falls among elderly persons living in the community. N Engl J Med 1988;319:1701–1707.
30. Agostini JV, Tinetti ME. Drugs and falls: rethinking the approach to medication risk in older adults. J Am Geriatr Soc 2002;50:1744–1745.
31. Leipzig RM, Cumming RG, Tinetti ME. Drugs and falls in older people: a systematic review and meta-analysis: II. Cardiac and analgesic drugs. J Am Geriatr Soc 1999;47:40–50.
32. Leipzig RM, Cumming RG, Tinetti ME. Drugs and falls in older people: a systematic review and meta-analysis: I. Psychotropic drugs. J Am Geriatr Soc 1999;47:30–39.
33. Alexander NB. Gait disorders in older adults. J Am Geriatr Soc 1996;44:434–451.
34. Bloem BR, Gussekloo J, Lagaay AM, et al. Idiopathic senile gait disorders are signs of subclinical disease. J Am Geriatr Soc 2000;48:1098–1101.
35. Sudarsky L. Geriatrics: gait disorders in the elderly. N Engl J Med 1990;322:1441–1446.
36. Dawson-Hughes B, Harris SS, Krall EA, Dallal GE. Effect of calcium and vitamin D supplementation on bone density in men and women 65 years of age or older. N Engl J Med 1997;337:670–676.
37. Dhesi JK, Jackson SH, Bearne LM, et al. Vitamin D supplementation improves neuromuscular function in older people who fall. Age Ageing 2004;33: 589–595.
38. Montero-Odasso M, Schapira M, Varela C, et al. Gait velocity in senior people. An easy test for detecting mobility impairment in community elderly. J Nutr Health Aging 2004;8:340–343.
39. Montero-Odasso M, Schapira M, Soriano ER, et al. Gait velocity as a single predictor of adverse events in healthy seniors aged 75 years and older. J Gerontol A Biol Sci Med Sci 2005;60:1304–1309.

40. Nutt JG, Marsden CD, Thompson PD. Human walking and higher-level gait disorders, particularly in the elderly. Neurology 1993;43:268–279.
41. Hough JC, McHenry MP, Kammer LM. Gait disorders in the elderly. Am Fam Physician 1987;35: 191–196.
42. Moreland JD, Richardson JA, Goldsmith CH, et al. Muscle weakness and falls in older adults: a systematic review and meta-analysis. J Am Geriatr Soc 2004;52:1121–1129.
43. Bloem BR, Gussekloo J, Lagaay AM, et al. Idiopathic senile gait disorders are signs of subclinical disease. J Am Geriatr Soc 2000;48:1098–1101.
44. Woo J, Ho SC, Yu AL. Walking speed and stride length predicts 36 months dependency, mortality, and institutionalization in Chinese aged 70 and older. J Am Geriatr Soc 1999;47:1257–1260.
45. Carey BJ, Potter JF. Cardiovascular causes of falls. Age Ageing 2001;30(Suppl 4):19–24.
46. Lipsitz LA. Orthostatic hypotension in the elderly. N Engl J Med 1989;321:952–957.
47. Montero-Odasso M, Schapira M, Duque G, et al. Gait disorders are associated with non-cardiovascular falls in elderly people: a preliminary study. BMC Geriatr 2005;5:15.
48. Perell KL, Nelson A, Goldman RL, et al. Fall risk assessment measures: an analytic review. J Gerontol A Biol Sci Med Sci 2001;56:M761–M766.
49. Mathias S, Nayak US, Isaacs B. Balance in elderly patients: the "get-up and go" test. Arch Phys Med Rehabil 1986;67:387–389.
50. Podsiadlo D, Richardson S. The timed "Up & Go": a test of basic functional mobility for frail elderly persons. J Am Geriatr Soc 1991;39:142–148.
51. Bischoff HA, Stahelin HB, Monsch AU, et al. Identifying a cut-off point for normal mobility: a comparison of the timed 'up and go' test in community-dwelling and institutionalised elderly women. Age Ageing 2003;32:315–320.
52. Berg K, Norman KE. Functional assessment of balance and gait. Clin Geriatr Med 1996;12:705–723.
53. Berg KO, Wood-Dauphinee SL, Williams JI, et al. Measuring balance in the elderly: validation of an instrument. Can J Public Health 1992;83(Suppl 2): S7–S11.
54. Tinetti ME. Performance-oriented assessment of mobility problems in elderly patients. J Am Geriatr Soc 1986;34:119–126.
55. Montero-Odasso M. The value of gait velocity test for high-functioning populations. J Am Geriatr Soc 2006;54(12):1949–1950.
56. Gass M, Dawson-Hughes B. Preventing osteoporosis-related fractures: an overview. Am J Med 2006;119:S3–S11.
57. Gillespie LD, Gillespie WJ, Robertson MC, et al. Interventions for preventing falls in elderly people. Cochrane Database Syst Rev 2003;CD000340.
58. Yoshikawa S, Nakamura T, Tanabe H, et al. Osteomalacic myopathy. Endocrinol Jpn 1979;26:65–72.
59. Schott GD, Wills MR. Muscle weakness in osteomalacia. Lancet 1976;1:626–629.
60. Montero-Odasso M, Duque G. Vitamin D in the aging musculoskeletal system: an authentic strength preserving hormone. Mol Aspects Med 2005;26:203–219.
61. Vandervoort AA. Aging of the human neuromuscular system. Muscle Nerve 2002;25:17–25.
62. Sorensen OH, Lund B, Saltin B, et al. Myopathy in bone loss of ageing: improvement by treatment with 1 alpha-hydroxycholecalciferol and calcium. Clin Sci (Lond) 1979;56:157–161.
63. Pfeifer M, Begerow B, Minne HW, et al. Effects of a short-term vitamin D and calcium supplementation on body sway and secondary hyperparathyroidism in elderly women. J Bone Miner Res 2000; 15:1113–1118.
64. Johansen A, Harding K, Evans R, et al. Trauma in elderly people: what proportion of fractures are a consequence of bone fragility? Arch Gerontol Geriatr 1999;29:215–221.
65. Ross PD, Davis JW, Epstein RS, et al. Pre-existing fractures and bone mass predict vertebral fracture incidence in women. Ann Intern Med 1991;114: 919–923.
66. Wasnich RD, Davis JW, Ross PD. Spine fracture risk is predicted by non-spine fractures. Osteoporos Int 1994;4:1–5.
67. Chan GK, Duque G. Age-related bone loss: old bone, new facts. Gerontology 2002;48:62–71.
68. Bischoff HA, Stahelin HB, Dick W, et al. Effects of vitamin D and calcium supplementation on falls: a randomized controlled trial. J Bone Miner Res 2003;18:343–351.
69. Lips P, Graafmans WC, Ooms ME, et al. Vitamin D supplementation and fracture incidence in elderly persons. A randomized, placebo-controlled clinical trial. Ann Intern Med 1996;124:400–406.
70. Latham NK, Anderson CS, Lee A, et al. A randomized, controlled trial of quadriceps resistance exercise and vitamin D in frail older people: the Frailty Interventions Trial in Elderly Subjects (FITNESS). J Am Geriatr Soc 2003;51:291–299.
71. Chapuy MC, Arlot ME, Duboeuf F, et al. Vitamin D3 and calcium to prevent hip fractures in the elderly women. N Engl J Med 1992;327:1637–1642.
72. Chapuy MC, Pamphile R, Paris E, et al. Combined calcium and vitamin D3 supplementation in elderly women: confirmation of reversal of secondary

hyperparathyroidism and hip fracture risk: the Decalyos II study. Osteoporos Int 2002;13:257–264.
73. Trivedi DP, Doll R, Khaw KT. Effect of four monthly oral vitamin D3 (cholecalciferol) supplementation on fractures and mortality in men and women living in the community: randomised double blind controlled trial. BMJ 2003;326:469.
74. Gallagher JC. The effects of calcitriol on falls and fractures and physical performance tests. J Steroid Biochem Mol Biol 2004;89–90:497–501.
75. Bischoff-Ferrari HA, Dawson-Hughes B, Willett WC, et al. Effect of Vitamin D on falls: a meta-analysis. JAMA 2004;291:1999–2006.
76. Kenny AM, Biskup B, Robbins B, et al. Effects of vitamin D supplementation on strength, physical function, and health perception in older, community-dwelling men. J Am Geriatr Soc 2003;51:1762–1767.
77. Graafmans WC, Ooms ME, Hofstee HM, et al. Falls in the elderly: a prospective study of risk factors and risk profiles. Am J Epidemiol 1996;143:1129–1136.
78. Dhesi JK, Jackson SH, Bearne LM, et al. A rationale for vitamin D prescribing in a falls clinic population. Age Ageing 2002;31(4):267–271.

10
Non-Pharmacological Treatments for Falls and Fractures

Stephen R. Lord, Jacqueline C.T. Close, and Catherine Sherrington

There is now strong evidence to support interventions in the prevention of falls in older people. Strategies shown to successfully reduce falls in randomized controlled trials (RCT) include exercise, occupational therapy interventions incorporating education and home hazard modification, psychotropic medication withdrawal, expedited cataract extraction, cardiac pacing for carotid sinus hypersensitivity, and targeted multi-factorial interventions. Some trials in nursing homes have found that hip protectors, if worn, prevent hip fractures. However, poor compliance is a major issue limiting the effectiveness of this intervention. This chapter describes and discusses the non-pharmacological approaches to the prevention of falls and fall-related injuries in older people, and emphasizes the strategies shown to be effective in a range of population groups.

Exercise

Exercise is the most tried and tested approach to falls prevention, and has been shown to be successful as a single intervention strategy in community-dwelling populations. It is also effective in residential- and aged-care facilities when part of multi-factorial interventions. Exercise covers a wide range of physical tasks (e.g., balance, strength, flexibility) delivered in numerous formats. Though there are many health and social benefits from a range of exercise regimes, the evidence supports balance training as an effective intervention to impact significantly on falls rates.

Home-Based Exercise Programs

The *Otago Exercise Programme* is a regimen of home exercises using a combination of strength and balance exercises supplemented with a walking program. It is designed to be individually prescribed by a trained professional, undertaken 2–3 times per week, and progressed over time. This program has been evaluated in a series of RCTs. In the original study, among women aged over 80 years *(1)*, there was a significant reduction in falls over a 12-month period (between group difference = 0.47, 95% confidence interval [CI] 0.04–0.90). At the end of a second year (with 69% of intervention and 74% of control group continuing from the original study), the reduction in falls rates remained significant (relative risk [RR] 0.69, 95% CI 0.49–0.97 *[2]*).

Further evaluation of the *Otago Exercise Programme* was undertaken in an RCT with community-dwelling older people. But this time, the program was delivered by a community nurse (trained by a physiotherapist) *(3)*. In a controlled trial, it was also repeated in routine health care settings *(4)*. Again, falls were reduced with both these approaches (incident rate ratio [IRR] 0.54, 95% CI 0.32–0.90 and IRR 0.70, 95% CI 0.59–0.84, respectively). Subsequent meta-analysis and economic evaluation of the *Otago Exercise Programme* demonstrated that maximum benefits are achieved by targeting people aged 80 years and over, and those with a history of falls *(4)*. The meta-analysis also showed that fall-related injuries were reduced by 35% (IRR 0.65, 95% CI 0.53–0.81).

The role of strength training in falls prevention is less clear. In a well-designed and executed RCT of older people recently discharged from hospital *(5)*, seated quadriceps strengthening exercises failed to reduce falls rates and was associated with a significant risk of musculoskeletal injury (RR 3.6, 95% CI 1.5–8.0).

Group Exercise Programs

Several studies have investigated the effectiveness of a group exercise approach to falls reduction. This is an important concept, as many older people enjoy the socialization and opportunity to leave the home that a group exercise program offers. Group exercises may be individualized and tailored to the needs of the older person or involve all participants undertaking the same exercises and at the same intensity. Not all programs are progressed over time, which may limit the benefits of exercise. A range of exercise programs has been trialed in a number of settings, and have targeted populations ranging from the fit/healthy end to the frailer end of the spectrum.

Several studies have found that group exercise programs that combine balance, strength, and functional components can prevent falls *(6–12)*. Most have been individually tailored and progressive. Many include supplementary home exercises. For example, Skelton et al. *(6)* used exercises based on the Otago program, and reduced falls when compared to an attention control group (IRR 0.69, 95% CI 0.50–0.96). Similarly, Barnett et al. found that group-based balance and strength exercises significantly reduced falls in community-dwelling people (IRR 0.60, 95% CI 0.36–0.99) *(7)*. A cluster randomized trial targeting residents of retirement villages and hostels tested a 12-month group exercise program designed to address falls risk factors and improve physical functioning *(8)*. This intervention resulted in a 22% reduction in falls in the intervention group (IRR 0.78, 95% CI 0.62–0.99).

Tai Chi programs have also been effective in preventing falls. The first study in this area by Wolf et al. *(11)*, found that Tai Chi was successful in increasing the time to first fall (unadjusted RR 0.63, 95% CI 0.45–0.89). A similar study in a population that had not been involved in strenuous activity in the previous 3 months *(12)* also showed reduced fall rates after adjustments for co-variates (RR 0.46, 95% CI 0.26–0.8).

Wolf et al. also used a cluster-randomized trial of congregate living facilities to target more impaired older adults with a 48-week Tai Chi program *(13)*. With this selected population, there was no significant reduction in falls, but a trend towards improvement (RR 0.75, 95% CI 0.52–1.08). It seems that this population were unable to adequately perform the exercises to obtain the same level of benefit gained by the younger, fitter subjects in the other trials.

There have also been a number of trials that have failed to show benefits of exercise in preventing falls *(14–19)*. Comparisons with successful trials suggest that this may be owing to low adherence to interventions, exercises being insufficiently challenging to balance, and a failure to progress exercise over time.

Visual Interventions

As visual loss is often correctable in older people *(20–22)*, simple intervention strategies such as regular eye examinations, use of correct prescription glasses, cataract surgery, and the removal of tripping hazards in the home and public places have the potential to prevent falls in older people. Bi- and multi-focal glasses have been identified as a risk factor for falls in community-dwelling older people *(23)*, which indicates that the use of single lens distance glasses instead of bi- or multi-focal glasses in higher-risk situations such as negotiating stairs, walking outside the home, and using public transport may also reduce the risk of falling.

Three RCTs have evaluated the efficacy of discrete visual interventions in preventing falls *(9,24,25)*. The first involved 1090 subjects aged 70 years and over, and used a factorial design to assess the independent effects of interventions aimed at vision improvement, home hazard reduction, and group exercise *(9)*. The visual improvement intervention comprised a referral to the participant's usual eye-care provider if the participant had impaired vision (poor visual acuity, decreased stereopsis, and/or reduced field of vision) and he or she was not already receiving treatment for this problem. The eye-care provider was also given the screening assessment results. Those randomized to the visual intervention had an estimated reduction of 4.4% in the annual falls rate (rate ratio for time to first fall = 0.89, 95% CI 0.75–1.04), a difference that did not reach statistical significance.

Two related trials have examined the effects of expedited cataract surgery in reducing fall rates. The first study involving 306 women aged 70 years and over *(24)* examined the efficacy of cataract surgery on the first eye. Subjects were randomized to either expedited (approximately 4 weeks) or routine (12-month wait) surgery. Vision, visual disability, physical activity levels, anxiety, depression, and balance confidence improved significantly in the operated group at the 6-month retest. And over the 12 months of follow-up, the fall rate in the operated group was reduced by 34% compared with the controls (IRR 0.66, 95% CI 0.45–0.96). Although the number of cases was few—four subjects in the operated group (3%) and 12 (8%) in the control group—this trial also demonstrated that a falls-prevention intervention can be effective in reducing fractures ($p = 0.04$).

A follow-on study by the same group, aimed to determine if second eye cataract surgery leads to a further reduction in falls as well as measuring associated health gain *(25)*. 239 women over 70, who had been referred to a hospital ophthalmology department, with one unoperated cataract, were randomized to either expedited (approximately 4 weeks) or routine (12-month wait) surgery. Visual function (especially stereopsis), confidence, visual disability, and handicap all improved in the operated compared with the control group. Over 12 months of follow-up, the rate of falling was reduced by 32% in the operated group (IRR 0.68, 95% CI 0.39–1.19). This study planned for a larger sample size, where a 32% reduction would have reached statistical significance. Ironically, the success of the first trial prompted policy changes to expedite cataract surgery for all older people, effectively rendering recruitment of control subjects impossible.

Withdrawal of Psychoactive and Other Medications

Studies undertaken in both community and institutional settings have consistently found strong associations between falls and use of multiple medications *(26)* and centrally acting drugs (sedative/hypnotics, anti-depressants, and antipsychotics) *(27)*. Use of anti-inflammatory drugs, however, does not appear to be associated with increased risk of falls after controlling for the presence of arthritis *(28)*. Results of studies into use of anti-hypertensive medications have been contradictory, and a recent meta-analysis concluded that there was not sufficient evidence to consider the use of these drugs to be a risk factor for falls *(28)*.

Given the link between centrally acting medications and falls risk, one might reasonably expect that withdrawal of centrally acting medications would be of benefit. In a factorial RCT of gradual psychoactive medication withdrawal and home-based exercise, Campbell et al. *(29)* found a significant reduction in falls in the older community-dwelling people randomized to the medication withdrawal arms of the study. This is a very encouraging finding, as the risk of falling for those who completed the trial was reduced by 65% (relative hazard 0.34, 95% CI 0.16–0.74). However, there were considerable problems encountered in undertaking this study, which emphasizes how difficult it is for older people to stop using psychoactive medications. First, it proved very difficult to recruit subjects into the trial, with 400 of the 493 (81%) eligible subjects declining participation. Further, of the 48 subjects who agreed to participate and were randomized to the psychoactive withdrawal programs, only 17 (35%) completed the trial. Eight of the 17 subjects who successfully completed the trial also restarted taking psychoactive medications within 1 month of the completion of the study. Given the difficulties in undertaking this trial, it is clear that avoiding prescribing these drugs if clinically possible would be a preferred approach.

Psychosocial treatments are effective in the treatment of anxiety, depression, and sleep disturbances in older people, and as such provide alternatives or complementary approaches to the pharmacological management of these conditions. Simple behavioral and environmental interventions and the prescription of exercise also offer additional means of enhancing sleep quality in this group *(26)*.

Pacemaker Insertion for Treatment of Carotid Sinus Hypersensitivity (CSH)

Recent studies indicate that the cardio-inhibitory form of CSH, often cited as a cause of drop attacks and syncope, may be responsible for a significant proportion of the unexplained falls *(30)*. Prospective case-control studies have found that CSH (diagnosed by a 3-second period of asystole, a 50-mmHg drop in blood pressure, or both following carotid sinus massage) is present in one-third of patients admitted to hospital for falls *(31–33)*.

In response to this observation, Kenny et al. *(34)* conducted a RCT examining the benefits of detailed cardiovascular investigation of unexplained fallers presenting to an Emergency Department and insertion of a dual-chamber pacemaker for those shown to have the cardio-inhibitory form of CSH. Of 3384 subjects who had a history of "non-accidental" falls, 1624 (48%) agreed to, or were suitable for, carotid sinus massage, and of these, 283 (17%) were diagnosed with CSH. A total of 43 of these subjects declined further involvement in the study and 39 were on cardiovascular medications that could not be discontinued. In consequence, 175 subjects were randomized into the study. Over the period of the study, falls were reduced in the pacemaker group by two-thirds compared to the control group, and the paced group were significantly less likely to fall (odds ratio [OR] 0.42; 95% CI 0.23–0.75).

With such a substantial reduction in falls, the case is well made for appropriate cardiovascular assessment, including carotid sinus massage, for those people with recurrent unexplained falls and syncope. However, the applicability of these findings beyond this small population of fallers is questionable. The potential neurological complications should also not be overlooked and so informed consent is essential for this procedure *(35)*.

Reducing Hazards in the Home

Most homes contain potential hazards, and many older people attribute their falls to trips or slips inside the home or immediate home surroundings. However, the existence of home hazards alone is insufficient to cause falls. The interaction between an older person's physical abilities and their exposure to environmental stressors appears to be more important *(36)*.

Three studies have targeted interventions focused on at-risk groups. Cumming et al. *(37)* conducted a study among 530 community-dwellers, most of whom had been recently hospitalized. The intervention group received a home visit by an occupational therapist who assessed the home for environmental hazards and facilitated any necessary home modifications. There was no significant reduction in falls in the intervention group as a whole. There was however a significant reduction in the rate of falls among those who had fallen in the year prior to the study (RR 0.64, 95% CI 0.50–0.83). Falls in this group were significantly reduced both inside and outside of the home, suggesting that the home modifications alone may not have been the major factor in the reduction in falls rates. Other aspects of the occupational therapy intervention, which included advice on footwear and behavior, may have played an important role.

The Falls-HIT trial specifically addressed home modifications, and reported a significant reduction in falls *(38)*. This study involved 361 people with mobility limitations who had recently been discharged from hospital. The intervention consisted of home assessment and recommendations in addition to training in the use of mobility aids. At 1-year follow-up, the intervention group had 31% fewer falls than the control group (IRR 0.69, 95% CI 0.51–0.97), with sub-group analysis revealing that the intervention was particularly effective in those with a history of multiple falls (IRR 0.63, 95% CI 0.43–0.94).

The third RCT involved a factorial design in 391 community-dwelling people aged 75 years and over with visual acuity of 6/24 or worse 40 *(39)*. The participants received an occupational therapy (OT)-delivered home assessment and modification program ($n = 100$), an exercise program prescribed at home by a physiotherapist plus vitamin D supplementation ($n = 97$), both interventions ($n = 98$), or social visits ($n = 96$). Fewer falls occurred in the group randomized to the home safety program (IRR 0.59, 95% CI 0.42–0.83), where 90% complied partially or completely with one or more of the OT recommendations.

Reducing hazards in the home does not appear to be an effective falls prevention strategy in the general older population and those at low risk of falls *(36)*. However, home hazard reduction is effective if targeted to older people with a history of falls and vision and mobility limitations. The effectiveness of home safety interventions may depend on/be maximized by improved transfer abilities or other behavioral changes. Environmental assessment and modification by trained individuals also appears to contribute to the success of multi-faceted falls prevention programs in at-risk groups. Solutions to potential barriers to an individual's adoption of home modifications, such as education and financial assistance, need to be considered and addressed.

Multi-Factorial Interventions

Multi-factorial interventions involve identifying a range of risk factors associated with falls and interventions based on the identified risk profile. Multi-factorial interventions have been shown to be effective in a number of settings, and it is worth noting that in hospitals and residential aged care facilities, only multi-factorial interventions have been shown to be effective in preventing falls. This is perhaps a reflection of the frailty of these populations and the multiple risk factors present.

The first successful evaluation of a multi-factorial intervention program conducted by Tinetti et al. was published in 1994 and used targeted risk factors as a means of identifying an at-risk population and guiding intervention *(40)*. Interventions included: medication adjustment, behavioral change recommendations, education and training, and home exercise programs. During the 1-year follow-up period, 47% of the control group fell compared with only 35% of the intervention group ($p = 0.04$). The adjusted incidence ratio for falling in the intervention group as compared with the control group was 0.69 (95% CI 0.52–0.90).

A large randomized trial of a multi-factorial falls prevention program undertaken by Wagner et al. *(41)* showed some benefits of targeted intervention strategies. This study involved 1559 members of a Health Maintenance Organization (HMO). One group received a home-based assessment conducted by a nurse and follow-up interventions (targeting inadequate exercise, alcohol use, medication use, and hearing and visual impairments). A second group received a general health promotion nurse visit, and the third group received usual care. The intervention group experienced significantly fewer falls than the usual care group over the first year of follow-up. However, differences between the nurse assessment with follow-up intervention group and the general health promotion nurse visit group were not significant. Benefits were not well maintained in the second year of follow-up, with no difference in falling rates between the groups at this time. This suggests the need for ongoing monitoring of and intervention for falls risk factors.

Several falls prevention programs have used group education sessions. In a randomized trial involving 3182 independently living HMO members aged 65 and over, Hornbrook et al. *(42)* found that a home assessment and advice on modifications followed by a group education, exercise, and discussion program reduced falls by 11%. However, Reinsch et al. *(43)* found that a general non-targeted education program involving classes on exercise, relaxation, and health and safety topics was not effective in preventing falls among community-dwellers attending senior citizens centers.

There is some evidence of the efficacy of home-based health and disability screening for older people. Although these programs have broader aims than reducing falls, they can involve the identification of risk factors for falling. Carpenter et al. *(44)* conducted a randomized trial involving 539 people aged 75 and over. The intervention group were visited and assessed by volunteers at regular intervals. Participants who developed increasing disability were referred to their family doctor for interventions as required. The number of falls reported by the control group doubled between the first and last interview, but remained the same for the intervention group. However, another study *(45)* found only a trend to a decreased falls rate following one screening visit by a physician's assistant or nurse then two follow-up visits by trained volunteers. Potential problems identified by the screening tool were addressed with referral and/or advice. A letter outlining findings and recommendations followed the screening visit.

Patients presenting to the Emergency Department represent an easily identifiable high-risk population. A study by Close et al. *(46)* looked specifically at older people presenting to the Emergency Department with a fall. The authors found that a medical and occupational therapy assessment and subsequent tailored intervention resulted in a significant decrease in fall rates over a 1-year period. A substantial reduction in the risk of falling (OR 0.39, 95% CI 0.23–0.66) and the risk of recurrent falls (OR 0.33, 95% CI 0.16–0.68) was reported. The intervention also had a significant impact on functional ability when compared to usual care. Similar results have been reported by Davison et al., again highlighting the benefits of a multi-faceted approach to intervention in the Emergency Department setting *(47)*.

Preventing Falls in Hospital Patients

Two RCTs have evaluated the effects of multi-faceted falls prevention programs in hospital settings. Haines et al. *(48)* developed a targeted, multi-factorial intervention falls prevention program and evaluated this in an RCT among 626 patients of three sub-acute wards in Melbourne, Australia. Interventions included a falls risk alert card with information brochure, an exercise program, an education program, and hip protectors. Participants in the intervention group experienced 30% fewer falls than participants in the control group. This difference was significant (P = 0.045), but not until after 45 days of observation. The results, though positive, have limited value when extrapolating to acute and other sub-acute settings where length of stay is considerably less.

Encouraging findings regarding the effectiveness of interventions for preventing falls in hospitals have also been reported by Healy et al. *(49)*, who conducted a cluster RCT in matched pairs of eight aged care wards and associated community units of a district general hospital in northern England. The intervention involved a care plan for patients identified at risk of falling, with targeted interventions addressing visual impairment, medication use, low or high blood pressure, abnormal urine test results, immobility, and poor footwear. The intervention also considered a bedrail risk/benefit assessment, bed height, simple environmental modifications, and patients' position in the ward. Compared with baseline fall rates, falls were significantly reduced only in the intervention wards, with a significant between-group difference (RR 0.71, 95% CI 0.55–0.90).

More work is required with respect to preventing falls in hospitals. Research has concentrated on aged care and rehabilitation wards, yet older people are cared for in many different wards in a hospital. So a failure to address the issue at a hospital level will reduce the potential benefits of introducing a hospital-wide approach to falls prevention.

Preventing Falls in Nursing Home Residents

There have been several RCTs investigating falls prevention programs in residential aged care facilities. Three RCTs have found that multi-faceted programs can decrease falls. Jensen et al. *(50)* conducted a cluster RCT among 439 residents of nine residential care facilities in Sweden. An 11-week multi-disciplinary program of general and resident-specific tailored strategies was found to significantly reduce falls during a 34-week follow-up period (adjusted IRR 0.60, 95% CI 0.50–0.73). This program involved educating staff, modifying the environment, implementing exercise programs, supplying and repairing aids, reviewing drug regimens, providing hip protectors, having post-fall problem-solving conferences, and guiding staff. A sub-group analysis of this study showed that only people with a Mini-Mental State Examination Score of greater than 18 benefited from the intervention, thus leaving open the question as to the value of intervention in those with cognitive impairment and dementia.

Becker et al. *(51)* conducted a cluster RCT among 981 long-stay residents of six nursing homes and found a lower incidence density ratio of falls in the intervention group compared with the control group over a 12-month period (RR 0.55, 95% CI 0.41–0.73). A total of 52% of the control group were fallers compared with 37% of the intervention group (RR 0.75, 95% CI 0.57–0.98). The intervention involved staff training and feedback, information provision and education for residents, environmental adaptations, exercise (balance exercises and progressive resistance training with ankle weights and dumbbells), and hip protectors. Interestingly, intervention effects were not apparent before 6 months, and the authors suggested that it may have taken this long for improvement in the mediating variables (physical performance, staff adherence, and environmental adaptations) to take effect.

In an earlier cluster RCT of multi-faceted programs in residential aged care, Ray et al. *(52)* studied 482 residents who had previously fallen. Seven pairs of nursing homes were randomized to receive either no intervention or a program that involved structured individual assessment (of environmental safety, wheelchair use, psychotropic drug use, and transfers and ambulation) by medical, nursing, and OT professionals. At posttest there was a mean reduction of 19% in the proportion of recurrent fallers in the intervention homes. Greater effects were evident for homes with a higher compliance with recommendations, and for residents with three or more previous falls.

However, not all RCTs have found an improvement in the intervention arm. Kerse et al. *(53)* reported an increased fall rate following a trial that involved altering existing staff resources and implementing individualized fall-risk management for residents (IRR 1.34, 95% CI 1.06–1.72). This intervention was less intensive than the three other RCTs conducted in residential care settings and the authors suggested that by diverting staff resources, low-intensity interventions may be worse than usual care. In the only RCT of a comprehensive post-fall assessment by a nurse practitioner with physician referral, Rubenstein et al. *(54)* found that although this approach reduced hospitalizations and hospital stays, it did not significantly reduce the rate of falls.

Preventing Hip Fractures With Hip Protectors

The likelihood that a fall will result in a fracture can be reduced by changing the interaction between the person and the surface on which they fall. This can be undertaken by modifying the surface or by placing a barrier between the person and the hard surface. Hip protectors are designed to fulfil the latter role.

Hip protectors are designed to absorb energy and to transfer load from the bone to the surrounding soft tissues *(55)*. The original hip protectors *(56)* incorporated a firm outer shell and an inner foam section. Other versions are made of dense plastic without an outer shell *(57)*. Hip protectors either fit into pockets of underwear or are built into underwear. The earliest study of hard shell hip protectors was a RCT among 701 residents of a nursing home *(56)*. The risk of fracture was significantly decreased in the intervention group (RR 0.44). Although eight members of the intervention group suffered hip fractures, none were wearing the hip protectors at the time of fracture. A further study in Sweden *(58)* tested a different model of hip protector and also found a decreased fracture rate among residents of a randomly selected nursing home that was offered hip protectors compared with a control nursing home (RR 0.33).

Unfortunately subsequent research into the efficacy and practicality of hip protector use has been less encouraging. The Cochrane review on this topic *(59)* found that pooling of data from five individually randomiszd trials conducted in residential care settings (1426 participants) showed no statistically significant reduction in hip fracture incidence (RR 0.83, 95% CI 0.54–1.24), and that two individually randomized studies that recruited community-dwelling elderly people showed no indication of a reduction in the incidence of hip fractures (RR 1.11, 95% CI 0.65–1.90). Furthermore, a more recent cluster-randomized trial *(60)* among residents of 127 aged care facilities (4117 occupied beds) also showed a slight increase in fracture rates in the group assigned hip protectors (RR 1.05, 95% CI 0.77–1.43).

Given the current data, many geriatric specialists feel that when worn correctly, hip protectors may prevent hip fractures. The majority of fractures in intervention groups of hip protector studies occur while the hip protector is not being worn or is incorrectly positioned. A recent study compared protected and unprotected falls among high-risk nursing home residents and found hip fractures were reduced by more than one-third in protected falls compared with unprotected falls *(61)*. Thus, poor compliance appears to markedly limit hip protector effectiveness. For example, O'Halloran et al. *(60)* found initial acceptance of the hip protectors at only 37%, and adherence fell to only 20% at 72 weeks. Other studies have found that many potential participants decline involvement (e.g., 79% declined in Birks et al. *[62]*). Key reasons for poor compliance include: discomfort, the extra effort needed to wear the device, urinary incontinence, and physical difficulties/illnesses. In some settings, cost may also be a barrier to hip protector use *(63)*.

Hip protectors do not decrease the risk of other fractures such as pelvic fractures *(64)*, but have been found to improve falls self-efficacy *(65)*. Despite their limitations, hip protectors can be useful clinically as a hip fracture prevention strategy among those at high risk of falls who are willing and able to wear them.

Conclusions

There is now good evidence to support the effectiveness of falls prevention programs. By using assessments based on evidence-based risk factors amenable to correction, it is possible to intervene in those most likely to benefit from targeted intervention strategies. Balance training has been shown to be an effective single intervention in the prevention of falls. However, a multi-factorial approach is needed in higher-risk individuals, such as those in hospital or residential care and those presenting to the emergency department as a result of a fall.

Poor compliance has been highlighted as an issue limiting the effectiveness of hip protectors, and more evidence is needed on the acceptability of interventions shown to be effective but not as yet evaluated outside of the research setting. There is now preliminary evidence to support falls prevention as a means of fracture prevention. However, to have a meaningful impact on fracture rates, it is imperative that bone health and falls prevention are considered together. Comparative studies are also required to establish the clinical effectiveness and cost efficiency of the interventions on offer.

References

1. Campbell AJ, Robertson MC, Gardner MM, Norton RN, Tilyard MW, Buchner DM. Randomised controlled trial of a general practice programme of home based exercise to prevent falls in elderly women. BMJ 1997;315:1065–1069.
2. Campbell AJ, Robertson MC, Gardner MM, Norton RN, Buchner DM. Falls prevention over 2 years: a randomized controlled trial in women 80 years and older. Age Ageing 1999;28:513–518.
3. Robertson MC, Devlin N, Gardner MM, Campbell AJ. Effectiveness and economic evaluation of a nurse delivered home exercise programme to prevent falls. 1: Randomised controlled trial. BMJ 2001;322:697–701.
4. Robertson MC, Gardner MM, Devlin N, McGee R, Campbell AJ. Effectiveness and economic evaluation of a nurse delivered home exercise programme to prevent falls. 2: Controlled trial in multiple centres. BMJ 2001;322:701–704.
5. Latham NK, Anderson CS, Lee A, et al. A randomized, controlled trial of quadriceps resistance exercise and vitamin D in frail older people: the Frailty Interventions Trial in Elderly Subjects (FITNESS). J Am Geriatr Soc 2003;51:291–299.
6. Skelton D, Dinan S, Campbell M, Rutherford O. Tailored Group Exercise (FaME) reduces falls in community dwelling older frequent fallers (an RCT) (research letter). Age Ageing 2005;34(6): 636–639.
7. Barnett A, Smith B, Lord SR, Williams M, Baumand A. Community-based group exercise improves balance and reduces falls in at-risk older people:

a randomised controlled trial. Age Ageing 2003;32: 407–414.

8. Lord SR, Castell S, Corcoran J, et al. The effect of group exercise on physical functioning and falls in frail older people living in retirement villages: a randomized, controlled trial. J Am Geriatr Soc 2003;51:1685–1692.
9. Day L, Fildes B, Gordon I, Fitzharris M, Flamer H, Lord S. Randomised factorial trial of falls prevention among older people living in their own homes. BMJ 2002;325:128.
10. Buchner DM, Cress ME, de Lateur BJ, et al. The effect of strength and endurance training on gait, balance, fall risk, and health services use in community-living older adults. J Gerontol 1997;52: M218–M224.
11. Wolf SL, Barnhart HX, Kutner NG, McNeely E, Coogler C, Xu T. Reducing frailty and falls in older persons: an investigation of Tai Chi and computerized balance training. Atlanta FICSIT Group. Frailty and Injuries: Cooperative Studies of Intervention Techniques. J Am Geriatr Soc 1996;44:489–497.
12. Li F, Harmer P, Fisher KJ, et al. Tai Chi and fall reductions in older adults: a randomized controlled trial. J Gerontol 2005;60:M187–M194.
13. Wolf SL, Sattin RW, Kutner M, O'Grady M, Greenspan AI, Gregor RJ. Intense tai chi exercise training and fall occurrences in older, transitionally frail adults: a randomized, controlled trial. J Am Geriatr Soc 2003;51:1693–1701.
14. Bunout D, Barrera G, Avendano M, et al. Results of a community-based weight-bearing resistance training programme for healthy Chilean elderly subjects. Age Ageing 2005;34:80–83.
15. Carter ND, Khan KM, McKay HA, et al. Community-based exercise program reduces risk factors for falls in 65- to 75-year-old women with osteoporosis: randomized controlled trial. Can Med Assoc J 2002;167:997–1004.
16. Lord SR, Ward JA, Williams P, Strudwick M. The effect of a 12-month exercise trial on balance, strength, and falls in older women: a randomized controlled trial. J Am Geriatr Soc 1995;43: 1198–1206.
17. Morgan RO, Virnig BA, Duque M, Abdel-Moty E, Devito CA. Low-intensity exercise and reduction of the risk for falls among at-risk elders. J Gerontol 2004;59:M1062–M1067.
18. Reinsch S, MacRae P, Lachenbruch PA, Tobis JS. Attempts to prevent falls and injury: a prospective community study. Gerontologist 1992;32:450–456.
19. Steinberg M, Cartwright C, Peel N, Williams G. A sustainable programme to prevent falls and near falls in community dwelling older people: results of a randomised trial. J Epidemiol Community Health 2000;54:227–232.
20. Teilsch JM, Sommer A, Witt K, Katz J, Royall RM. Blindness and visual impairment in an American urban population: The Baltimore Eye Survey. Arch Ophthalmol 1990;108:286–290.
21. Attebo K, Ivers RQ, Mitchell P. Refractive errors in an older population: the Blue Mountains Eye Study. Ophthalmology 1999:106;1066–1072.
22. Jack CI, Smith T, Neoh C, Lye M, McGalliard JN. Prevalence of low vision in elderly patients admitted to an acute geriatric unit in Liverpool: elderly people who fall are more likely to have low vision. Gerontology 1995;41:280–285.
23. Lord SR, Dayhew J, Howland A. Multifocal glasses impair edge contrast sensitivity and depth perception and increase the risk of falls in older people. J Am Geriatr Soc 2002;50:1760–1766.
24. Harwood RH, Foss AJE, Osborn F, Gregson RM, Zaman A, Masud T. Falls and health status in elderly women following first eye cataract surgery: a randomised controlled trial. Br J Ophthalmol 2005;89;53–59.
25. Foss AJ, Harwood RH, Osborn F, Gregson RM, Zaman A, Masud T. Falls and health status in elderly women following second eye cataract surgery: a randomised controlled trial. Age Ageing 2006;35:66–71.
26. Lord SR, Sherrington C, Menz H, Close JCT. *Falls in older people: risk factors and strategies for prevention, second edition.* Cambridge, UK: Cambridge University Press, 2007.
27. Leipzig RM, Cumming RG, Tinetti ME. Drugs and falls in older people: a systematic review and meta-analysis. I. Psychotropic drugs. J Am Geriatr Soc 1999;47:30–39.
28. Leipzig RM, Cumming RG, Tinetti ME. Drugs and falls in older people: a systematic review and meta-analysis II. Cardiac and analgesic drugs. J Am Ger Soc 1999;47:40–50.
29. Campbell AJ, Robertson MC, Gardner MM, Norton RN, Buchner DM. Psychotropic medication withdrawal and a home based exercise programme to prevent falls: results of a randomised controlled trial. J Am Geriatr Soc 1999;47:850–853.
30. Ward C, McIntosh S, Kenny R. Carotid sinus hypersensitivity—a modifiable risk factor for fractured neck of femur. Age Ageing 1999;28: 127–133.
31. Davies AJ, Kenny RA. Falls presenting to the accident and emergency department: types of presentation and risk factor profile. Age Ageing 1996;25:362–366.

32. Richardson DA, Bexton RS, Shaw FE, Kenny RA. Prevalence of cardioinhibitory carotid sinus hypersensitivity in patients 50 years or over presenting to the accident and emergency department with "unexplained" or "recurrent" falls. Pacing Clin Electrophysiol 1997;20:820–823.
33. Davies A, Steen N, Kenny R. Carotid sinus hypersensitivity is common in older patients presenting to an accident and emergency department with unexplained falls. Age Ageing 2001;30:289–293.
34. Kenny R, Richardson D, Steen N, Bexton R, Shaw F, Bond J. Carotid sinus syndrome: a modifiable risk factor for nonaccidental falls in older adults (SAFE PACE). J Am College Cardiol 2001;38: 1491–1496.
35. Richardson D, Bexton R, Shaw F, Steen N, Bond J, Kenny R. Complications of carotid sinus massage—a prospective series of older patients. Age Ageing 2000;29:413–417.
36. Lord SR, Menz HB, Sherrington S. Home environment risk factors for falls in older people and the efficacy of home modifications. Age Ageing 2006; 35-S2:ii55–ii59.
37. Cumming RG, Thomas M, Szonyi G, et al. Home visits by an occupational therapist for assessment and modification of environmental hazards: a randomized trial of falls prevention. J Am Geriatr Soc 1999;47:1397–1402.
38. Nikolaus T, Bach M. Preventing falls in community-dwelling frail older people using a home intervention team (HIT): Results from the randomised falls-HIT trial. J Am Geriatr Soc 2003;51: 300–305.
39. Campbell AJ, Robertson MC, La Grow SJ, et al. Randomised controlled trial of prevention of falls in people aged > or =75 with severe visual impairment: the VIP trial. BMJ 2005;331:817–925.
40. Tinetti ME, Baker DI, McAvay G, et al. A multifactorial intervention to reduce the risk of falling among elderly people living in the community. New Engl J Med 1994;331:821–827.
41. Wagner EH, LaCroix AZ, Grothaus L, et al. Preventing disability and falls in older adults: a population-based randomized trial. Am J Public Health 1994;84: 1800–1806.
42. Hornbrook MC, Stevens VJ, Wingfield DJ, Hollis JF, Greenlick MR, Ory MG. Preventing falls among community-dwelling older persons: results from a randomized trial. Gerontologist 1994;34:16–23.
43. Reinsch S, MacRae P, Lachenbruch PA, Tobis JS. Attempts to prevent falls and injury: a prospective community study. Gerontologist 1992;32:450–456.
44. Carpenter G, Demopoulos G. Screening the elderly in the community: controlled trial of dependency surveillance using a questionnaire administered by volunteers. BMJ 1990;300:253–256.
45. Fabacher D, Josephson K, Pietruszka F, Linderborn K, Morley J, Rubenstein L. An in-home preventive assessment programme for independent older adults. J Am Geriatr Soc 1994;42:630–638.
46. Close J, Ellis M, Hooper R, Glucksman E, Jackson S, Swift C. Prevention of falls in the elderly trial (PROFET): a randomised controlled trial. Lancet 1999;353:93–97.
47. Davison J, Bond J, Dawson P, Steen IN, Kenny RA. Patients with recurrent falls attending Accident & Emergency benefit from multifactorial intervention—a randomised controlled trial. Age Ageing 2005;34:162–168.
48. Haines TP, Bennell KL, Osborne RH, Hill KD. Effectiveness of targeted falls prevention programme in subacute hospital setting: randomised controlled trial. BMJ 2004;328:676.
49. Healey F, Monro A, Cockram A, Adams V, Heseltine D. Using targeted risk factor reduction to prevent falls in older in-patients: a randomised controlled trial. Age Ageing 2004;33:390–395.
50. Jensen J, Lundin-Olsson L, Nyberg L, Gustafson Y. Fall and injury prevention in older people living in residential care facilities: a cluster randomized trial. Ann Int Med 2002;136:733–741.
51. Becker C, Kron M, Lindemann U, et al. Effectiveness of a multifaceted intervention on falls in nursing home residents. J Am Geriatr Soc 2003; 51:306–313.
52. Ray WA, Taylor JA, Meador KG, et al. A randomized trial of a consultation service to reduce falls in nursing homes. JAMA 1997;278:557–562.
53. Kerse N, Butler M, Robinson E, Todd M. Fall prevention in residential care: a cluster, randomized, controlled trial. J Am Geriatr Soc 2004;52: 524–531.
54. Rubenstein LZ, Robbins AS, Josephson KR, Schulman BL, Osterweil D. The value of assessing falls in an elderly population. A randomized clinical trial. Ann Int Med 1990;113:308–316.
55. Mills N. The biomechanics of hip protectors. Proceedings of the Institution of Mechanical Engineers. Part H. J Engineering Med 1996;210: 259–266.
56. Lauritzen JB, Petersen MM, Lund B. Effect of external hip protectors on hip fractures. Lancet 1993;341:11–13.
57. Wallace RB, Ross JE, Huston JC, Kundel C, Woodworth G. Iowa FICSIT trial: the feasibility of elderly wearing a hip joint protective garment to reduce hip fractures. J Am Geriatr Soc 1993;41: 338–340.

58. Ekman A, Mallmin H, Michaelsson K, Ljunghall S. External hip protectors to prevent osteoporotic hip fractures. Lancet 1997;350:563–564.
59. Parker M, Gillespie L, Gillespie W. *Hip protectors for preventing hip fractures in the elderly*. Chichester, UK: John Wiley & Sons, 2004.
60. O'Halloran P, Cran G, Beringer T, et al. A cluster randomised controlled trial to evaluate a policy of making hip protectors available to residents of nursing homes. Age Ageing 2004;33:582–588.
61. Forsen L, Sogaard A, Sandvig S, Schuller A, Roed U, Arstad C. Risk of hip fracture in protected and unprotected falls in nursing homes in Norway. Inj Prev 2004;10:16–20.
62. Birks Y, Porthouse J, Addie C, et al. Primary Care Hip Protector Trial Group. Randomized controlled trial of hip protectors among women living in the community. Osteoporos Int 2004;15: 701–706.
63. van Schoor N, Deville W, Bouter L, Lips P. Acceptance and compliance with external hip protectors: a systematic review of the literature. Osteoporos Int 2002;13:917–924.
64. Cameron ID. Hip protectors: Prevent fractures but adherence is a problem. BMJ 2002;324:375–376.
65. Cameron I, Stafford B, Cumming R, et al. Hip protectors improve falls self efficacy. Age Ageing 2000;29:57–62.

11
Medical Treatment of Age-Related Osteoporosis: Present and Future

Steven Boonen

Introduction

The expected rise in 80-year-old and over men and women in populations throughout the world will increase the incidence of senile osteoporosis in the coming decades *(1)*. The consequent rise in fractures may be even greater than currently predicted, as there is evidence to suggest that the rate of increase is greater than that accounted for by the demographic changes alone *(2)*. Additionally, unlike younger age groups, where women are predominantly affected, men aged over 65 years are also at significantly increased risk of fracture *(3)*. Osteoporotic fractures are associated with reduced quality of life and increased morbidity and mortality, particularly in the 80-year-old and over age group *(4)*. Hip fractures, which are considered the most debilitating type of fracture with the greatest adverse economic impact, occur most frequently in this elderly population *(5,6)*. Despite the contribution that fractures, particularly hip fractures, make to the public health burden, strategies for early diagnosis and appropriate treatment are not widely implemented in this age group; action is necessary to reverse the spiraling trend of increased fractures caused by the aging population.

Bone Turnover as a Major Determinant of Bone Strength in Old Age

Bone remodelling, where bone is resorbed by osteoclasts and reformed by osteoblasts, occurs throughout life *(7)*. Evidence from prospective studies, using markers of bone formation and bone resorption, indicates that an excessive rate of bone remodeling is one of the major determinants of bone loss *(8–10)* (Figure 11.1). For example, in one study in older women, higher levels of bone resorption markers were associated with a significantly faster rate of bone loss at the total hip *(9)*. This bone loss continues during aging and may even be accelerated in individuals over the age of 80 (Figure 11.2) *(8)*. Excessive bone remodeling leads to changes in micro-architecture with accumulation of microdamage and some degree of hypomineralization *(12,13)*, resulting in bone fragility.

Increased bone turnover is partly caused by decreased levels of estrogen and by vitamin D deficiency (or insufficiency). Women over 80 years old typically have very low levels of circulating estradiol (average 6.3 pg/mL), and this low exposure to endogenous estrogen has been shown to contribute to age-related bone loss; in prospective studies, elderly individuals with estradiol levels in the lowest quartile were found to have a twofold increase in their risk of hip and vertebral fracture *(14–16)*. Aging is also associated with vitamin D deficiency/insufficiency, which can lead to secondary hyperparathyroidism and parathyroid hormone (PTH)-induced bone loss *(17)*. In addition, insufficient levels of vitamin D may increase the risk of falls—another risk factor for fractures in the very elderly *(18)*.

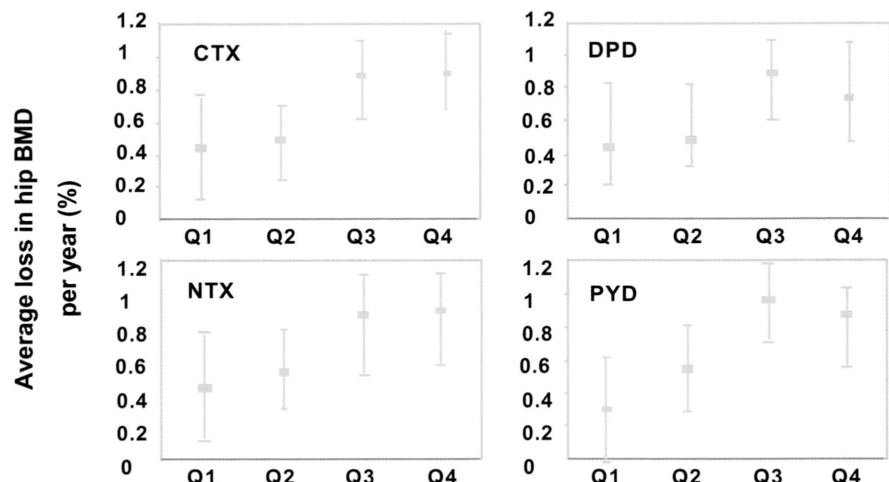

FIGURE 11.1. Mean age-adjusted percentile loss in total hip BMD per year (±95% CI) by quartile of urine markers of bone resorption. A test for trend across the quartiles yielded a p value of 0.004 for N-telopeptides (NTX), 0.025 for C-telopeptides (CTX), 0.007 for free pyridinolines (PYD), and 0.026 for free deoxypyyridinoline (DPD) (From Bauer et al. *[9]*).

Fracture Incidence and Outcome in the Elderly

Hip fracture is the most serious outcome of senile osteoporosis. The demand for hospital resources by patients with hip fracture is disproportionate to that seen with all other fracture types *(19)*, and an increased risk of death has been documented as well *(20,21)*. The incidence of hip fracture rises exponentially in women aged 80 years and over, and approximately 60% of patients with hip frac-

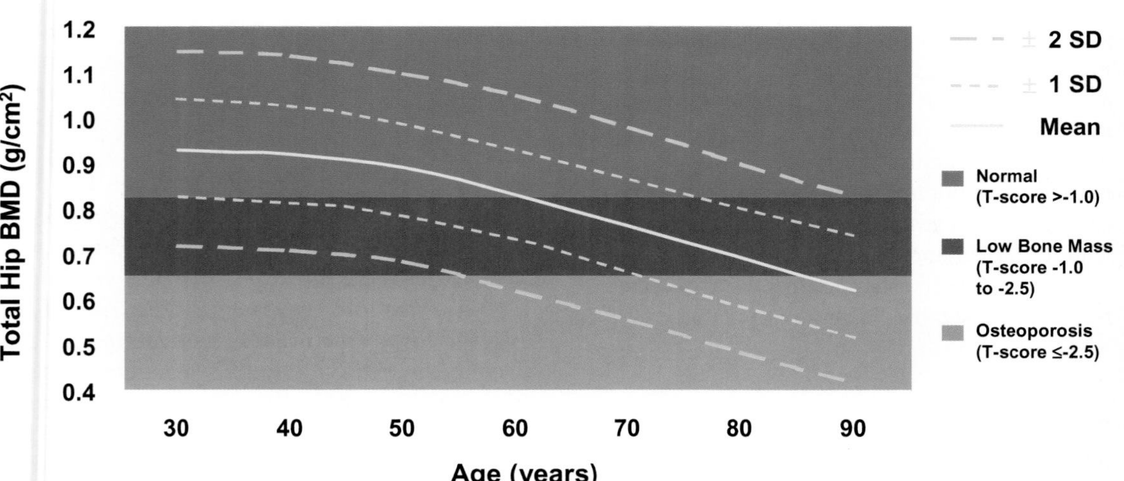

FIGURE 11.2. Changes in total hip BMD with age. (From Meunier et al. *[8]*).

tures are found in this age group *(22–24)*. However, this increase in hip fracture with age has considerable regional variation *(25–28)*. In one study there were greater than fourfold and 13-fold differences in age-standardized risk of hip fracture amongst men and women, respectively, between different centees *(25)*.

Vertebral fractures continue to increase with age in both men and women as well *(29–31)*. For example, in the Longitudinal Aging Study Amsterdam (LASA), 52.3% of women ($n = 65$) and 41.8% of men ($n = 79$) over 80 years had one or more vertebral deformities—compared with 21.7 and 24.2%, respectively, in the younger age group of 65 to 69 years *(32)*. Although the overall impact of vertebral fractures is relatively small in the elderly population compared with hip fracture and other age-related morbidities *(33)*, they are associated with functional limitations and impaired well being, and preventative measures should be implemented. In men and women, fractures of the proximal humerus, forearm, and upper limb fractures increase with age as well *(34,35)*. These fractures are associated with less morbidity compared with hip fractures, but they are associated with reduced quality of life and contribute to the substantial cost of fracture in the elderly population.

Intervention in Senile Osteoporosis

Calcium and Vitamin D Supplementation

Calcium and vitamin D are crucial for bone health throughout life, and deficiencies are widespread in older and institutionalized adults *(36)*. These deficiencies contribute to the increasing prevalence of osteoporosis with age *(37,38)*. Calcium deficiency can be caused by a poor intake and/or less efficient absorption from the intestine, either passively or by vitamin D-mediated active transport *(39)*. In the Study of Osteoporotic Fractures (SOF, $n = 5452$), calcium absorption decreased from 34.3% in persons aged 69 to 74 years to 28.8% in those aged 85 years or more. As calcium absorption decreased, the risk for hip fracture was increased, although this correlation was not significant for other non-vertebral fractures *(40)*.

Low calcium stimulates the secretion of PTH in order to increase the production of 1,25 dihydroxyvitamin D (physiologically active form of vitamin D). PTH maintains calcium homeostasis and normocalcemia, and regulates bone remodeling. The associated increases in bone turnover leads to an increase in fracture rate regardless of bone mineral density (BMD) *(41–44)*. Vitamin D has a central role in calcium homeostasis and maintenance of bone. In the SOF study, the increased relative risk (RR) for hip fracture in individuals with serum vitamin D levels less than or equal to 57 nmol/L was 2.1 (adjusted for age and weight), when compared with higher levels of vitamin D *(15)*. Dietary deficiency of vitamin D is common, and the biosynthesis of 1,25 dihydroxyvitamin D decreases owing to insufficient sunlight exposure and decreased functional capacity of the skin in housebound and geriatric patients *(22)*.

Vitamin D has also been associated with muscular strength and propensity to fall *(45)*. Increases were observed in the size and number of muscle fibers in elderly women with a 3-month supplementation of 1-α hydroxyvitamin D [46]. A recent study showed that 25-hydroxyvitamin D levels correlate with physical activity, balance, gait speed, and thigh muscle strength *(47)*. There is, therefore, considerable evidence to suggest that an adequate dietary intake of calcium and vitamin D in the very elderly will attenuate secondary hyperparathyroidism, help to maintain bone mass and strength, improve muscle strength, and reduce fracture risk.

In a number of studies, PTH levels were reduced by approximately 30% in individuals receiving vitamin D or its active metabolites when compared with controls *(48–52)* and this was associated with reduced bone turnover *(53)* and increased BMD *(54)*. In another study in nursing home residents ($n = 142$), supplementation resulted in a 15% decrease in PTH with a concomitant reduction in bone resorption *(55)*. It appears that combined calcium and vitamin D supplementation results in greater reductions in the levels of serum PTH than with either agent alone, and this is particularly evident in patients with severe vitamin D deficiency or low calcium intake at baseline (48).

Elderly women exhibited significant improvements in musculoskeletal function, and the risk of falling decreased by 49% after 3 months of treatment with calcium and vitamin D *(56)*. In another study, calcium (600 mg/day) and vitamin D (10,000 IU/week) supplementation reduced the risk of falling by 27% after 2 years in elderly people with low baseline serum 25-hydroxyvitamin D levels of 25–90 nmol/L *(57)*. In contrast, other studies have failed to show a significant reduction in falls with calcium and vitamin D supplementation *(58)*. In a meta-analysis of double-blind randomized controlled trials of vitamin D supplementation in subjects with stable health states, the risk of falling was reduced by 22% compared with calcium alone or placebo *(59)*. In elderly women with a recent hip fracture (n = 150; mean age: 81 years), a reduction in falls and fractures was recently observed with calcium and vitamin D as well *(60)*.

Femoral neck, lumbar spine, and/or neck BMD increased by 4–6% in individuals receiving combination supplementation, and this was accompanied by decreases in bone resorption markers *(61–63)*. In a subgroup of women in the 2-year Decalyos II study, femoral neck BMD remained relatively unchanged (mean = 0.29 ± 8.63% per year) during treatment with calcium and vitamin D, whereas it decreased in the placebo group (mean = −2.36 ± 4.92% per year) *(64)*.

The impact of calcium and vitamin D on fracture risk has been studied in community-based and institutionalized populations (Table 11.1). Two randomized placebo-controlled studies of individuals in institutions, and two of elderly male and female community residents without documented osteoporosis, have demonstrated a positive impact of calcium and vitamin D supplementation on fracture risk. In the Decalyos I randomized placebo-controlled study in ambulatory institutionalized women (n = 3270; mean age 84 years) with severe calcium and vitamin D deficiencies, the RR of hip fracture and all non-vertebral fractures fell by 43 and 32%, respectively, after 18 months of calcium (1200 mg/day) and vitamin D3 (800 IU/day) supplementation. After 36 months, hip and non-vertebral fracture risk were reduced by 29 and 24%, respectively *(62,65)* (Figure 11.3). A similar reduction in the risk of hip fracture was observed in Decalyos II (n = 639; mean age 85.2 years), where 79% of individuals had a calcium intake of less than 800 mg/day and

TABLE 11.1. Overview of Randomized Controlled Clinical Trials of Long-Term Calcium and Vitamin D in the Prevention of Fractures *(68)*

Source	Study population	Trial design	Dosing: Calcium (mg/day)	Dosing: Vitamin D (IU/day)	Duration (months)	Incidence of fractures (treatment vs control) [p value]: Any non-vertebral	Incidence of fractures (treatment vs control) [p value]: Hip
Studies in institutionalized patients							
(62)	3,270 F, mean age 84 years	vs placebo	1,200	800	18	66 vs 97 [0.015]	21 vs 37 (0.043)
(64)	639 F, mean age 85.2 years	vs placebo	1,200	800	24	17.8 vs 17.9% [NS]	6.9 vs 11.1% (0.07)
Studies in community-dwelling patients							
(58)	3,314 F, mean age 77 years[a]	vs no treatment	1,000	800	median 25	4.4 vs 4.6%	0.6 vs 0.9%
(68)	2,638, 85% F, aged ≥70 years[b]	vs placebo	1,000	800	24–62	12.6 vs 12.7%	3.5 vs 3.1%
(67)	5,073 M and F, mean age 74 years	vs placebo[c]	1,000	400	42	6.4 vs 7.9%	Not reported
(50)	389 M and F, mean age 71 years	vs placebo	500	700	36	5.6 vs 12.9%	0 vs 1
(73)	36,282 F, mean age 62.4 years	vs placebo	100	400	median 84	Not reported	1.0 vs 1.1%

[a] Patients had a least one self-reported risk factor for osteoporosis. Patients in both groups received a leflet providing information on calcium intake and fall prevention.
[b] Patients had ≥ prior low-trauma fractures. Results cited are new low-trauma fractures.
[c] Control patients were offered an environmental and health program aimed at preventing fractures.

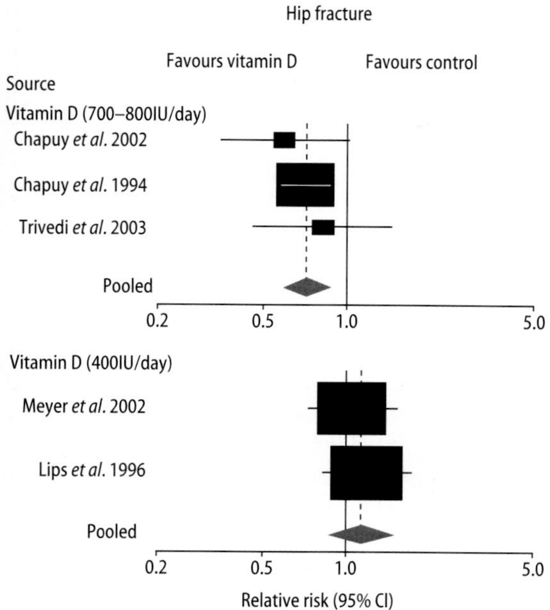

FIGURE 11.3. Forest plots showing differences in hip and non-vertebral fracture risk between in vitamin D supplemented patients at different doses (700–800 IU/day, *[64,65,140]* and 400 IU/day *[75,141]*) and the control groups (From Bischoff-Ferrari et al. *[72]*).

a serum 25-hydroxyvitamin D of less than 50 nmol/L *(64)*.

Studies of supplementation of individuals in the community have demonstrated smaller reductions in fracture risk, but the baseline deficiencies of calcium and vitamin D were less severe. A significant reduction in non-vertebral fractures was seen in individuals receiving calcium and vitamin D compared with placebo, but this was largely caused by a reduction in ankle and radius fractures *(66)*. In a non-randomized trial of elderly community residents ($n = 9605$) on supplementation, fracture risk was reduced by 16% compared with controls *(67)*. In contrast to these studies, three other trials demonstrated no reduction in fracture risk. In the RECORD trial of elderly men and women with a previous low-trauma fracture ($n = 5292$), there was no difference in the occurrence of new fractures between those receiving either supplementation or placebo *(68)*. Similar negative results were obtained for a trial of oral vitamin D3 and calcium for prevention of a secondary fracture in women with at least one risk factor for hip fracture *(58)*, and in the Women's Health Initiative (WHI) trial *(59)*. However, these studies, in particular WHI, involved younger individuals often with less severe, if any, deficiencies of calcium and vitamin D, living in the community and generally free of disability. The conflicting results are likely to be caused, at least in part, by a lack of targeting to those who do have insufficiencies. The available evidence suggests that supplements should be directed to those individuals with known, or at most risk of, insufficiencies; unrestricted supplementation in the community may be unnecessary *(69,70)*. It has been suggested that supplementation with vitamin D in older, as well as younger, adults should be implemented when serum 25-hydroxyvitamin D is less than 50 nmol/L *(71)*, as it causes much greater decreases in PTH levels and physical function than when serum 25-hydroxyvitamin D is above this level *(55)*.

In addition to targeting of the supplementation, using the appropriate dose may be critical as well. Currently, the US recommended daily allowance is 1200 mg/day for calcium and 400 IU/day for vitamin D for those over 50 years of age *(72)*. European guidelines for this age group are calcium at 800 mg/day and 400 IU/day of vitamin D for those over 65 years age *(73)*. However, meta-analyses of vitamin D supplementation have indicated that a dose of 800 IU/day is required to produce optimum benefit in terms of a reduction in fracture risk and falling *(74)*. The authors of the WHI report acknowledged that a dosage of vitamin D of 400 IU/day used in their study may have been insufficient to produce a response *(75)*. Similarly, in another study, supplementation with 400 IU/day of vitamin D alone had no evident benefit *(76)* (Figure 11.3). In addition to the dose of vitamin D, it is essential to combine vitamin D with calcium, particularly in elderly individuals. A Cochrane review concluded that elderly people would benefit most from a combination of calcium and vitamin D supplementation *(77)*. More recently, an indirect comparison of randomized controlled trials of vitamin D versus placebo and vitamin D plus calcium versus placebo indicated that adequate calcium additions are necessary for optimum clinical efficiency with vitamin D supplementation (77a). No safety concerns have been raised with this type of supplementation at the levels normally administered (calcium: 1–1.2 g/day; vitamin D3: 800 U/day).

Finally, compliance with calcium and vitamin D supplementation is also essential, as the effects will not persist after calcium and vitamin D supplements have been discontinued *(63,78)*. In recent community-based fracture studies, compliance was reported to be only 40–60% *(58,68,73)*, but individuals who live in institutions achieve higher rates of compliance and more positive benefits *(62,64,65)*.

Pharmaceutical Intervention

Although calcium and vitamin D are essential to prevent bone loss and fractures in older individuals, elderly patients with documented osteoporosis need calcium, vitamin D, and pharmacologic intervention (anti-resorptives, teriparatide, or strontium ranelate) *(69)*. These interventions will provide benefit to elderly patients on top of the benefit already provided by calcium and vitamin D. There is now considerable evidence that even in very elderly patients, pharmaceutical intervention to prevent bone loss remains effective and reduces the risk of fracture and associated morbidity, mortality, and economic consequences. The available therapies for the treatment of osteoporosis such as bisphoshonates, calcitonin, raloxifene, teriparatide, and strontium ranelate have different characteristics and may have treatment outcomes in the elderly. Many elderly patients with established osteoporosis have multiple comorbid conditions such as gastrointestinal disease *(79)* and renal insufficiency *(80)*. Therefore, it is important that administered drugs are not only effective in this population but also safe.

Bisphosphonates

The use of bisphosphonates in preventing bone loss and fractures is well established. However, there is limited data on the effects of these agents in individuals of advanced age with osteoporosis. In women over 80 years of age with documented osteoporosis (a femoral neck T score of less than −2.5 or at least one prevalent vertebral fracture), the efficacy of risedronate in reducing fracture risk was demonstrated using a post-hoc pooling of data from three randomized double-blind controlled 3-year fracture endpoint trials (Hip Intervention Programme [HIP], Vertebral Efficacy with Risedronate Therapy—Multinational [VERT-MN], and VERT North America [VERT-NA]) *(81–83)*. In individuals treated with risedronate ($n = 704$; 2.5 or 5 mg/day) the risk of new vertebral fractures was 81% lower than for those treated with placebo ($n = 688$, $p < 0.001$) after 1 year. As with younger patients, the magnitude of the risk reduction associated with risedronate was larger in the first year of treatment of patients 80 years and over, but the efficacy was still apparent after 3 years of treatment (44% lower than placebo, $p = 0.003$) *(79)* (Figure 11.4, Table 11.2). In this analysis of patients 80 years and over, risedronate was well tolerated and had a safety profile similar to that of placebo *(79)*.

In the VERT and HIP trials, a statistically significant reduction in non-vertebral fractures with risedronate treatment had been demonstrated in patients over a wide range of ages *(81–84)*. However, in patients aged 80 years or more, a treatment effect on non-vertebral fractures was not seen *(79)* (Figure 11.4, Table 11.2). Currently, there is little evidence to support the efficacy of bisphosphonates in reducing the risk of non-vertebral fractures in women 80 years of age or older, as these women have not been recruited in most studies. In the HIP trial of risedronate, women aged 70–79 years with osteoporosis and

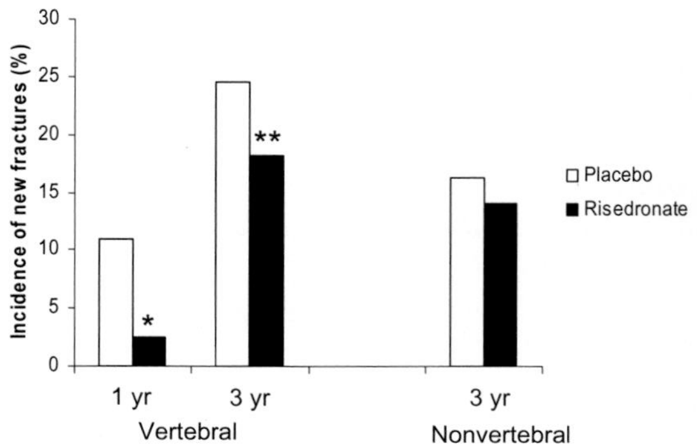

FIGURE 11.4. Reduction in incidence of vertebral and non-vertebral fracture in patients treated with risedronate over 1 and 3 years (Adapted from Boonen et al. *[79]*).

TABLE 11.2. Overview of Randomized Placebo-Controlled Clinical Trials of Pharmaceutical Anti-Osteoporotic Agents in the Prevention of Fractures in Elderly Patients

Source	Study population	Agent[a]	Dose/day	Duration (months)	Incidence of fractures (treatment vs control)	
					Vertebral	Non-vertebral
(79)	1392 F, age ≥80 years (mean 83 years)[b]	risedronate	oral 2.5 or 5 mg	12	2.5 vs 10.9%, [$p < 0.001$]	—
(79)	1392 F, age ≥80 years (mean 83 years)[b]	risedronate	oral 2.5 or 5 mg	36	18.2 vs 24.6%, [$p = 0.003$]	14.0 vs 16.2% [NS]
(102)	244 F, age ≥75 years (mean 78 years)[c]	teriparatide	sc 20 μg	median 19	5.2 vs 15.1%, [$p < 0.050$]	3.2 vs 4.2% [NS]
(109)	1488 F, age ≥80 years (mean 83 years)[d]	strontium ranelate	oral 2 g	12	3.5 vs 8.3%, [$p = 0.002$]	4.0 vs 6.8% [$p = 0.027$]
(109)	1488 F, age ≥80 years (mean 83 years)[d]	strontium ranelate	oral 2 g	36	19.1 vs 26.5% [$p = 0.013$]	19.7 vs 14.2% [$p = 0.011$]

[a] All patients received calcium and vitamin D supplementation.
[b] 84% of patients had one or more prevalent vertebral fracture.
[c] All patients had at least one moderate or two mild atraumatic vertebral fractures.
[d] All patients had osteoporosis with at least one prevalent vertebral fracture or a femoral neck BMD ≤0.600 g/cm² (Hologic).

women aged 80 years and over with at least one non-skeletal risk factor for hip fracture or a low BMD were assessed. No non-vertebral fracture risk reduction was observed in women over 80. But a proportion of these women may not have been osteoporotic, as most of them had not been selected on the basis of low BMD *(83)*. However, even in the pooled data analysis from the HIP, VERT-MN, and VERT-NA trials in patients over 80 with documented osteoporosis, non-vertebral fracture risk reduction was not observed. Because these women had a severe degree of osteoporosis (as expected for their age), the lack of treatment effect on non-vertebral fracture risk cannot be attributed to a lesser extent of skeletal fragility in these very elderly patients. The apparent lack of treatment efficacy in these patients cannot be ascribed to a more pronounced effect of calcium and vitamin D supplementation in patients over 80 either, because, in placebo-treated elderly patients, changes in bone turnover markers were similar to those observed in patients aged less than 80 years *(79)*.

The impact of age on the anti-fracture efficacy of alendronate was recently analyzed using data from a subset of individuals who had been enrolled in the Fracture Intervention Trials (FIT) and had documented osteoporosis. There was no evidence for an effect of age on the significant reductions in the RR for clinical fractures in those on alendronate (5 mg/day for 2 years followed by 10 mg/day for 1 to 2.5 years) compared with placebo. In fact, the absolute risk reductions for both vertebral and hip fractures in women aged 75 to 85 years with low BMD actually increased with age, supporting an increase in the cost-effectiveness of bisphosphonate treatment in older patients. However, a limitation of these analyses was the maximum age of women at entry to the FIT study (80 years); despite aging during the trial, women over 80 years accounted for less than 8% of the patient-years on which the analysis was based *(85)*. With alendronate treatment, long-term safety data have been reported *(86)*, but the safety profile in patients 80 years old has hardly been addressed.

Overall, it would seem that bisphosphonate treatment efficacy and safety is not affected by age. However, no compelling evidence currently exists to support the efficacy of bisphosphonates in reducing the risk of non-vertebral fractures in women aged 80 years or more.

Estrogen Replacement Therapy (ERT)

The positive effects of ERT on bone mass at different sites, including hip, in early postmenopausal women are undisputed *(87,88)*. Approximately 10–15% of skeletal mass is estrogen-dependent, implying that this amount of bone is rapidly lost in peri-/post-menopausal women or later in life when ERT is discontinued *(87,89)*. In various cross-sectional analyses of older women, neither bone density *(90)* nor the reduction in hip fracture incidence was preserved in those who had discontinued ERT *(91–93)*. In a prospective cohort study (n = 9704, 65 years or over), the RR for hip fracture was lower among current estrogen users (RR 0.6, 95% confidence interval [CI] 0.36, 1.02) than among those who had never used estrogen. However, previous use of estrogen, regardless of duration, did not significantly impact the risk for fractures *(94)*. In one case-control study of 1327 women aged 50–81 years with hip fracture, the risk of further hip fracture was decreased in both current and former users of hormone replacement therapy (HRT) *(95)*.

To prevent initial hip fractures in old age, ERT may have to be initiated peri-menopausally and maintained throughout life. In a meta-analysis of ERT in elderly women, the protection against hip fracture waned with age *(96)*, and at present it is not clear whether the benefits of ERT would outweigh the risks of thromboembolism, endometrial and breast cancer, and cardiovascular complications associated with long-term use of HRT. Thus, estrogen is unlikely to be useful as an anti-osteoporotic strategy to prevent fractures in the very elderly population.

Selective Estrogen Receptor Modulators (SERMs)

Currently, no specific trials with SERMs have been reported in patients aged 80 years or more. The large 3-year Multiple Outcomes of Raloxifene Evaluation (MORE) trial investigated the effect on raloxifene on post-menopausal women aged 31–80 years. Raloxifene increased BMD in the femoral neck and in the spine, and the risk of vertebral fracture was reduced. The risk of non-vertebral fracture was only reduced by raloxifene in a subgroup of women with severe vertebral fractures at baseline. Its use in a population aged 80 years or more with or without a history of fracture has yet to be established *(97,98)*.

Teriparatide

Teriparatide is an anabolic agent that stimulates bone turnover, with a positive bone balance resulting in increased bone mass and improvements in bone architecture *(99–101)*. The effectiveness of teriparatide has been demonstrated for vertebral and non-vertebral fracture in post-menopausal women, but it has not been extensively studied in individuals 80 years and over.

Data from the randomized multi-center double-blind placebo-controlled Fracture Prevention Trial (FPT) compared the relative treatment effect of teriparatide in women younger than 75 years ($n = 841$) and those older than 75 years ($n = 244$) on markers of bone turnover, BMD, risk of fractures, adverse events, and the incidence of hypercalcemia. Increases in bone-specific alkaline phosphatase (BSAP) were similar in both age groups within 1 month, supporting early bone formation with teriparatide regardless of age; these increases in BSAP were apparent up to 1 year. The increase in femoral neck BMD (<75 years: 9.1%; ⩾75 years: 9.2%) compared with placebo was also similar in both age groups. In addition, there were no significant treatment-by-age interactions for bone turnover markers, height loss, hypercalcemia, or hyperuricemia.

In a more recent analysis *(102)*, the relative effect of teriparatide in reducing the incidence of vertebral and non-vertebral fragility fractures was statistically indistinguishable in women aged 75 years and over and those aged less than 75 years. However, a significant reduction in non-vertebral fractures compared with placebo could not be documented in the group of women over 75 years of age (Table 11.2), because only a small number of women in this age group had a non-vertebral fracture and the analysis was not sufficiently powered to assess non-vertebral fracture risk reductions in this age group. There were no increases in the frequency of treatment-emergent adverse events in this older age group *(102)*.

Overall, the data from these analyses show that the safety and efficacy of teriparatide in post-menopausal women with osteoporosis is not affected by age. Because of its ability to stimulate cancellous and cortical bone formation and to partly restore the micro-architecture of the bone, teriparatide is a new advance in the treatment of age-associated osteoporosis, particularly in those with severe osteoporosis and existing fractures.

Strontium Ranelate

Currently, most agents available for the treatment of osteoporosis either inhibit bone resorption, which is accompanied by a subsequent reduction in bone formation *(103)*, or enhance bone formation *(104)*. Evidence suggests that strontium ranelate dissociates these two processes, such that bone formation continues to be active during inhibition of bone resorption *(105)*.

In two international phase III randomized placebo-controlled double-blind studies (the Spinal Osteoporosis Therapeutic Intervention [SOTI] and Treatment Of Peripheral Osteoporosis [TROPOS]), substantial reductions were reported in both vertebral and non-vertebral fractures, including hip fractures, over 1, 3, and 5 years in post-menopausal women aged 50 to 100 years following administration of strontium ranelate *(106–108)*.

A pre-planned analysis of the intent to treat 80- to 100-year-old population (n = 1488) of these studies showed that the relative risk reduction for vertebral fracture was 59% (RR 0.41; 95% CI 0.22; 0.75, $p = 0.002$) after 1 year and 32% (RR 0.68; 95% CI 0.50; 0.92, $p = 0.013$) after 3 years, compared with placebo. For non-vertebral fractures, including hip fractures, there were substantial reductions of 41% (RR 0.59; 95% CI 0.37; 0.95, $p = 0.027$) after 1 year and 31% (RR 0.69; 95% CI 0.52; 0.92, $p = 0.011$) after 3 years (Figure 11.5, Table 11.2). The major non-vertebral fractures of hip, wrist, pelvis and sacrum, ribs-sternum, clavicle, or humerus combined led to a

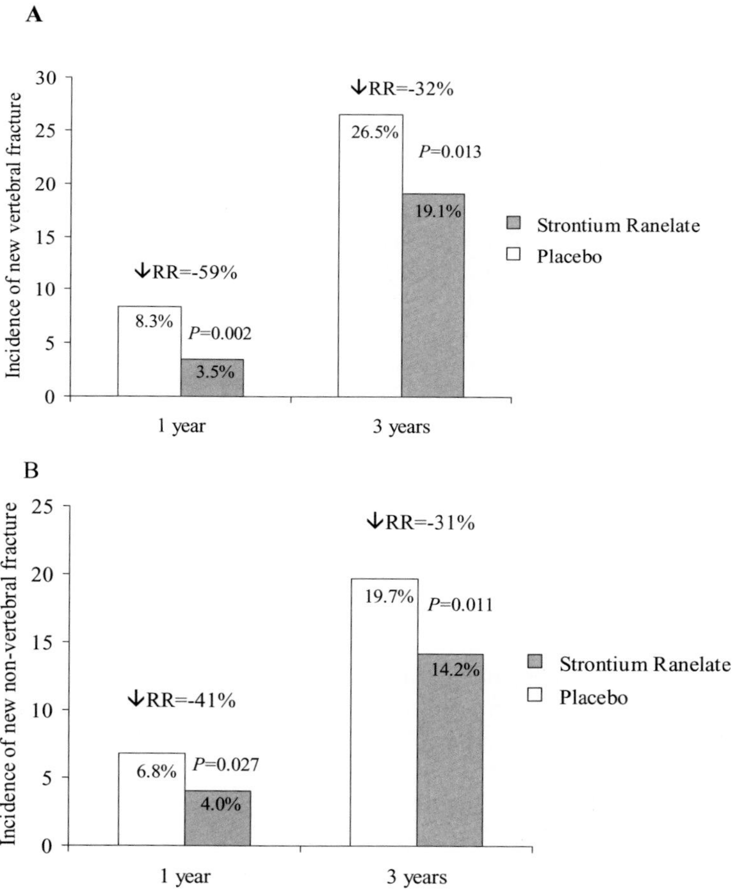

FIGURE 11.5. Reduction of vertebral **(A)** and non-vertebral **(B)** fracture risk over 1 and 3 years with strontium ranelate in patients aged 80 years or more. (From Seeman et al. *[109]*).

RR compared with placebo of 37% ($p = 0.003$) after 3 years *(109)*.

It was recently demonstrated that, over 5 years, strontium ranelate continues to be effective and significantly reduces the risk of vertebral fracture and non-vertebral fracture in elderly patients, with a safety profile similar to that in younger patients *(110)*. To date, strontium ranelate is the only anti-osteoporotic treatment to demonstrate an early and long-term sustained reduction in vertebral and non-vertebral fractures, in patients over 80.

Current and Future Management of Senile Osteoporosis

Although a number of guidelines for diagnosis and treatment of elderly patients at risk for osteoporosis and fracture have been presented *(22,111–113)*, osteoporosis continues to be under-diagnosed and under-treated. In general, there is a lack of awareness of the incidence of osteoporosis and its potentially devastating outcomes in the very elderly population.

Treatment of osteoporosis in older patients depends on ensuring bone strength and reducing falls. The incidence of fracture in individuals with osteoporosis is compounded by the increase in falls in both elderly men and women, and evidence-based guidelines to help prevent falls exist *(114,115)*. However, implementation of relatively simple fall-prevention measures and BMD screening for high-risk individuals is not widespread.

In recent years there have been considerable advances in establishing effective pharmaceutical agents and non-pharmaceutical intervention methods for reducing fracture risk in osteoporosis, but treatment is still rare even in patients with a previous fracture. Reported treatment rates for osteoporosis in elderly persons vary from 5–69% *(116)*, and this decreases with age *(117)*. It is clear that routine screening and preventative measures have not been incorporated into primary care practice *(118)*, and even many orthopedic surgeons do not see the need to investigate or treat osteoporosis in elderly patients, even after a hip fracture has occurred *(119)*. In one study, conducted in women and men aged 80–89 years, only 2.4 and 1.4%, respectively, had BMD scans following hip or vertebral fracture. And only 37.2 and 1.2%, respectively, were treated following any first fracture, despite the increased risk of further fracture (Figure 11.6) *(120)*. In one study, patients who were managed as specified by guidelines following a fracture were younger (mean of 68.6 years compared with 73.5 years) and less likely to have additional risk factors of low weight, or hip or wrist fracture *(117)*. Similarly, elderly stroke patients have an increased risk of hip fracture, but measures to prevent bone loss are rarely implemented for these patients *(121)*.

Surprisingly, even supplementation with calcium and vitamin D is relatively rare in elderly patients following a fracture. In a recent report, only 6% of 170 patients (mean age: 80 years) were treated with calcium, 3% with vitamin D, and 0% with alendronate at admission with hip fracture; the corresponding figures were 7, 4, and 2% at discharge *(122)*. Indeed, elderly patients discharged with pneumonia were just as likely to receive calcium, vitamin D, and/or anti-resorptive therapy as those with hip fracture *(123)*. It is evident that prevention and treatment policies vary between institutions, regions, and countries, but implementation of such policies appears to be universally low.

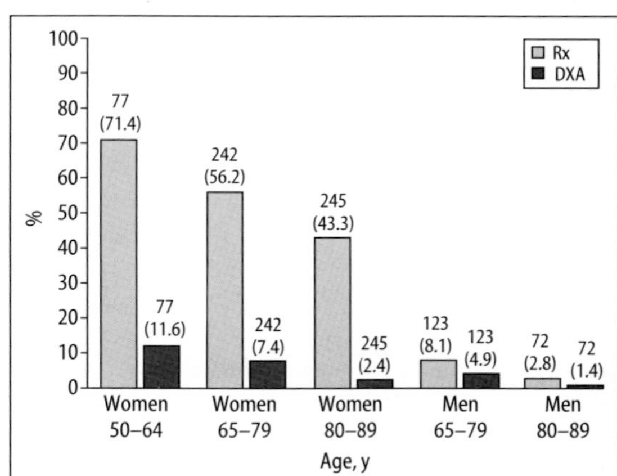

FIGURE 11.6. Number (percentage of women and men by age category who had BMD measurements or received pharmacological treatment for hip and vertebral fractures combined. Rx = pharmacological treatment, DXA = dual X-ray absorptiometry. (From Feldstein et al. *[117]*).

There is an urgent need to increase awareness of osteoporosis in old age, both among patients and physicians. Educational efforts should convince physicians that treating senile osteoporosis and reducing fracture risk in the elderly and the associated benefits are achievable with current treatment options. As discussed in this chapter, the efficacy of agents like teriparatide, risedronate, and strontium ranelate in reducing fracture risk in elderly patients with documented osteoporosis has been well established in clinical trials. However, many elderly patients do not receive treatment, as it is perceived that it is too late to alter the course of the disease. Patient selection for intervention has been based almost entirely on bone-related risk factors for treatment, including a prevalent fracture, but routine BMD measurements with dual-energy X-ray absorptiometry (DXA) at the hip and spine in very elderly individuals are often not encouraged *(122)*. Moreover, low BMD—although a major risk factor for fractures in elderly persons—is generally not sufficient on its own to predict fractures *(124–126)*. In a recent study only between 10–40% of fractures met the criteria for DXA-defined osteoporosis (BMD of 2.5 standard deviations below normal for young adults) *(127)*, and this large overlap in BMD between individuals with and without fracture is particularly marked in old age *(128)*. In addition to non-density related aspects of bone strength, falling is a major risk factor for fractures, especially appendicular fractures *(112,124–126)*. For predicting hip fracture, risk factors for falls and low BMD act as independent and additive risk factors *(129)*. The question is whether the reduction in fracture risk in the very elderly could potentially be optimized by combining bone-directed strategies with fall-directed strategies.

Finally, secondary prevention of hip fractures should become an integral part of the management of individuals who sustain hip fractures. One option is the prescription of medications that lower the risk of hip fracture. Such therapies that are currently available include calcium and vitamin D supplementation, alendronate, risedronate, and strontium ranelate. However, the rate of use of these therapies among patients with hip fractures is low. Despite the fact that proven, efficacious drugs are now available for the treatment of osteoporosis, osteoporosis continues to be under-diagnosed and under-treated in the elderly, even after hip fracture. One of the many reasons why clinicians do not consistently initiate treatment for osteoporosis even after a hip fracture might be the fact that all of these drugs have been tested for primary prevention of hip fractures. There is an urgent need for studies to evaluate either pharmacologic or non-pharmacologic measures aimed at secondary prevention of hip fractures.

Summary

Osteoporotic fractures are an extremely common health problem in the elderly, with the incidence projected to rise as longevity increases, unless preventive policies are initiated. Recent evidence indicates that treating osteoporosis in this population and the associated benefits are achievable with current treatment options. In elderly patients, bone loss can be inhibited and fracture risk reduced by calcium and vitamin D supplementation, and pharmaceutical intervention with agents such as bisphosphonates, teriparatide, and strontium ranelate. Nevertheless, osteoporosis in old age continues to be under-diagnosed and under-treated.

References

1. Ettinger MP. Aging bone and osteoporosis: strategies for preventing fractures in the elderly. Arch Intern Med 2000;163:2237–2246.
2. Palvanen M, Kannus S, Niemi S, et al. Secular trends in the osteoporotic fractures of the distal humerus in elderly women. Eur J Epidemiol 1998; 14:159–164.
3. Colón-Emeric CS, Pieper CF, Artz MB. Can historical and functional risk factors be used to predict fractures in community-dwelling older adults? Development and validation of a clinical tool. Osteoporos Int 2002;13:955–961.
4. Melton LJ, Kan SH, Frye MA, et al. Epidemiology of vertebral fractures in women. Am J Epidemiol 1989;129:1000–1011.
5. Autier P, Haentjens P, Bentin J, et al. for the Belgium Hip Fracture Study Group. Costs induced by hip fractures: a prospective controlled study in Belgium. Osteoporos Int 2000;11:373–380.

6. Cooper C, Campion G, Melton LJ. Hip fracture in the elderly: a worldwide projection. Osteoporos Int 1992;2:285–289.
7. van der Meulen MC, Beaupe GS, Carter DR. Mechanobiologic influences in long bone cross-sectional growth. Bone 1993;14:635–642.
8. Meunier PJ, Delmas PD, Eastell R, et al. International Committee for Osteoporosis Clinical Guidelines. Diagnosis and management of osteoporosis in postmenopausal women: clinical guidelines. Clin Ther 1999;21:1025–1044.
9. Bauer DC, Sklarin PM, Stone KL, et al. Biochemical markers of bone turnover and prediction of hip bone loss in older women: the study of osteoporotic fractures. J Bone Miner Res 1999;14: 1404–1410.
10. Cummings SR, Black DM, Nevitt MC, et al. Bone density at various sites for prediction of hip fractures: the Study of Osteoporotic Fractures Research Group. Lancet 1993;341:72–75.
11. Heaney RP. Is the paradigm shifting? Bone 2003;33:457–465.
12. Garnero P, Hausherr E, Chapuy MC, et al. Markers of bone resorption predict hip fracture in elderly women: the EPIDOS Prospective Study. J Bone Miner Res 1996;11:1531–1538.
13. Mori S, Harruff R Ambrosius W, Burr DB. Trabecular bone volume and microdamage accumulation in the femoral heads of women with and without femoral neck fractures. Bone 1997;21: 521–526.
14. Ettinger B, Pressman A, Sklarin P, et al. Associations between low levels of serum estradiol, bone density, and fractures among elderly women: the Study of Osteoporotic Fractures. J Clin Endocrinol Metab 1998;83:2239–2243.
15. Cummings SR, Browner WS, Bauer D, et al. Endogenous hormones and the risk of hip and vertebral fractures among older women. Study of Osteoporotic Fractures Research Group. N Engl J Med 1998;339:733–738.
16. Stone K, Bauer DC, Black DM, et al. Hormonal predictors of bone loss in elderly women: a prospective study. J Bone Miner Res 1998;13: 1167–1174.
17. Seeman E. Osteoporosis II: pathogenesis of bone fragility in women and men. Lancet 2002;359: 1841–1850.
18. Lips P. Vitamin D deficiency and secondary hyperparathyroidism in the elderly: consequences for bone loss and fractures and therapeutic implications. Endocr Rev 2001;22:477–501.
19. Garraway WM, Stauffer RN, Kurland LT, et al. Limb fractures in a defined population II: orthopedic treatment and utilization of health care. Mayo Clin Proc 1979;54:708–713.
20. Barrett JA, Baron JA, Beach ML. Mortality and pulmonary embolism after fracture in the elderly. Osteoporos Int 2003;14:889–894.
21. Kanis JA, Oden A, Johnell O, et al. The components of excess mortality after hip fracture. Bone 2003;32:468–473.
22. Eastell R, Reid DM, Compston J, et al. Secondary prevention of osteoporosis: when should a non-vertebral fracture be a trigger for action. Q J Med 2001;94:575–597.
23. Boockvar KS, Halm EA, Litke A, et al. Hospital readmissions after hospital discharge for hip fracture: surgical and nonsurgical causes and effects on outcome. J Am Geriatr Soc 2003;51:300–403.
24. Donaldson LJ, Cook A, Thompson RG. Incidence of fractures in a geographically defined population. J Epidemiol Community Health 1990;44: 241–245.
25. Elffors I, Allander E, Kanis JA, et al. The variable incidence of hip fracture in Southern Europe: The MEDOS study. Osteoporos Int 1994;4:253–263.
26. Kanis JA, Johnell O, Oden A, et al. Risk of hip fracture according to the World Health Organization Criteria for Osteopenia and Osteoporosis. Bone 2000;27:585–590.
27. Johnell O, Gullberg B, Allander E, et al. The apparent incidence of hip fracture in Europe: a study of National Register sources. Osteoporos Int 1992;2: 248–254.
28. Walker-Bone K, Dennison E, Cooper C. Epidemiology of osteoporosis. Rheum Dis Clin North Amer 2001;27:1–18.
29. European Prospective Osteoporosis Study (EPOS) Group. Incidence of vertebral fracture in Europe: results from the European Prospective Osteoporosis Study (EPOS). J Bone Miner Res 2002;29: 517–522.
30. Kenny A, Taxel P. Osteoporosis in older men. Clin Cornerstone 2000;2:45–51.
31. Scane SC, Sutcliffe AM, Francis RM. The sequelae of vertebral crush fractures in men. Osteoporos Int 1994;4:89–92.
32. Pluijm SMF, Tromp AM, Smit JH, et al. Consequences of vertebral deformities in older men and women. J Bone Miner Res 2000;15:1564–1572.
33. Kanis JA, Oden A, Johnell O, et al. Excess mortality after hospitalisation for vertebral fracture. Osteoporos Int 2004;15:108–112.
34. Kelsey JL, Browner WS, Seeley DG, et al. Risk factors for fractures of the distal forearm and proximal humerus. Am J Epidemiol 1992;135: 477–489.

35. Ismail AA, Pye SR, Cockerill WC, et al. Incidence of limb fracture across Europe: results from the European Prospective Osteoporosis Study (EPOS). Osteoporos Int 2002;13:565–571.
36. Chapuy MC, Preziosi P, Maamer M, et al. Prevalence of vitamin D insufficiency in an adult normal population. Osteoporos Int 1997;7:439–443.
37. Heaney RP. Calcium in the prevention and treatment of osteoporosis. J Intern Med 1992;231: 169–180.
38. Heaney RP. The importance of calcium intake for lifelong skeletal health. Calcif Tiss Int 2002;70: 70–73.
39. Heaney RP, Gallagher JC, Johnston CC, et al. Calcium nutrition and bone health in the elderly. Am J Clin Nutr 1982;36 (Suppl):986–1013.
40. Ensrud KE, Duong T, Cauley JA, et al. Low fractional calcium absorption increases the risk for hip fracture in women with low calcium intake. Ann Intern Med 2000;132:345–353.
41. Quesada JM, Coopmans W, Ruiz B, et al. Influence of vitamin D on parathyroid function in the elderly J Clin Endocrinol Metab 1992;75:494–501.
42. Boonen S, Broos P, Verbeke G, et al. Calciotropic hormones and markers of bone remodelling in age-related (type II) femoral neck osteoporosis: alterations consistent with secondary hyperparathyroidism-induced bone resorption. J Gerontol A Biol Sci Med Sci 1997;52:M286–M293.
43. Boonen S, Vanderschueren D, Cheng XG, et al. Age-related (type II) femoral neck osteoporosis in men: biochemical evidence for both hypovitaminosis D- and androgen deficiency-induced bone resorption. J Bone Miner Res 1997;12: 2119–2126.
44. Garnero P, Sornay-Rendu E, Claustrat B, et al. Biochemical markers of bone turnover, endogenous hormones and the risk of fractures in postmenopausal women: the OFELY study. J Bone Miner Res 2000;15:1526–1536.
45. Bischoff HA, Stahelin HB, Urscheler N, et al. Muscle strength in the elderly: its relation to vitamin D metabolites. Arch Phys Med Rehabil 1999;80:54–58.
46. Sorensen OH, Lund B, Saltin B, et al. Myopathy in bone loss of ageing: improvement by treatment with 1-alpha-hydroxy cholecalciferol and calcium. Clin Sci (Lond) 1979;56:157–161.
47. Gerdhem P, Ringsberg KA, Obrant KJ, et al. Association between 25-hydroxy vitamin D levels, physical activity, muscle strength and fractures in the prospective population-based OPRA Study of Elderly Women. Osteoporos Int 2005;16: 1425–1431.
48. Lips P, Duong T, Oleksik A, et al. A global study of vitamin D status and parathyroid function in postmenopausal women with osteoporosis: baseline data from the multiple outcomes of raloxifene evaluation clinical trial. J Clin Endocrinol Metab 2001;86:1212–1221.
49. Brazier M, Kamel S, Maamer M, et al. Markers of bone remodelling in the elderly subject: effects of vitamin D insufficiency and its correction. J Bone Miner Res 1995;10:1753–1761.
50. Dawson-Hughes B, Harris SS, Krall EA, et al. Rates of bone loss in postmenopausal women randomly assigned to one of two dosages of vitamin D. Am J Clin Nutr 1995;61:1140–1145.
51. Malabanan A, Veronikis IE, Holick MF. Redefining vitamin D insufficiency. Lancet 1998;351: 805–806.
52. McKane WR, Khosla S, Egan KS, et al. Role of calcium intake in modulating age-related increases in parathyroid function and bone resorption. J Clin Endocrinol Metal 1996;81:1699–1703.
53. Ooms ME, Roos JC, Bezemer PD, et al. Prevention of bone loss by vitamin D supplementation in elderly women: a randomized double-blind trial. J Clin Endocrinol Metab 1995;80:1052–1058.
54. Grados F, Brazier M, Kamel S, et al. Prediction of bone mass density variation by bone remodelling markers in postmenopausal women with vitamin D insufficiency treated with calcium and vitamin D supplementation. J Clin Endocrinol Metab 2003;88:5175–5179.
55. Lips P, Wiersinga A, van Ginkel FC, et al. The effect of vitamin D supplementation on vitamin D status and parathyroid function in elderly subjects. J Clin Endocrinol Metab 1988;67:644–650.
56. Bischoff HA, Stahelin HB, Dick W, et al. Effects of vitamin D and calcium supplementation on falls: a randomized controlled trial. J Bone Miner Res 2003;18:343–351.
57. Flicker L Macinnis RJ, Stein MS, et al. Should older people in residential care receive vitamin D to prevent falls? Results of a randomized trial. J Am Geriatr Soc 2005;53:1881–1888.
58. Porthouse J, Cockayne C, King C, et al. Randomised controlled trial of calcium and supplementation with cholecalciferol (vitamin D_3) for prevention of fractures in primary care. BMJ 2005;330:1003–1008.
59. Bischoff-Ferrari HA, Dawson-Hughes B, Willett WC, et al. Effect of vitamin D on falls: a meta-analysis. JAMA 2004;291:1999–2006.
60. Harwood RH, Sahota O, Gaynor K, et al. A randomised, controlled comparison of different calcium and vitamin D supplementation regimens

in elderly women after hip fracture: the Nottingham Neck of Femur (NoNOF) Study. Age Ageing 2004;33:45–51.

61. Adams JS, Kantorovich V, Wu C, et al. Resolution of vitamin D insufficiency in osteopenic patients results in rapid recovery of bone mineral density. J Clin Endocrinol Metab 1999;84:2729–2730.
62. Chapuy MC, Arlot ME, Duboeuf, et al. Vitamin D_3 and calcium to prevent hip fractures in elderly women. N Engl J Med 1992;327:1637–1642.
63. Prestwood KM, Pannullo AM, Kenny AM, et al. The effect of a short course of calcium and vitamin D on bone turnover in older women. Osteoporos Int 1996;6:314–319.
64. Chapuy MC, Pamphile R, Paris E, et al. Combined calcium and vitamin D_3 supplementation in elderly women: confirmation of reversal of secondary hyperparathyroidism and hip fracture risk: the Decalyos II study. Osteoporos Int 2002; 13:257–264.
65. Chapuy MC, Arlot ME, Delmas PD, et al. Effect of calcium and cholecalciferol treatment for three years on hip fractures in elderly women. BMJ 1994;308:1081–1082.
66. Dawson-Hughes B, Harris SS, Krall EA, et al. Effect of calcium and vitamin D supplementation on bone density in men and women 65 years of age or older. N Engl J Med 1997;337:670–676.
67. Larsen ER, Mosekilde L, Foldspang A. Vitamin D and calcium supplementation prevents osteoporotic fractures in elderly community dwelling residents: a pragmatic population-based 3-year intervention study. J Bone Miner Res 2004;19: 370–378.
68. The RECORD Trial Group. Oral vitamin D and calcium for secondary prevention of low-trauma fractures in elderly people: a randomised placebo-controlled trial. Lancet 2005;365:1621–1628.
69. Boonen S, Vanderschueren D, Haentjens P, et al. Calcium and vitamin D in the prevention and treatment of osteoporosis—a clinical update. J Int Med 2006;259:539–552.
70. Boonen S, Bischoff-Ferrari A, Cooper C, et al. Addressing the musculoskeletal components of fracture risk with calcium and vitamin D: a review of the evidence. Calcif Tissue Int 2006;78: 257–270.
71. Bischoff-Ferrari HA, Dietrich T, Orav EJ, et al. Higher 25-hydroxyvitamin D concentrations are associated with better lower-extremity function in both actuve and inactive persons aged ⩾60 y. Am J Clin Nutr 2004:80;752–758.
72. Yates AA, Schlicker SA, Suitor CW. Dietary reference intakes: the new basis for recommendations for calcium and related nutrients, B vitamins and choline. J Am Diet Assoc 1998;98:699–706.
73. European Commission. Report on osteoporosis in the European community—action for prevention. http://www.osteofound.org/publications/pdf/eu_report_98.pdf, 1998, date accessed: 9/5/2006.
74. Bischoff-Ferrari HA, Willett WC, Wong JB, et al. Fracture prevention with vitamin D supplementation: a meta-analysis of randomized controlled trials JAMA 2005;294:2257–2264.
75. Jackson RD, LaCroix AZ, Gass M, et al. Calcium plus vitamin D supplementation and the risk of fractures. N Engl J Med 2006;354:669–683.
76. Lips P, Graafmans WC, Ooms ME, et al. Vitamin D supplementation and fracture incidence in elderly persons: a randomized, placebo-controlled clinical trial. Ann Intern Med 1996;124:400–406.
77. Gillespie WJ, Avenell A, Henry DA, et al. Vitamin D and vitamin D analogues for preventing fractures associated with involutional and postmenopausal osteoporosis. Cochrane Database Syst Rev 2001;(1):CD000227.

77a. Boonen S, Lips P, Bouillon R, et al. Need for additional calcium to reduce the risk of hip fracture with vitamin D supplementation: evidence from a comparative meta-analysis of randomized controlled trials. J Clin Endocrinol Metab 2007;92:1415–1423.

78. Dawson-Hughes B, Harris SS, Krall EA, et al. Effect of withdrawal of calcium and vitamin D supplements on bone mass in elderly men and women. Am J Clin Nutr 2000;72:745–750.
79. Boonen S, McClung MR, Eastell R, et al. Safety and efficacy of risedronate in reducing fracture risk in osteoporotic women aged 80 and older: implications for the use of antiresorptive agents in the old and oldest old. J Amer Geriatr Soc 2004;52: 1832–1839.
80. Lindeman RD, Tobin J, Shock NW. Longitudinal studies on the rate of decline in renal function with age. J Am Geriatr Soc 1985;33:278–285.
81. Harris ST, Watts NB, Genant HK, et al. for the Vertebral Efficacy with Risedronate Therapy (VERT) Study Group. Effects of risedronate treatment on vertebral and nonvertebral fractures in women with postmenopausal osteoporosis: a randomised controlled trial. JAMA 1999;282: 1344–1352.
82. Reginster J, Minne HW, Sorensen OH, et al. on behalf of the Vertebral Efficacy with Risedronate Therapy (VERT) Study Group. Randomized trial of the effects of risedronate on vertebral fractures in women with established postmenopausal osteoporosis. Osteoporos Int 2000;11:83–91.

83. McClung MR, Guesens P, Miller PD, et al. for the Hip Intervention Program Study Group. Effect of risedronate on the risk of hip fracture in elderly women. N Engl J Med 2001;344:333–340.
84. Eastell R, Barton I, Hannon RA, et al. Relationship of early changes in bone resorption to the reduction in fracture risk with risedronate. J Bone Miner Res 2003;18:1051–1056.
85. Hochberg MC, Thompson DE, Black DM, et al. Effect of alendronate on the age-specific incidence of symptomatic osteoporotic fractures. J Bone Miner Res 2005;20:971–976.
86. Tonino RP, Meunier PJ, Emkey R, et al. Skeletal benefits of alendronate: 7-year treatment of postmenopausal osteoporotic women. J Clin Endocrinol Metab 2000;85:3109–3115.
87. Lindsay R, Hart D, Clark D. The minimum effective dose of estrogen for prevention of postmenopausal bone loss. Obstet Gynecol 1984; 63:759–763.
88. Stevenson J, Cuat M, Gangar K, et al. Effects of transdermal versus oral hormone replacement therapy on bone density in spine and proximal femur in postmenopausal women. Lancet 1990; 335:265–269.
89. Heaney R. Estrogen-calcium interactions in the postmenopause: a quantitative description. Bone Miner 1990;11:67–84.
90. Felso D, Zhang Y, Hannan M, et al. The effect of postmenopausal estrogen therapy on bone density in elderly women. N Engl J Med 1993;329: 1141–1146.
91. Weiss N, Ure C, Ballard J, et al. Decreased risk of fractures of the hip and lower forearm with postmenopausal use of estrogen. N Engl J Med 1980; 303:1195–1198.
92. Paganini-Hill A, Ross R, Gerkins V, et al. Menopausal estrogen therapy and hip fractures. Ann Intern Med 1981;95:28–31.
93. Kiel D, Felson D, Anderson J, et al. Hip fracture and the use of estrogens in postmenopausal women—The Framingham Study. N Engl J Med 1987;317:1169–1174.
94. Cauley JA, Seeley DG, Ensrud K, et al. Estrogen replacement therapy and fractures in older women. Ann Intern Med 1995;122:9–16.
95. Michaëlsson K, Baron JA, Farahmand BY, et al. Hormone replacement therapy and risk of hip fracture: population based case-control study. Br Med J 1998;316:1858–1863.
96. Torgerson DJ, Bell-Syer SE. Hormone replacement therapy and prevention of nonvertebral fractures: a meta-analysis of randomized trials. JAMA 2001;285:2891–2897.
97. Ettinger B, Black DM, Mitlak BH, et al. Reduction of vertebral fracture risk in postmenopausal women with osteoporosis treated with raloxifene: results from a 3-year randomized clinical trial. Multiple Outcomes of Raloxifene Evaluation (MORE) Investigators. JAMA 1999;282:637–645.
98. Delmas PD, Genant HK, Crans GG, et al. Severity of prevalent fractures and the risk of subsequent vertebral and nonvertebral fractures: results from the MORE trial. Bone 2003;33: 522–532.
99. Lindsay R, Nieves J, Formica C, et al. Randomized controlled study of effect of parathyroid hormone on vertebral-bone mass and fracture incidence among postmenopausal women on oestrogen with osteoporosis. Lancet 1997;350:550–555.
100. Dempster DW, Cosman F, Parisien M, et al. Anabolic actions of parathyroid hormone on bone. Endocr Rev 1993;14:690–709.
101. Marcus R, Wang O, Satterwhite J, et al. The skeletal response to teriparatide is largely independent of age, initial bone mineral density, and prevalent vertebral fractures in postmenopausal women with osteoporosis. J Bone Miner Res 2003;18: 18–23.
102. Boonen S J, Marin F, Mellstrom D, et al. Safety and efficacy of teriparatide in elderly women with established osteoporosis: bone anabolic therapy from a geriatric perspective. J Am Geriatri Soc 2006;54:782–789.
103. Eastell R. Treatment of postmenopausal osteoporosis. N Engl J Med 1998;338:736–746.
104. Neer RM, Arnaud CD, Zanchetta JR, et al. Effect of parathyroid hormone (1–34) on fractures and bone mineral density in postmenopausal women with osteoporosis. New Engl J Med 2001;344: 1434–1441.
105. Marie PJ. Optimizing bone metabolism in osteoporosis: insight into the pharmacologic profile of strontium ranelate. Osteoporos Int 2003;14 (Suppl 3):S9–S12.
106. Meunier PJ, Roux C, Seeman E, et al. The effects of strontium ranelate on the risk of vertebral fracture in women with postmenopausal osteoporosis. N Engl J Med 2004;350:459–468.
107. Reginster JY, Seeman E, De Vernejoul MC, et al. Strontium ranelate reduces the risk of non vertebral fractures in postmenopausal women with osteoporosis: Treatment Of Peripheral Osteoporosis (TROPOS) Study. Endocrinol Metab 2005; 90:2816–2822.
108. Reginster JY, Meunier PJ, Roux C, et al. Strontium ranelate: an anti-osteoporotic treatment demonstrated vertebral and nonvertebral anti-fracture

efficacy over 5 years in post-menopausal osteoporotic women. Osteoporos Int 2006;17 (Suppl 2): S14(OC24).

109. Seeman E, Vellas B, Benhamou CL, et al. Strontium ranelate reduces the risk of vertebral and non-vertebral fractures in women aged eighty years and over. J Bone Miner Res 2006;21:1113–1120.
110. Seeman E, Vellas B, Benhamou CL, et al. Sustained 5-year vertebral and non-vertebral fracture risk reduction with strontium ranelate in elderly women with osteoporosis. Osteoporos Int 2006; 18:1–13(OC39).
111. Gourlay M, Richy F, Reginster JY. Strategies for the prevention of hip fracture. Am J Med 2003;115:309–317.
112. Lee SH, Dargent-Molina P, Bréart G, for the EPIDOS Group. Risk factors for fractures of the proximal humerus: results from the EPIDOS prospective study. J Bone Miner Res 2002;17:817–825.
113. Cadarette SM, Jaglal SB, Kreiger N, et al. Development and validation of the Osteoporosis Risk Assessment Instrument to facilitate selection of women for bone densitometry. Can Med Assoc J 2000;162:1289–1294.
114. American Geriatrics Society, British Geriatrics Society, and American Academy of Orthopaedic Surgeons Panel on Fall Prevention. Guideline for the prevention of falls in older persons. J Am Geriatr Soc 2001;49:664–672.
115. Close JC, McMurdo ME on behalf of the British Geriatrics Society Falls and Bone Health Section. Falls and bone health services for older people. Age Ageing 2003;32:494–496.
116. Briancon D, de Gaudemar JB, Forestier R. Management of osteoporosis in women with peripheral osteoporotic fractures after 50 years of age: a study of practices. Joint Bone Spine 2004;71:128–130.
117. Feldstein A, Elmer PJ, Orwoll E, et al. Bone mineral density measurement and treatment for osteoporosis in older individuals with fractures. Arch Intern Med 2003;163:2165–2172.
118. Birge SJ, Morrow-Howell N, Proctor EK. Hip fracture. Clin Geriatr Med 1994;10:589–609.
119. Sheehan J, Mohamed F, Reilly M, Perry IJ. Secondary prevention following fractured neck of femur: a survey of orthopaedic surgeons practice. Irish Med J 2000;93:105–107.
120. Feldstein AC, Nichols GA, Elmer PJ, et al. Older women with fractures: patients falling through the cracks of guideline-recommended osteoporosis screening and treatment. J Bone Joint Surg Am 2003;85-A:2294–2302.
121. Poole KE, Reeve J, Warburton EA. Falls, fractures, and osteoporosis after stroke. Time to think about protection? Stroke 2002;33:1432–1436.
122. Kamel HK, Hussain MS, Tariq S, et al. Failure to diagnose and treat osteoporosis in elderly patients hospitalized with hip fracture. Am J Med 2000; 109:326–328.
123. Bahl S, Coates PS, Greenspan SL. The management of osteoporosis following hip fracture: have we improved our care? Osteoporos Int 2003; 14:884–888.
124. Cummings SR, Nevitt MC. Falls. N Engl J Med 1994;331;87,873.
125. Greenspan SL, Myers ER, Maitland LA, et al. Fall severity and bone mineral density as risk factors for hip fracture in ambulatory elderly. JAMA 1994;271:128–133.
126. Greenspan SL, Myers ER, Kiel DP, et al. Fall direction, bone mineral density, and function: Risk factors for hip fracture in frail nursing home elderly. Am J Med 1998;104:539–545.
127. Stone KL, Seeley DG, Lui L-Y, et al. BMD at multiple sites and risk of fracture of multiple types: long-term results from the Study of Osteoporotic Fractures. J Bone Miner Res 2003; 18:1947–1954.
128. Marshall D, Johnell O, Wedel H. Meta-analysis of how well measures of bone mineral density predict occurrence of osteoporotic fractures. BMJ 1996;312:1254–1259.
129. Cummings SR, Nevitt MC, Browner WS, et al., The Study of Osteoporotic Fractures Research Group. Risk factors for hip fractures in white women. N Engl J Med 1995;332:767–773.

12
Treatment of Osteoporosis in Long-Term Care

Gustavo Duque and Louise Mallet

Introduction

The major determinants of admission at long-term care institutions (LTCI) include severe disability, poor social/familial support, advanced cognitive impairment, and either sequelae or end stages of chronic diseases such as Alzheimer's disease, diabetes, and heart and renal failure. All these conditions have made elderly patients unable to cope with their life in the community *(1)*, requiring a higher amount of assistance for their activities of daily living. LTCI offer a set of care measures that attempt to improve their patients' quality of life and provide relief to caregivers and families.

Osteoporosis is one of the major health problems among LTC residents, and is considered one of the major "Geriatric Syndromes" because its incidence increases with age, and because it predisposes to the occurrence of fractures and disability. In fact, despite evidence that osteoporosis is highly prevalent in LTCI, it remains under-diagnosed and under-treated *(2–4)*. This is unfortunate because the higher incidence of osteoporotic fractures *(4)* has a significant impact on quality of care and, most importantly, on patient quality of life and mortality. Even if a diagnosis of osteoporosis was made more appropriately in the LTCI, the effectiveness of various treatment approaches used in non-institutionalized seniors have not been established in the LTC population *(5)*. In this chapter, we will review the current considerations that should be made concerning the treatment of osteoporosis in LTCI. A comprehensive review of the literature will be made, followed by a series of recommendations about the treatment of osteoporosis in LTCI, taking into account the particularities of the LTC population.

The Particular Characteristics of the LTC Environment

The high prevalence of osteoporosis in LTCI has been demonstrated by studies assessing the World Health Organization criteria *(3)*. This prevalence goes from 50% of men and up to 80–85% in women *(6,7)*. However, not all bone mineral density (BMD) decrements are necessarily owing uniquely to long-term nursing home stays, but to disease, dysfunction, and disability that ultimately leads to admission *(6)*. In a prospective cohort of white female nursing home residents (n = 1427) over 18 months *(8)*, a total of 223 osteoporotic fractures occurred among 180 women. Low BMD and transfer dependence were the most significant for fractures. In addition, among residents dependent in transfer, those with a BMD below the median had a more than threefold increase in fracture risk when compared with other residents dependent in transfer. These and other recent reports *(9–11)* highlighted the importance of dependence in transfer as a risk factor for osteoporosis in this population independently of their BMD *(12)*.

Osteoporotic fractures in LTCI have a significant economic impact, considering that the amount of assistance as well as the medical care of their complications is much more expensive than prevention measures for fractures. For instance, a study of nursing home residents in

Maryland found that in the month following a fracture, those who experienced fractures were hospitalized more than 15 times as often as those who did not *(13)*. This significant burden on the health system also has an important impact on medical expenditures and health budgets, representing 28.2% of total expenditures for the treatment of osteoporotic fractures in the American population *(14)*.

How to Diagnose Osteoporosis in LTCI

The diagnosis of osteoporosis in community-dwelling populations is usually made after consideration of risk factors and the quantification of BMD. The combination of both assessments identifies patients who are at high risk of fractures. In settings where BMD is not available, the use of other risk factors, including past history of fracture, may provide enough evidence to recommend treatment independently of BMD results *(15,16)*. This concept is particularly relevant for LTCI for several reasons, because bone density testing may not be practical owing to the difficulty in mobilizing patients for transport to a facility with bone density equipment, and the technical difficulties associated with patients' mobility or behavioral problems that interfere with BMD testing. Finally, the performance of a BMD has not been shown to modify physicians' therapeutic decision-making in the treatment of osteoporosis. Gupta and Arnos *(17)* have shown that only 49% of 136 postmenopausal women in a nursing home population had BMD measurements. Of these 66 women, 31 (47%) had osteoporosis, 21 (32%) had osteogenic BMD, and 14 (21%) had normal BMD. Most importantly, only 55% of patients with documented osteoporosis were being treated, which illustrates the under-use of both diagnostic and therapeutic approaches for osteoporotic patients in nursing homes even although BMD results showed a decrease in bone mass, which clearly correlates with fracture risk.

In a recent study, Colon-Emeric et al. *(3)* found that factors associated with any bone protection (medication or hip protectors) in institutionalized populations included female gender and no urban/suburban location. In contrast, residents with esophagitis, peptic ulcer disease, and alcohol abuse were less likely to receive treatment.

Looking for an alternative approach for the assessment of bone density and/or risk of fractures in institutionalized patients, Elliot et al. used ultrasound to quantify bilateral calcaneal BMD in 49 institutionalized women aged 68–100 years and correlated them with their serum vitamin D levels *(18)*. Using this more mobile diagnostic method, which does not rely on ionizing radiation, the authors found that osteoporosis was highly prevalent (59%) and poorly documented in the patient's medical record. However, ultrasound also has a number of limitations as a diagnostic method for osteoporosis, such as the operator's experience and the variability between different machines. Nevertheless, it may be a good alternative to BMD for the diagnosis and, in some cases, the follow-up of patients with osteoporosis in nursing homes because of its usefulness for screening purposes, with sensitivities and specificities of 70–85% *(18)*.

In summary, osteoporosis is clearly under-diagnosed and under-treated in LTCI. Considering the implications that osteoporotic fractures have on patients morbidity and mortality, it is mandatory to establish a unified approach to identify patients at risk and to treat them appropriately. From a diagnostic point of view, it should be based on a combination of patient risk factors, clinical findings (kyphosis, clinical fractures), radiological findings, and height reduction. The therapeutic decision-making will be reviewed further in this chapter.

Who Should Be Treated?

A national panel of nursing home experts in the United States developed a set of specific care processes associated with better outcomes for general medical conditions, including osteoporosis *(19)*. In their report, Saliba et al. discussed potential indicators before completing confidential ballots rating validity (process associated with improved outcomes), feasibility of measurement (with charts or interviews), feasibility of implementation (given staffing resources in average community LTCI), and importance (expected benefit and prevalence in LTCIs). Among the 114 quality indicators identified during this exercise, seven were specifically suggested for osteoporosis (Table 12.1).

TABLE 12.1. Quality Indicators for the Management of Medical Conditions in Nursing Home Residents

Topic	NH indicator	Note
On admission to the NH	ALL female residents should be offered both calcium and vitamin D and weight-bearing exercises within 1 month.	Exclude if advanced dementia or poor prognosis Feasibility of measurement questionable
Mobilization	IF a NH resident is bedfast, then mobilization should be attempted unless there is a contraindication.	Feasibility of measurement questionable
Calcium/vitamin D for osteoporosis	IF a NH resident has osteoporosis, then calcium and vitamin D supplements should be prescribed within 1 month of admission or of a new diagnosis of osteoporosis.	Exclude if advanced dementia or poor prognosis
Treatment of new osteoporosis	IF a NH resident is newly diagnosed with osteoporosis, then he or she should be offered pharmacologic treatment within 3 months of diagnosis.	Exclude if advanced dementia or poor prognosis
Calcium/vitamin D for corticosteroid use	IF a NH resident is taking corticosteroids for more than 1 month, then the resident should also be offered calcium and vitamin D.	
Identifying secondary osteoporosis	IF a NH resident has a new diagnosis of osteoporosis, then, during the initial evaluation period, medications should be reviewed as possibly contributing to osteoporosis.	Exclude if advanced dementia or poor prognosis
Exercise therapy for new fracture	IF an ambulatory NH resident has an osteoporotic fracture diagnosed, then some form of physical therapy should be prescribed within 1 month.	Exclude if advanced dementia or poor prognosis

NH, nursing home.
Adapted from *(19)*.

Additionally, one of their conclusions was that despite these clear recommendations and quality markers, only 55% of women with osteoporosis in LTCI are receiving calcium and only 42% are receiving vitamin D, maybe the most simple and harmless methods of intervention for osteoporosis in LTCI. Considering that osteoporotic fractures are a marker of poor quality of care in LTCI, it is interesting that the use of preventive measures in the institutions was quite low.

The fact that osteoporosis is being undertreated in institutionalized elderly patients is well documented *(17,20)*. This is probably owing to the fact that there are virtually no clinical trials of treatment in LTCI. Recently, a symposium was held in the province of Quebec (Canada) to discuss the issue of under-diagnosis and undertreatment of osteoporosis in LTCI *(21)*. They conclude that most of the decisions made by providers in the LTCI are based on the length of treatment versus patient life expectancy and/or prognosis, compliance, tolerability, pharmacoeconomics, and finally prevention of polypharmacy.

Length of Treatment Versus Patient Life Expectancy and/or Prognosis

The mean survival time of institutionalized elderly patients varies from site to site, because of the complexity of the concurrent diseases, quality of care, and mean age. In Canadian LTCI, the average length of stay is about 2.5 years *(23)*. Initial reports on the time required by osteoporosis treatment to have an effect on fracture prevention has been questioned after new evidence has demonstrated that increases in BMD could be achieved within 6 months of initiating treatment, and that fracture rates start to decrease after the first year in most cases *(24)*. In fact, recent studies using bisphosphonates have reported earlier effectiveness in fracture prevention *(25,26)*. Considering the average length of stay, the effectiveness of treatment and the catastrophic consequences of having a fracture in LTC patients, it is important to re-emphasize the importance of initiation osteoporosis treatment (both preventive and therapeutic) in this high-risk population. Finally, it should be emphasized that treatment for osteoporosis in elderly LTC residents will only be effective if concomitant assessments, prevention, and interventions of falls risk factors are simultaneously pursued. A complete review on the strategies for fall prevention is available in Chapters 9 and 10 of this book.

Adherence

Adherence to osteoporosis medications is an important problem in ambulatory elderly patients *(25,27)*. Approximately 20–30% of patients may abandon their treatment within 6–12 months after beginning therapy *(27)*. Reasons associated with non-adherence include side effects of medication, fear of side effects or other health risks, and not knowing the results of BMD test results. In LTCI, this should not represent a problem, because administration of medications is closely supervised by nursing staff and, in some cases, regular follow-up by pharmacists. Furthermore, reducing medication administration frequency to weekly or monthly eases the burden on nurses administering medications. No data is available regarding adherence of osteoporotic treatments in LTCI. However, re-evaluation of drug therapy should be done periodically, especially when LTC patients refuse to take their medications, or when nurses have to crush or modify the dosage form for the patient to take his medications.

Tolerability

Tolerability to osteoporosis treatment is generally good. To decrease constipation and flatulence associated with calcium, it is suggested to start with 500 mg of elemental calcium once a day for 1–2 weeks, and then increase to 500 mg of elemental calcium twice per day and then three times per day. Vitamin D has not been associated with side effects or toxicities *(28)*. In a study examining vitamin D and calcium deficiency in LTC residents, despite having been prescribed vitamin D and calcium, Hamid et al. *(29)* reported that most of the residents were not supplemented adequately with calcium and vitamin D. In several cases, it was owing to poor adherence, even in this institutionalized population.

Bisphosphonates are usually well tolerated if specific administration requirements are followed. These requirements include fasting, taking with a full glass of water, remaining in an upright position, and not taking any medications or food concomitantly. However, erosive esophagitis, at times severe, can develop, particularly if administration requirements are not followed properly. Bisphosphonates should be avoided in patients with esophageal strictures, achalasia, or untreated symptomatic acid reflux *(30)*. Use of oral bisphosphonates is not recommended in patients with severe renal impairment. According to package inserts, alendronate is not recommended for use in patients with a creatinine clearance less than 35 mL/minute *(31)*, and risedronate is not recommended in patients with a creatinine clearance less than 30 mL/minute *(32)*. However, recent study *(33)* has shown that they can be safely administered at reduced doses in patients with 15 mL/minute, although the efficacy of reduced dosing on fracture reduction has not been established.

Pharmacoeconomics

Preventing and treating osteoporosis in LTCI may represent an economic burden to their already limited budgets if the cost of medications and the time needed to administer the medications by nurses are the only factors taken into consideration. However, this should be looked at in a different perspective. Vertebral, or more importantly, hip fractures, represent an enormous burden for institutions and society because of numerous factors such as use of analgesic treatments, functional and cognitive deterioration, and use of more nursing staff without considering that fractures are indicators of bad quality of management *(19)*. Finally, as suggested by Haentjens et al. *(34)*, preventing and treating osteoporosis in order to prevent hip fractures in LTCI is cost effective when all the mentioned considerations are made.

Polypharmacy or Appropriate Use of Medication

The average number of medications in LTC patients in Quebec is 7.5 *(22)*. Physicians working in LTCI should periodically review the indications of the medications prescribed to their patients at and after admission. A systematic medication review should be done with the physician, pharmacist, and other members of the team as needed. Additionally, a list of medical problems should be included in the patient's chart to document any new active medical problem.

Polypharmacy is a term that should be deleted from the scientific literature and should be replaced by "appropriate use of medication." If there is a clear indication, osteoporosis treatment should be maintained in LTC residents. Discontinuation of osteoporosis treatment in LTC residents may have important health consequences. It is well documented that discontinuation of vitamin D, calcium, and even bisphosphonates is followed by changes in bone markers that suggest an increase in bone resorption, which will affect bone mass and predispose to fractures *(35)*. The benefits of preventing a fracture in patients with indications for treatment surpass the considerations for discontinuation of treatment.

Treatment of Osteoporosis in Nursing Homes

General Guidelines

- Co-morbidities, risk factors, and life expectancy should be considered before initiating treatment.
- ALL patients admitted in LTCI should be evaluated for BOTH falls and non-fall-related risk of fractures. Interventions targeting identified risk factors should be implemented. A plan of action regarding discontinuation of medications that can induce falls should be implemented.
- Bed-ridden residents unable to mobilize should be excluded from treatment of osteoporosis. However, considering that they are still at risk for fractures that occur with transfer from bed to chair or even lifting, vitamin D supplementation may be considered as an effective preventive measure for fractures if the patient can swallow medications.
- The resident's opinion and/or that of the responsible party for health care decisions must be always considered (advantages and disadvantages) regarding treatment option for osteoporosis.

Screening

- Even though screening for BMD for all residents 65 years and older has been recommended, logistical considerations often preclude from implementing this in clinical practice. Considering the age and functionality of patients admitted at LTCI, it is often impossible to have a BMD done in this population. If possible, patients with risk factors should be assessed for osteoporosis.

Laboratory Tests

- There is no evidence to indicate that biochemical bone markers are useful in this type of setting.
- Secondary causes for osteoporosis should be ruled out with the following: serum calcium, albumin, serum phosphorus, alkaline phosphatase, thyroid stimulating hormone (TSH), serum creatinine and protein electrophoresis.
- Serum levels of vitamin D, parathyroid hormone (PTH), and active forms of vitamin D are not recommended on a routine basis. These tests should be done in severe cases, in patients not responsive to usual treatment, or in patients with severe renal impairment.

Indications for Starting Treatment

- Patients with risk factors for osteoporosis even though BMD is unknown or not done because of logistical problems.
- Osteoporosis detected by densitometry.
- Previous history of osteoporotic fractures.
- Patients with new fractures (vertebral and non-vertebral).

Treatment

Non-Pharmacological Interventions (Table 12.2)

A number of studies have demonstrated that non-pharmacological interventions are effective for reducing the number of fractures in elderly

Table 12.2. Non-Pharmacologic Intervention in Individuals with Low Bone Density

Smoking cessation
Cutting down on alcohol consumption
Regular weight-bearing and strengthening exercises
Drinking coffee with milk
Avoiding medications known to decrease bone mass
Ensuring a well-balanced diet
Fall assessment and implementing interventions to decrease risk of falling
Recommending hip protectors for individuals willing to wear them

Adapted from *(21)*.

patients *(36)*. In some (but not all) clinical trials, the use of hip protectors has been shown to save money while preventing hip fractures and improving quality of life in LTC residents. Compliance has been low in all previous studies *(37)*, and it is not well documented which hip protector is the best to use.

Pharmacological Interventions (Table 12.3 and Table 12.4)

Calcium and vitamin D supplements should be prescribed for institutionalized elderly residents to decrease or prevent the risk of osteoporotic fractures, including hip fractures *(21)*. Recent studies have shown that vitamin D may not be effective for the prevention of falls and fractures in elderly population; however, these studies were done either in ambulatory dwelling elderly patients *(38,39)* or using a dose of vitamin D that was sub-therapeutic *(40)*.

It has been suggested that dietary intake of calcium and sun exposure could provide adequate levels of vitamin D in elderly patients; however, Vecino et al. measured vitamin D levels in an ambulatory elderly population in Quebec *(41)* and found that despite dietary supplementation with vitamin D and appropriate sun exposure, the prevalence of either vitamin D deficiency or insufficiency in this ambulatory elderly population was 35%.

Furthermore, there is evidence that vitamin D supplementation at a dose of 800 IU/day reduces the risk of falls through improvements of muscle strength *(42)*. Preparations of vitamin D can be used from 10,000 IU a week, 50,000 IU every month, or 150,000 IU every 3 months. In LTCI, this can decrease nursing time in terms of medication administrations without affecting its efficacy or toxicity *(28)*.

Calcium supplementation should be part of preventive strategy in osteoporosis management. A total elemental calcium intake of 1500 mg/day is recommended for nursing home residents. There are many preparations or forms of calcium supplementation available on the market. These preparations may vary in the type of salt, the amount of elementary calcium, the costs, and the absorption rates. Calcium carbonate is the most frequently used calcium supplement because it contains 40% of element calcium and is the least expensive. Calcium carbonate requires an acidic environment for best absorption; it should be taken with meals for optimal absorption. Elderly patients may have decrease gastric secretion, and a number of them are simultaneously taking acid-reducing medications.

Calcium citrate may be an alternative for some patients. It contains 24% of elemental calcium per tablet but it does not need an acidic environment to be absorbed. However, it is more expensive than calcium carbonate. Dosage should be divided throughout the day to facilitate adherence, because the tablets size are quite large, making it difficult for some patients to swallow. Liquid formulations are available, but the taste may be a problem for some patients. Chewable preparations are also available as well as combination preparation with vitamin D. A common side effect of calcium is constipation. It can be decreased by slowly titrating the dose from once daily for a few weeks to twice then three times daily.

Calcium supplement can decrease the absorption of quinolones, tetracyclines, or levothyroxine if administered concurrently. Managing this drug interaction can be done by spacing the time of administration of calcium by at least 2 hours.

Table 12.3. Treatment of Osteoporosis: Calcium and Vitamin D Supplements

Calcium
1500 mg/day for all LTC residents
Vitamin D3
800 UI/day for all LTC residents

From *(21)*.

Bisphosphonates

Alendronate, risedronate, and most recently, ibandronate have been approved for prevention and treatment of post-menopausal osteoporosis. Several studies *(3,43,44)* have recently found differing patterns of prescription for anti-resorptive medications in nursing facility residents and community-dwelling elderly patients. They reported that LTCI residents are less likely to receive bisphosphonate treatment and more likely to receive calcitonin, which is known to have a weak effect in fracture reduction.

Only one randomized controlled trial has been done in elderly osteoporotic women residing in LTCI, and found that alendronate (10 mg po daily) *(45)* increased BMD in both spine and femoral neck with good tolerance when compared with placebo. The incidence of fractures did not reach statistical significance though because of the limited number of patients and limited follow-up period.

Additionally, several major trials reporting variable effects according to sub-groupings by age were found. The Fracture Intervention Trial (FIT), *(46)* which did not analyze an elderly population, showed that after 3 years of therapy the rate of new vertebral fractures was reduced in 47% of the alendronate group compared to the placebo group. Similarly, a 51% reduction in hip fractures was seen. The Hip Intervention Trial (HIP) *(47)* in older populations showed a higher BMD in the treated group after 6 months and a reduction in the incidence of fractures of 41% in the treated group. Although studies comparing the benefits of different bisphosphonates have shown contradictory results, the clinician should consider the period of time required to obtain not only a gain in BMD but also an effective reduction in the number of fractures. The recent REAL study *(26)* showed that patients receiving risedronate have lower rates of hip and non-vertebral fractures during their first year of therapy than patients receiving alendronate. However, this study did not include patients living in LTCI. Although tolerance and adherence have improved since the development of once-weekly dosing, there are still some limitations in adherence. Pamidronate infusion or newer bisphosphonates such as yearly zoledronic acid by injection may be a solution in the future.

Proper instructions should be followed by the patient to decrease the risk for esophagitis. Patients must take their bisphosphonates on an empty stomach with a full glass of water, then remain in an upright position and avoid food, beverage, and other medications for at least 30 minutes. For these reasons, bisphosphonates are inappropriate for bed-ridden patients or patients at risk of aspiration. Additionally, side effects are not frequent and include headache, flushing, and muscle pain.

Calcitonin

Calcitonin has the advantage of being easy to administer and has a good tolerability profile. Side effects include nasal dryness, nose bleeds, and occasional nasal ulceration. It is administered as a nasal spray, and proper technique of administration should be used to assure efficacy. The nozzle should be kept in a straight line with the nasal passage, and nostrils should be alternated with each dose. It does not have any significant effect on the incidence of non-vertebral fractures, which are by large the most important events to be prevented in LTCI. Currently, calcitonin is only recommended for the relief of pain associated with vertebral fractures *(48)*. It should be prescribed for short-term use.

Estrogens

Results from the Women's Health Initiative *(49)* showed a clinically significant protective effect of estrogens against hip fractures. However, this study also demonstrated that the overall risks from estrogen use exceeded the benefits. Considering the mean age of the LTCI population, and the negative risk/benefit analysis, estrogens are not appropriate for the treatment of osteoporosis in LTCI. Patients being admitted to LTCI already on estrogens should be reassessed.

Selective Estrogen Receptor Modulators (SERMs)

Hansdottir et al. *(50)* evaluated the effect of raloxifene on markers of bone turnover in older women living in LTCI. They showed that raloxifene did reduce bone turnover, but no evaluation on fracture incidence was done. The safety of raloxifene in older populations remains to be determined.

TABLE 12.4. Pharmacological Treatment of Osteoporosis in LTCI

Consider:
• Mental and nutritional status
• Risk of falls and fractures
• Mobility
• Previous treatments for osteoporosis
• Other medical conditions and medications
• Patient's opinion (if competent)
Indications
Bisphosphonates
• Patient at high risk of fractures:
• Risk factors
• Previous fractures
• Low BMD (<–2.5 SD) (if available)
SERMs
• Second choice if intolerance to bisphosphonates
• Female residents
Calcitonin
• Analgesic treatment of symptomatic vertebral fractures
PTH
• Not tested in LTCI
• Approved only for post-menopausal ambulatory women with osteoporosis
Strontium Ranelate
• Not tested in LTCI
• Potential good alternative to anti-resorptives

LCTI, long-term care institution; BMD, bone mineral density; SD, standard deviation; SERM, selective estrogen receptor modulator; PTH, parathyroid hormone.
Adapted from (*21*).

Anabolic Treatment

Teriparatide is indicated for the management of individuals at high risk for fractures, including subjects who are younger than age 65 and who have low BMD measurements *(51)*. No studies using PTH in older populations have been pursued, and no reports of ongoing studies are available. Furthermore, PTH is a costly treatment, which needs to be administered subcutaneously on a daily basis.

Finally, strontium ranelate is a new alternative that has shown its effectiveness in the prevention of non-vertebral fractures, including hip fractures *(52)*. Although the effectiveness of strontium has not been assessed in institutionalized patients, the fact that it has an anabolic effect as well as an easy way of administration as a soluble powder makes it an excellent alternative to other medications with difficult administration, such as bisphosphonates and PTH.

Conclusion

Institutionalized older adults are the population at higher risk for both falls and fractures. Interventions oriented to prevent their occurrence should include a complete assessment at admission, medication review, risk assessment, and non-pharmacological interventions. Concerning pharmacological approach, all patients at risk should receive both calcium and vitamin D. And, if tolerated and indicated, pharmacological treatment with either anti-resorptive or anabolics should be started.

References

1. Medina-Walpole A, Katz PR. Nursing Home Care. In: *Hazzard's principles of geriatric medicine and gerontology, fifth edition*, Halter JB, Ouslander J, Tinetti ME, et al. (Eds.). New York: McGraw Hill, 2003,pp. 973–986.
2. Ooms ME, Vlasman P, Lips P, et al. The incidence of hip fractures in independent and institutionalized elderly people. Osteoporos Int 1994;4:6–10.
3. Colon-Emeric C, Lyles KW, Levine DA, et al. Prevalence and predictors of osteoporosis treatment in nursing home residents with known osteoporosis or recent fracture. Osteoporos Int 2007;18: 553–559.
4. Wallace RB. Bone health in nursing home residents. JAMA 2000;284:1018–1019.
5. Cheng HY. Evidence-based prescribing of antiresorptive therapy for female nursing home residents with osteoporosis: how good is the evidence? J Am Geriatr Soc 2006;54:375–376.
6. Beaupre LA, Jones CA, Saunders LD, et al. Best practices for elderly hip fracture patients. A systematic overview of the evidence. J Gen Intern Med 2005;20:1019–1025.
7. Cooper C, Campion G, Melton LJ III. Hip fractures in the elderly: a world-wide projection. Osteoporos Int 1992;2:285–289.
8. Chandler JM, Zimmerman SI, Girman CJ, et al. Low bone mineral density and risk of fracture in white female nursing home residents. JAMA 2000;284: 972–977.
9. Greenspan SL, Myers ER, Kiel DP, et al. Fall direction, bone mineral density, and function: risk factors for hip fracture in frail nursing home elderly. Am J Med 1998;104:539–545.
10. Gloth FM 3rd. Osteoporosis in long term care. Part 1 of 2: recognizing bone and beyond. Director 2004;12:175–176, 179–180.

11. Broe KE, Hannan MT, Kiely DK, et al. Predicting fractures using bone mineral density: a prospective study of long-term care residents. Osteoporos Int 2000;11:765–771.
12. Zimmerman SI, Girman CJ, Buie VC, et al. The prevalence of osteoporosis in nursing home residents. Osteoporos Int 1999;9:151–157.
13. Zimmerman S, Chandler JM, Hawkes W, et al. Effect of fracture on the health care use of nursing home residents. Arch Intern Med 2002;162:1502–1508.
14. Ray NF, Chan JK, Thamer M, et al. Medical expenditures for the treatment of osteoporotic fractures in the United States in 1995: report from the National Osteoporosis Foundation. J Bone Miner Res 1997;12:24–35.
15. Hajjar RR, Kamel HK. Osteoporosis for the home care physician. Part 1: etiology and current diagnostic strategies. J Am Med Dir Assoc 2004;5:192–196.
16. Schousboe JT, Ensrud KE, Nyman JA, et al. Universal bone densitometry screening combined with alendronate therapy for those diagnosed with osteoporosis is highly cost-effective for elderly women. J Am Geriatr Soc 2005;53:1697–1704.
17. Gupta G, Aronow WS. Underuse of procedures for diagnosing osteoporosis and of therapies for osteoporosis in older nursing home residents. J Am Med Dir Assoc 2003:4:200–202.
18. Elliott ME, Binkley NC, Carnes M , et al. Fracture risks for women in long-term care: high prevalence of calcaneal osteoporosis and hypovitaminosis D. Pharmacotherapy 2003;23:702–710.
19. Saliba D, Solomon D, Rubenstein L, et al. Quality indicators for the management of medical conditions in nursing home residents. J Am Med Dir Assoc 2004;5:297–309.
20. Kamel HK. Underutilization of calcium and vitamin D supplements in an academic long-term care facility. J Am Med Dir Assoc 2004;5:98–100.
21. Duque G, Mallet L, Roberts A, et al. Quebec Symposium for the Treatment of Osteoporosis in Long-Term Care. To treat or not to treat, that is the question: proceedings of the Quebec Symposium for the Treatment of Osteoporosis in Long-term Care Institutions, Saint-Hyacinthe, Quebec, November 5, 2004. J Am Med Dir Assoc 2006;7:435–441.
22. Bergman H, Montambault J. Services d'hébergement. In: *Précis pratique de gériatrie, second edition*, Arcand M, Hébert R (Eds.). St-Hyacinthe: Edisem, Paris: Maloine, 1997.
23. Bischoff-Ferrari HA, Willett WC, Wong JB, et al. Fracture prevention with vitamin D supplementation: a meta-analysis of randomized controlled trials, JAMA 2005;293:2257–2264.
24. Roux C, Seeman E, Eastell R, et al. Efficacy of risedronate on clinical vertebral fractures within six months. Curr Med Res Opin 2004;20:433–439.
25. Caro JJ, Ishak KJ, Huybrechts KF, et al. The impact of compliance with osteoporosis therapy on fracture rates in actual practice. Osteoporos Int 2004;15:1003–1008.
26. Silverman SL, Watts NB, Delmas PD, et al. Effectiveness of bisphosphonates on nonvertebral and hip fractures in the first year of therapy: the risedronate and alendronate (REAL) cohort study. Osteoporos Int 2007;18(1):25–34.
27. Papaioannou A, Kennedy CC, Dolovich L, et al. Patient adherence to osteoporosis medications. Problems, consequences and management strategies. Drugs Aging 2007;24:35–55.
28. Hathcock JN, Shao A, Vieth R, et al. Risk assessment for vitamin D. Am J Clin Nutr 2007;85(1):6–18.
29. Hamid Z, Riggs A, Spencer T, et al. Vitamin D deficiency in residents of academic long-term care facilities despite having been prescribed vitamin D. J Am Med Dir Assoc 2007;8:71–75.
30. Jachna CM, Shireman TI, Whittle J, et al. Differing patterns of antiresorptive pharmacotherapy in nursing facility residents and community dwellers. J Am Geriatr Soc 2005;53:1275–1281.
31. Fosamax (package insert). Whitehouse Station, NJ: Merck & Co, Inc; 2004.
32. Actonel (package insert). Cincinnati, Ohio: Procter & Gamble Pharmaceuticals; 2003.
33. Linnebur SA, Milchak JL. Assessment of oral bisphosphonate use in elderly patients with varying degrees of kidney function. Am J Geriatr Pharmacother 2004;2:213–218.
34. Haentjens P, Autier P, Barette M, et al. Belgian Hip Fracture Study Group. The economic cost of hip fractures among elderly women. A one-year, prospective, observational cohort study with matched-pair analysis. Belgian Hip Fracture Study Group. J Bone Joint Surg Am 2001;83-A:493–500.
35. Deane A, Constancio L, Fogelman I, et al. The impact of vitamin D status on changes in bone mineral density during treatment with bisphosphonates and after discontinuation following long-term use in post-menopausal osteoporosis. BMC Musculoskelet Disord 2007;8:3.

36. Lips P, Ooms ME. Non-pharmacological interventions. Baillieres Best Pract Res Clin Endocrinol Metab 2000;14:265–277.
37. Singh S, Sun H, Anis AH. Cost-effectiveness of hip protectors in the prevention of osteoporosis related hip fractures in elderly nursing home residents. J Rheumatol 2004;31:1607–1613.
38. Porthouse J, Cockayne S, King C, et al. Randomised controlled trial of calcium and supplementation with cholecalciferol (vitamin D3) for prevention of fractures in primary care. BMJ 2005;330:1003.
39. Grant AM, Avenell A, Campbell MK, et al., RECORD Trial Group. Oral vitamin D3 and calcium for secondary prevention of low-trauma fractures in elderly people (Randomised Evaluation of Calcium Or vitamin D, RECORD): a randomised placebo-controlled trial. Lancet 2005;365:1621–1628.
40. Jackson RD, LaCroix AZ, Gass M, et al. Women's Health Initiative Investigators. Calcium plus vitamin D supplementation and the risk of fractures, N Engl J Med 2006;354:669–683.
41. Vecino C, Gratton M, Kremer R, et al. The seasonal variance in serum levels of vitamin D determines a compensatory response by parathyroid hormone: study in an ambulatory elderly population in Quebec. Gerontology 2006;52:33–39.
42. Bischoff-Ferrari HA, Orav EJ, Dawson-Hughes B. Effect of cholecalciferol plus calcium on falling in ambulatory older men and women: a 3-year randomized controlled trial, Arch Intern Med 2006;166:424–430.
43. O'Connell MB. Prescription drug therapies for prevention and treatment of postmenopausal osteoporosis. J Manag Care Pharm 2006;12(6 Suppl A):S10–S19; quiz S26–S28.
44. Jachna CM, Shireman TI, Whittle J, et al. Differing patterns of antiresorptive pharmacotherapy in nursing facility residents and community dwellers. J Am Geriatr Soc 2005;53:1275–1281.
45. Greenspan SL, Schneider DL, McClung MR, et al. Alendronate improves bone mineral density in elderly women with osteoporosis residing in long-term care facilities. A randomized, double-blind, placebo-controlled trial. Ann Intern Med 2002;136:742–746.
46. Black DM, Cummings SR, Karpf DB, et al. Randomised trial of effect of alendronate on risk of fracture in women with existing vertebral fractures. Fracture Intervention Trial Research Group. Lancet 1996;348:1535–1541.
47. McClung MR, Geusens P, Miller PD, et al. Effect of risedronate on the risk of hip fracture in elderly women. Hip Intervention Program Study Group. N Engl J Med 2001;344:333–340.
48. Lyritis GP, Ioannidis GV, Karachalios T, et al. Analgesic effect of salmon calcitonin suppositories in patients with acute pain due to recent osteoporotic vertebral crush fractures: a prospective double-blind, randomized, placebo-controlled clinical study. Clin J Pain 1999;15:284–289.
49. Writing Group for the Women's Health Initiative Investigators. Risks and benefits of estrogen plus progestin in healthy post-menopausal women, JAMA 2002;288:321–333.
50. Hansdottir H, Franzson L, Prestwood K, et al. The effect of raloxifene on markers of bone turnover in older women living in long-term care facilities, J Am Geriatr Soc 2004;52:779–783.
51. Hodsman AB, Bauer DC, Dempster DW, et al. Parathyroid hormone and teriparatide for the treatment of osteoporosis: a review of the evidence and suggested guidelines for its use. Endocr Rev 2005;26:688–703.
52. Roux C. Antifracture efficacy of strontium ranelate in postmenopausal osteoporosis. Bone 2007; In press.

13
Fracture Care in the Elderly

Christopher M. Bono and Timothy Bhattacharyya

Introduction

Fractures are an unfortunate but common occurrence in the aged population. They are a result of the inevitable decline of a number of bodily systems including bone homeostasis, muscular strength, balance, dexterity, and, in some cases, psychological fitness. With the increasing elderly population resultant from longer life expectancies, the sheer number of fractures encountered by health care providers has necessitated closer evaluation of their treatment. This has in fact commanded attention as a distinct area of study within orthopedic traumatology and spinal surgery over the past few years.

A discussion of fractures in older persons must recognize the catastrophic influence of age-related osteoporosis on the skeleton. Such a discussion engages not only the culpability of osteoporosis for proclivity towards fracture, but also the technical challenges faced with attempts to mend the weakened bones. With age, osteoporosis insidiously converts normal rigid bones into veritable "empty egg shells" that can be crushed between one's fingers with little effort. In addition, a discussion of fracture treatment in older individuals would be remiss without acknowledging the associated co-morbidities that can make a surgical procedure risky to perform *(1)* or that may result from a delay in stabilization *(2,3)*.

A number of recent advancements in fracture care have had potential benefits for the elderly patient with osteoporosis. Vertebroplasty and kyphoplasty are minimally invasive surgical treatments for vertebral compression fractures that, despite the previous gold standard treatment of "benign neglect," left many of the afflicted with long-standing pain, disability, and co-morbidity *(4)*. Improvements in percutaneous fixation of extremity fractures aim to lessen the morbidity of surgical stabilization in this fragile population *(5)*. With recognition of compromised healing of osteoporotic bone *(6)*, the application of growth factors, such as bone morphogenetic proteins (BMPs), to accelerate fracture union and spinal arthrodesis may have a greater role in management of the injured older individual *(7–9)*.

Fixation Challenges in Osteoporotic Bone

The relationship between advanced age, decreased bone mineral density (BMD), and increased risk for fragility fractures has been well established. This will be discussed in other chapters of this book. Germane to the current discussion is the difficulty of manipulating, reducing, and stabilizing fragments of osteoporotic bone.

Fractures can be described by a number of important attributes. These include comminution (i.e., when the bone has fractured into many smaller fragments), involvement of an articular surface (i.e., joint), angulation (i.e., planar deformities), and displacement (i.e., how far apart the fragments are from each other). An important surgical principle of fracture treatment is to reverse these deformities in order to approximate normal alignment as best as possible. This requires manipulation of the bone fragments with metallic instruments to reduce displacement, correct angulation, and restore length. In normal bone, large forces can be applied with little concern of causing additional injury to the bone. In osteoporotic bone, such forces can have devastating and explosive effects on the bony architecture, which can render them unreconstructible.

Assuming that acceptable reduction can be achieved, the next surgical challenge is maintaining this reduction. Currently, this is most commonly achieved with the use of implants made either of stainless steel or titanium in the form of rods or plates. Screws are the primary mode of fixing rods or plates to the bone. In non-osteopenic specimens, screws readily achieve excellent purchase (i.e., hold) within bone. This is not the case, unfortunately, with osteoporotic bone. Early failure of fracture fixation in osteoporotic bone is most influenced by the degree of BMD loss *(10,11)*.

This difference can be appreciated by the following household analogy. When inserting a screw into a wall at home to anchor an object such as a picture frame or draperies, one can either hit a "good spot" or a "bad spot". A good spot would be directly over a wooden beam, representing normal bone (Figure 13.1A). The screw passes through the plasterboard to engage the underlying beam, which provides an excellent and stable anchor. A bad spot would miss the beam, placing the screw only in plasterboard. As it is turned, the threads advance the screw. However, once the screw head reaches the wall, subsequent turns never reach an endpoint, as the plasterboard crumbles around it (Figure 13.1B). Regardless of how many turns, the screw head can be plucked from the wall with one's fingertips. This disappointing tactile experience is uncannily similar to placing screws into osteoporotic bone. With the screw's incompetence to achieve its own purchase in bone, asking it to secure a plate for an unstable fracture becomes a futile request.

Despite this unencouraging picture, all is not hopeless. Metallic screws, rods, and plates are indeed still the most common method of fixation of osteoporotic fractures. Human ingenuity has somewhat conquered the plague of weakened bone by devising methods to augment fixation. So-called osteoporosis screws have been developed. These incorporate a threaded-cap, which can be applied to the far end of a screw, working more like a nut and bolt than a wood screw. Using the plasterboard analogy described previously, this would be similar to placing a toggle bolt that derives its stability from pressing against the inner surface of the wall. Another method is using bone cement, such as polymethylmethacrylate (PMMA), to augment the fixation strength of a screw. PMMA can be used in both long bones as well as the spine.

Changing the location of the fixation device can also aid in its ability to stabilize a fracture.

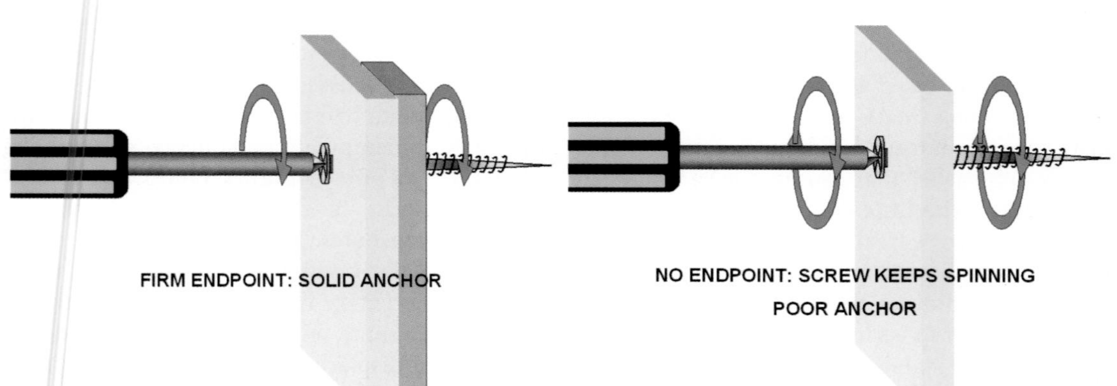

FIGURE 13.1. In normal bone, a screw achieves excellent purchase with a firm endpoint. Using the described analogy of inserting a screw in to a plaster wall, this would be analogous to "catching" the beam **(A)**. In contrast, inserting screws into osteoporotic bone yields no endpoint, analogous to "missing" the beam **(B)**. The screw can be turned indefinitely with no endpoint as it spins in place.

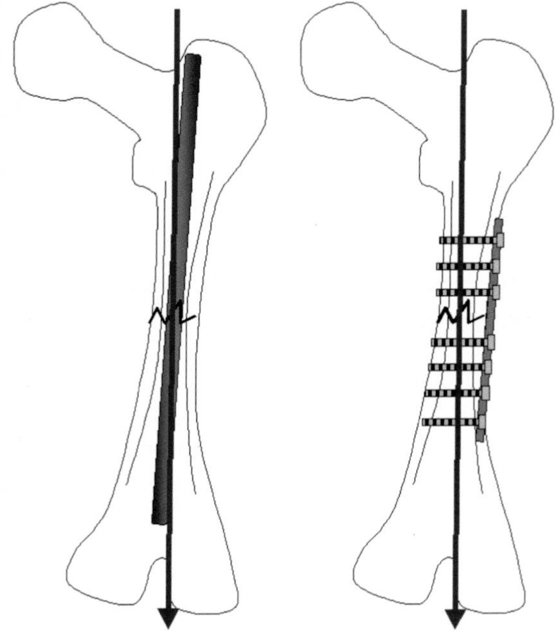

FIGURE 13.2. An intramedullary nail is better aligned with the weight-bearing axis of a bone (left), which may have advantages in osteoporotic patients. Plates and screws lie farther away from the weight-bearing axis (right).

Intramedullary nails, though not initially developed for osteoporotic bone, are inserted into the medullary cavity of long bones, such as the femur, tibia, and humerus. In contrast to plates, intramedullary devices are located closer to the weight-bearing axis of the bone (Figure 13.2). This allows the fracture ends of the bone to bear more of the load than would be allowed by a plate. Sliding hip screws rely on a similar principle in that they allow the broad cancellous surfaces of an intertrochanteric fracture to sustain the majority of the load. The primary function of the implant, therefore, is to keep the fragments aligned but not to bear load.

Finally, there are methods of treating fractures that do not rely on screw-based implants or fracture reduction. For example, most surgeons consider an arthroplasty (i.e., joint replacement) to be the treatment of choice for elderly patients with femoral neck fractures of the hip *(12)*. Such a treatment circumvents the need to reduce and stabilize a fracture, as it involves removal and replacement of the fractured segment of bone. Furthermore, the prosthesis is usually secured to the bone with PMMA cement, which is preferred over so-called press-fit fixation, in the setting of osteoporotic bone. Such a fixation method does not directly rely on bone density as much as screw, plate, or rod fixation. Another example is vertebral augmentation (i.e., kyphoplasty and vertebroplasty), in which PMMA cement is injected into the fractured vertebral body. Although fracture pain is presumably lessened by the stability of the PMMA in its hardened state, this is not dependent on reduction of the fracture. This treatment technique also avoids the plagues of attempting to stabilize spinal fractures with pedicle screws and rods, which have a tendency to loosen and fail in osteoporotic bone.

Timing of Fracture Treatment in the Elderly

The optimal time to stabilize fractures in older persons is a continuously debated topic. Influential factors include the anatomical region, the fracture's effect on ambulation, and the overall medical condition of the patient. It cannot be assumed that the indications to fix a fracture in a young person are the same in an elder person. Likewise, the importance of early fixation for some injuries is pronounced in older individuals who are more prone to medically decline with prolonged recumbency.

Hip Fractures

Hip fractures directly and immediately affect a patient's ability to ambulate. Non-operative management leaves patients recumbent, placing them at high risk for decubitus ulcers, thromboembolic events, and pulmonary decompensation. Furthermore, non-operative treatment has been shown to result in a higher mortality rate *(13)*. Most authors agree that surgery should not be delayed for a prolonged period of time to wait for "medical clearance" *(3)*. In fact, these patients are often most medically optimized at the time of presentation, as they tend to decline during their hospital stay.

For these reasons, hip fractures are preferably surgically treated within the first 2–4 days after injury. Some investigators have observed that surgery performed within 24 hours significantly reduces mortality rates *(2)*. Zuckerman et al. *(3)* found that delay in hip fracture fixation of more than 2 calendar days significantly increased the 1-year mortality rate in cognitively intact, ambulatory individuals. Most recently, the mortality rate was not found to be higher in elderly patients who underwent hip fracture treatment within 4 days of injury *(14)*. The current recommendation is to fix patients with hip fractures as early as medically allowable *(15)*.

Vertebral Fractures

Thoracic and lumbar compression fractures can have detrimental effects on quality of life, pulmonary function, and the ability to perform activities of daily living. Whereas hip fractures have immediately negative effects, vertebral compression fractures are more insidious, often occurring as occult injuries, and exhibit their effects gradually over time. As subsequent and multiple injuries are common, these effects can be cumulative.

With the introduction of vertebroplasty and kyphoplasty, an effective treatment for pain relief and restoration of function is available where none previously existed *(16–18)*. Despite its effectiveness, this tool must be used within a sound and balanced treatment algorithm that appreciates the natural history of fractures. Pain is relieved with observation alone in nearly two-thirds of cases. Within this group, pain relief is substantial within 6 weeks *(18a)*. As the procedure is not without complications, albeit rare ones, an algorithmic approach would likely avoid many unneeded surgeries. In contradistinction, persistently painful fractures can lead to physical deconditioning, emotional and psychological distress, and dependence on pain medication. Though the precise threshold is unknown, waiting too long to perform a kyphoplasty or vertebroplasty appears to lessen the chance that pain will be successfully ameliorated.

Odontoid fractures (also known as dens fractures) occur at the C2 vertebral level. They are very common in the elderly *(19)*. Some surgical techniques, such as odontoid screw fixation, have a high failure rate in patients with remote injuries *(20)*. Some authors have considered delayed or non-operative treatment as a risk factor for respiratory decline and death in the elderly *(21)*. Others have recognized that senile odontoid fractures, regardless of treatment method, is associated with a 10% mortality risk *(22)*. At the current time, there is no consensus of the optimal treatment method or timing of surgery.

Bone Healing Is Challenged in Osteoporotic Bone

The rate and quality of bone healing in osteoporotic patients is compromised compared to non-osteoporotic patients. This relationship has been demonstrated in a myriad of animal studies. Namking-Matthai *(23)* found femur fractures healed at slower rates and with poorer bone quality in ovariectomized rats. In a similar study, Meyer et al. *(24)* found the strength of fracture callus to be compromised in older, osteoporotic rats. Delayed fracture healing and poor rates of spinal fusion have been clinically observed in osteoporotic and elderly patients *(25)*.

The disadvantaged state of osteoporotic bone healing highlights the importance of optimizing blood supply to the fracture site. Modern techniques of fracture surgery include delicate handling of the surrounding soft tissues and avoidance of extensive periosteal stripping to expose the fracture site. This leads to less devitalization of the bone's blood supply and improves its healing potential.

Stabilization maneuvers that preserve the soft-tissue envelope surrounding a fracture are preferred. Intramedullary nails are an excellent example. They are inserted into the bone at a distance from the fracture site. They allow fracture reduction and stabilization without exposing the fracture itself. Percutaneous plating techniques also avoid direct exposure the fracture site. The plates are inserted in a subcutaneous manner, which are then stabilized percutaneously by locking screws (Figure 13.3A–D).

Biological Solutions

Adjunctive methods of promoting fracture healing and spinal fusion are rapidly advancing. These include growth factors that are introduced in or

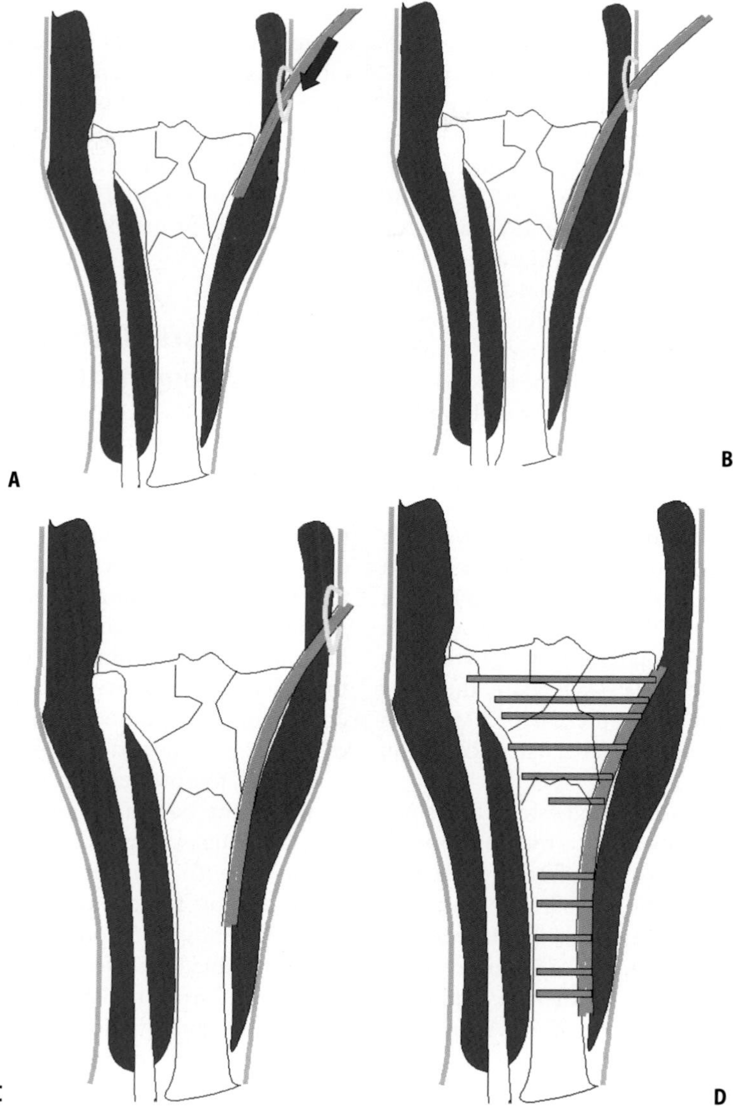

FIGURE 13.3. If closed reduction can be achieved, less invasive methods of plate fixation can be used in osteoporotic and elderly patients. In contrast to formal open fixation, these methods utilize smaller incision (arrow) in the skin through which a plate is introduced under the muscle (**A**). The plate is then slid along the periosteal surface (**B**) until it is in an acceptable position (**C**). The plate is then held in place with screws that are inserted in a percutaneous manner using specialized alignment guides (**D**).

around a fracture or spinal fusion site. The active components of these compounds are select human proteins that have been replicated by recombinant DNA technology. They are generally known as BMPs. At the time of this writing, there are two BMPs commercially available, which are BMP-7 (trade name is OP-1 from Stryker, Allendale, NJ) and BMP-2 (trade name is Infuse from Medtronic Sofamor-Danek, Memphis, TN).

BMPs have had demonstrable positive effects on fracture healing in an array of animal models. More importantly, they have shown higher rates of solid union when used for open tibia fractures and established tibial non-unions *(7,8)*. Although some animal data suggests that BMPs can aid in bone healing *(26)*, these beneficial effects have not been established in humans. However, many surgeons use BMPs in a so-called off-label manner for fracture healing enhancement.

The effects of these compounds in spinal fusion have been extensively investigated *(9,27–32)*. In some cases, they may be a viable alternative to autogenous iliac crest bone graft, the current gold standard material to produce spinal fusion. For example, BMP-2 placed on a collagen sponge inserted in a metallic cage for anterior lumbar interbody fusion has resulted in nearly a 100% fusion rate *(33)*. However, posterolateral lumbar fusion is more commonly performed in the elderly population. This type of fusion is markedly more challenged than anterior lumbar fusions, with rates typically ranging from 60–85% *(34)*. With the addition of BMP to autograft bone, fusion rates have been approximately 70% *(29)*. As a stand-alone material, BMPs have had varying results in human posterolateral fusion, with rates ranging from 55–100% *(30,31)*. To date, there are no clinical data denoting if the use of BMPs can overcome the inhibitory effects of osteoporosis on spinal fusion.

Recent animal data has suggested that some pharamacological agents used to treat osteoporosis may also have a positive effect on fracture healing. The best example of this is parathyroid hormone (PTH). In high doses, PTH seems to enhance fracture healing in rats *(35)*; however, the safety of such a high-dose regimen in humans is unknown. Even so, the role of PTH on bone healing in osteoporotic animals has yet to be determined. Other anti-osteoporotic agents, such as alendronate, have demonstrated clear inhibitory effects on spinal fusion healing *(36,37)* but not fracture healing *(38,39)*.

Electrical Stimulation

There is conflicting evidence concerning the efficacy of electrical stimulation on spinal fusion or fracture healing. In a recent systematic review, Resnick et al. *(40)* found no consistent evidence to support or contest the use of electrical stimulation devices to enhance spinal fusion. The use of stimulators seems to be more encouraging in extremity fractures, particularly tibia fractures *(41,42)*. Perhaps this is because the targeted bone is more subcutaneous, making it closer to the stimulation device in comparison to spinal fusion in which the targeted bone is much deeper. Notwithstanding these observations, there are no data, concerning the efficacy of electrical stimulation to enhance spinal fusion or fracture healing in the elderly or osteoporotic population.

Bone Fractures Differently in the Elderly Osteoporotic Person

Fundamentally, osteoporotic fractures (also known as fragility fractures) occur with low-energy mechanisms. This is in contrast to young, healthy bone, which requires a substantial amount of energy to cause it to fail. This is evident epidemiologically in that fractures in young patients occur most commonly from high-speed motor vehicle accidents, falls, and sporting injuries, whereas fractures in the elderly are more typically falls from standing or tripping. This difference influences the nature of fractures sustained in these two groups.

Beyond the mechanism of injury, the manner in which the bone fails also differs. Some of the most striking examples are tibial plateau fractures of the knee. In younger patients, fractures occur from abrupt forces delivered from the distal femoral condyles to the articular surface of the proximal tibia. These forces tend to shear a portion of the bone from the shaft or metaphysis. In the elderly, it is more typical to see a so-called articular depression fractures. The distal femoral condyles push into the proximal tibial, as they do in the younger patients, but the bone fails by crushing or compacting the cancellous bone beneath the articular surface (Figure 13.4). However, these "pure" examples are rare, with most injuries exhibiting varying proportions of depression and shear failure. The mechanism of injury for spinal fractures is also different in elderly and osteoporotic patients. Young vertebral bodies can sustain tremendous axial compressive loads. This can be likened to standing on top of an unopened can of soda. Provided one had excellent balance, one could support his or her weight on the can, which represents a normal, healthy vertebra. If the soda can was emptied, the same maneuver would result in the can being crushed. In fact, it may take much less than one's body weight to crush the can, which represents an osteoporotic vertebral body.

The morphology of fractures is different in the elderly as well. Osteoporotic fractures in the lumbar spine tend to have a so-called bow-tie appearance, in which the central portions of the bone are depressed (Figure 13.5). Compression fractures in the thoracic spine tend to be wedge-type fractures, likely because of the angular forces they sustain from pronounced kyphosis in older individuals. This trend has not been appreciated in normal, non-osteoporotic thoracolumbar fractures. Bursting-type fractures (in which the posterior vertebral body has been pushed into the spinal canal) are quite common in young patients, though fairly rare in older individuals.

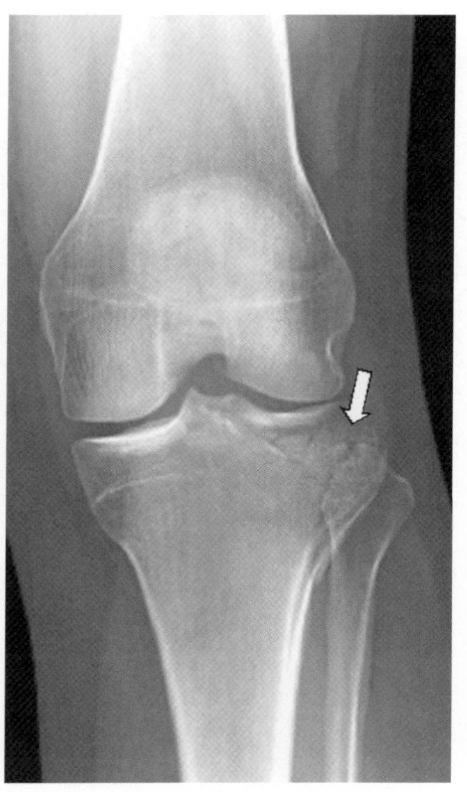

FIGURE 13.4. Anteroposterior radiograph of an osteoporotic depression fracture in an elderly patient.

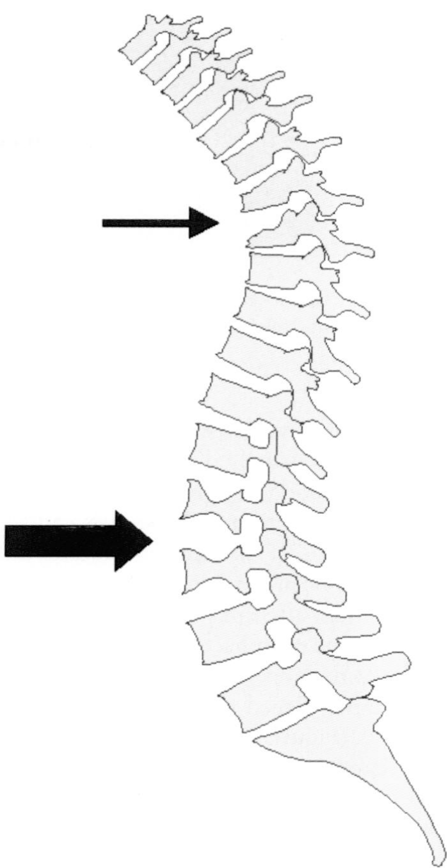

FIGURE 13.5. Wedge fractures are more common in the thoracic spine (small arrow), whereas central depression fractures are more frequent in the lumbar spine (large arrow). These patterns are likely the result of the mechanical alignment of the spine in these regions.

Specific Injuries and Treatment in the Elderly Patient

Hip Fractures

Hip fractures can be classified according to anatomic region. Femoral neck fractures occur within the confines of the hip capsule (Figure 13.6). The blood vessels that supply the femoral head and neck are also intracapsular and lie directly on the bone. Fracture displacement easily disrupts these vessels. Small amounts of displacement usually do not cause a vascular insult, so that minimally displaced fractures have a good chance of healing with appropriate internal fixation. Grossly dis-

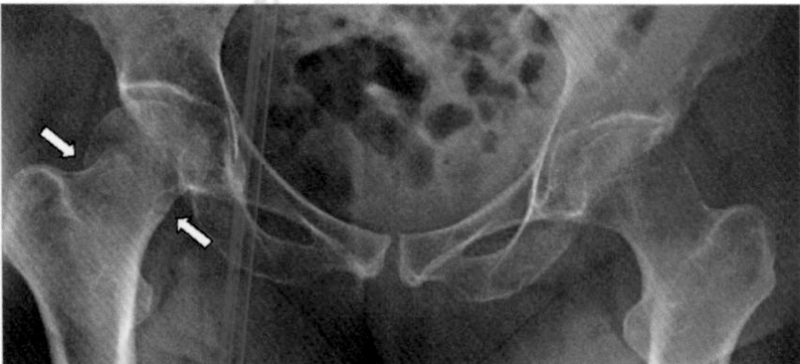

FIGURE 13.6. Femoral neck fractures occur within the hip capsule, which often disrupts the blood supply with substantial amounts of displacement.

placed fractures have a risk of non-union, as the blood vessels are usually disrupted. This leads to an insufficient blood supply to the fracture site. Furthermore, disruption of the vessels can lead to avascular necrosis of the femoral head. In elderly patients, it may be preferable to replace the injured bone rather than attempt to fix it.

Non-displaced or impacted fractures are treated with internal fixation. This is best achieved using multiple screws placed parallel to and within the femoral neck (Figure 13.7). Using a lag-type screw design, compression is created at the bone ends, which increases stability and promotes union. This procedure is minimally invasive, as the screws can be placed through percutaneous, stab-wound incisions, which incur little blood loss. Furthermore, they preserve the soft tissue envelope surrounding the fracture site. High-rates of union have been achieved using internal fixation of non- or minimally displaced femoral neck fractures.

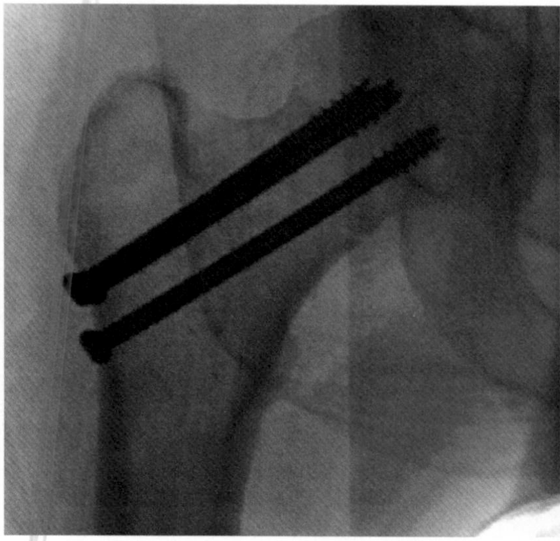

FIGURE 13.7. Femoral neck fractures that can be adequately reduced and have a reasonably good likelihood of healing can be fixed with three lag screws.

The treatment of displaced femoral neck fractures is more controversial. Options include reduction and internal fixation or prosthetic replacement. The advantage of reduction and internal fixation is that it can be performed through a limited incision with minimal blood loss. The major disadvantage is that, despite an anatomic reduction and stable fixation, the fracture may not heal. This can lead to significant pain, morbidity, and the necessity of additional surgery. Prosthetic replacement eliminates these concerns. However, it is a more extensive procedure with its own set of complications such as dislocation, loosening, and infection.

The current literature suggests that prosthetic replacement has advantages in the treatment of displaced femoral neck fractures in elderly individuals (Figure 13.8). It results in a lower

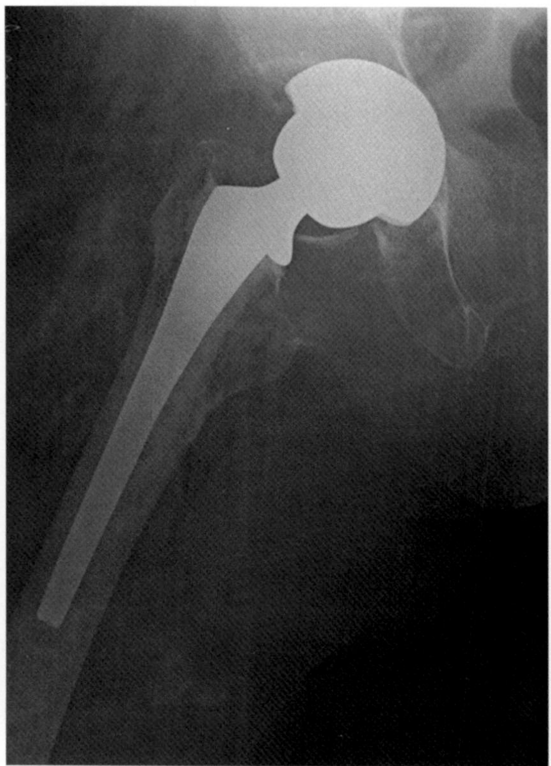

FIGURE 13.8. Displaced fractures have a poor likelihood of healing and are better treated by hemiarthroplasty replacement.

re-operation rate and better long-term hip function *(43,44)*. A recent randomized prospective study in healthy elderly patients showed that arthroplasty was more cost-effective than primary fixation of hip fractures *(45)*. Furthermore, this group demonstrated significantly better functional outcomes in those who underwent a total hip replacement (includes replacement of the hip socket) than those who underwent a hemiarthroplasty (replacement of the proximal femur only) *(45)*. These advantages must be considered in light of the pre-operative mental and functional level of the patient. Some studies have shown fewer complications with internal fixation versus hemiarthroplasty in non-ambulatory patients who have severe mental disorders *(43,44)*.

Intertrochanteric fractures occur within the broad cancellous region between the greater trochanter and the lesser trochanter (Figure 13.9).

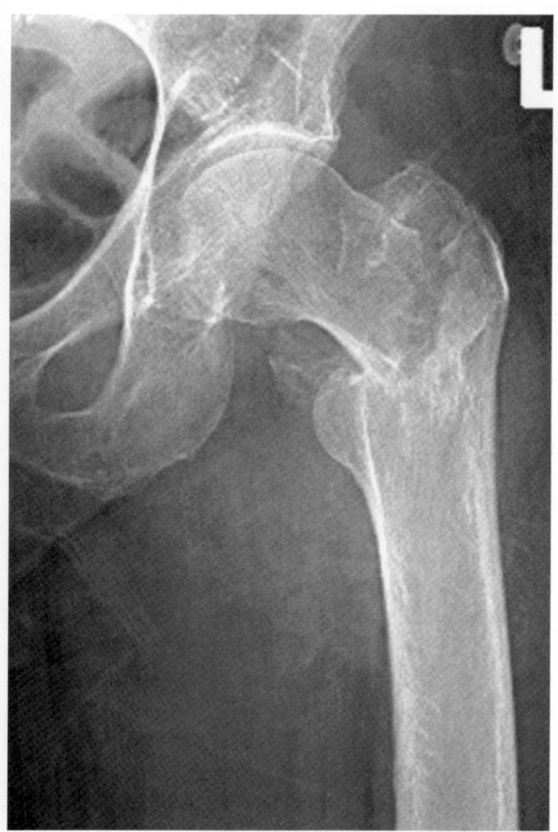

FIGURE 13.9. Intertrochanteric fractures lies outside the hip capsule and therefore have a good chance of healing. Reduction and internal fixation is usually successful.

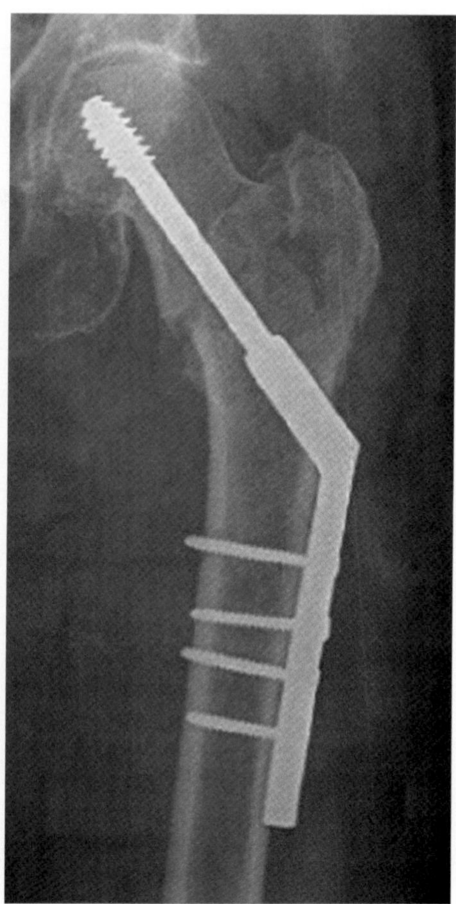

FIGURE 13.10. Stabilization of intertrochanteric fracture with a dynamic hip screw and plate (DHS).

These fractures are extracapsular. Displacement does not compromise the blood supply to the fracture site and therefore they have a much higher rate of healing than femoral neck fractures. Unfortunately, they are more prone to deformity, such as varus angulation and shortening. The treatment of intertrochanteric fractures is less controversial. Most surgeons agree that early internal fixation is optimal. However, what is not clear is the optimal device with which to repair these fractures.

Various methods of internal fixation are available including dynamic sliding hip screws (Figure 13.10) and intramedullary nail devices (Figure 13.11). Intramedullary devices have clear advantages for long bone injuries such as femur and tibia fractures and have replaced

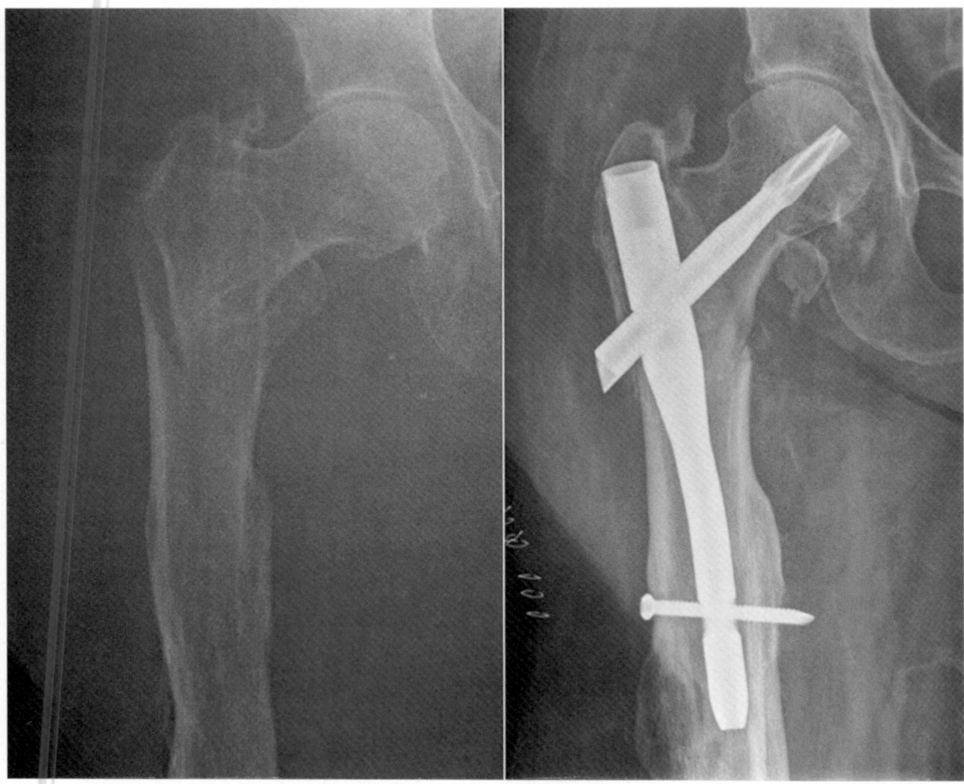

FIGURE 13.11. Stabilization of intertrochanteric fracture with an intramedullary hip screw.

plates and screws as the treatment of choice. A similar advantage of intramedullary devices over plate devices for hip fractures has not been as clearly shown. Some authors have found them to be reasonable alternatives, though complication rates might be higher *(46)*. Others *(47)* have found no difference in complication rates when compared to sliding hip screws, though it may offer advantages for particularly unstable fractures.

Thoracic and Lumbar Fractures

The most common vertebral injury in patients with osteoporosis is a thoracic or lumbar compression fracture. This injury can occur with very low energy mechanisms, such as picking up a bag of groceries, coughing, or sneezing. Pain can be acute in onset or insidious. Pain can resolve rather quickly or persist for long periods of time, with no reliable means of predicting which will occur.

The thoracolumbar spine is the most commonly involved region (T12–L1). Fractures can lead to pain, deformity (such as kyphosis or kyphoscoliosis), pulmonary compromise, and early gastrointestinal satiety *(48,49)*. Osteoporotic compression fractures can significantly diminish a patient's overall quality of life and ability to perform normal everyday activities.

Vertebroplasty was first introduced in Europe in the 1980s *(17)*. The technique involves percutaneous injection of PMMA into a fractured vertebral body. Vertebroplasty was introduced to the United States in the mid-1990s. With this, a variation of vertebroplasty was developed known as kyphoplasty *(18)*. Though similar in principle, kyphoplasty involves the additional insertion of various tools, including an inflatable bone tamp, which is intended to create a cavity in the vertebral body in which cement is inserted. An additional goal of the tamp is to restore the height of the compressed vertebra before insertion of cement (Figure 13.12).

The balloon tamp seems to have two main advantages. First, it offers the possibility of reversing vertebral compression height loss and kyphosis in some patients. This appears to be influenced by the acuity of the fracture, with older fractures exhibiting little correction in comparison to newer ones. Recent data has failed to show any clinical advantages of height restoration in terms of pain relief or functional outcomes. These shortcomings are dwarfed by the second, and perhaps more important advantage of cavity creation. High-pressure injections with vertebroplasty have lead to high rates of cement extrusion (between 20–70%). Creating a cavity for the PMMA placement, as is performed with kyphoplasty, has resulted in lower rates of cement extrusion (averaging approximately 9%) *(16,18,50)*. As cement extrusion can be associated with devastating complications such as pulmonary emboli, respiratory distress, and neural deficit, techniques to lessen this occurrence become increasingly important. Vertebroplasty proponents contend that the vast majority of cases of cement extrusion are clinically asymptomatic; kyphoplasty proponents denounce this philosophy as a game of Russian roulette. The disagreement is the fuel for ongoing debate between the two groups.

There is no consensus regarding the optimal time to augment osteoporotic vertebral compression fractures. One approach is to endure a period of 4–6 weeks of conservative treatment after the injury is sustained. This treatment can include bracing, rehabilitative therapy, and pharmacological pain management.

The main indication for vertebral augmentation is persistent pain from an unhealed osteoporotic compression fractures. This is noted best by increased bone edema recognized on T1-weighted

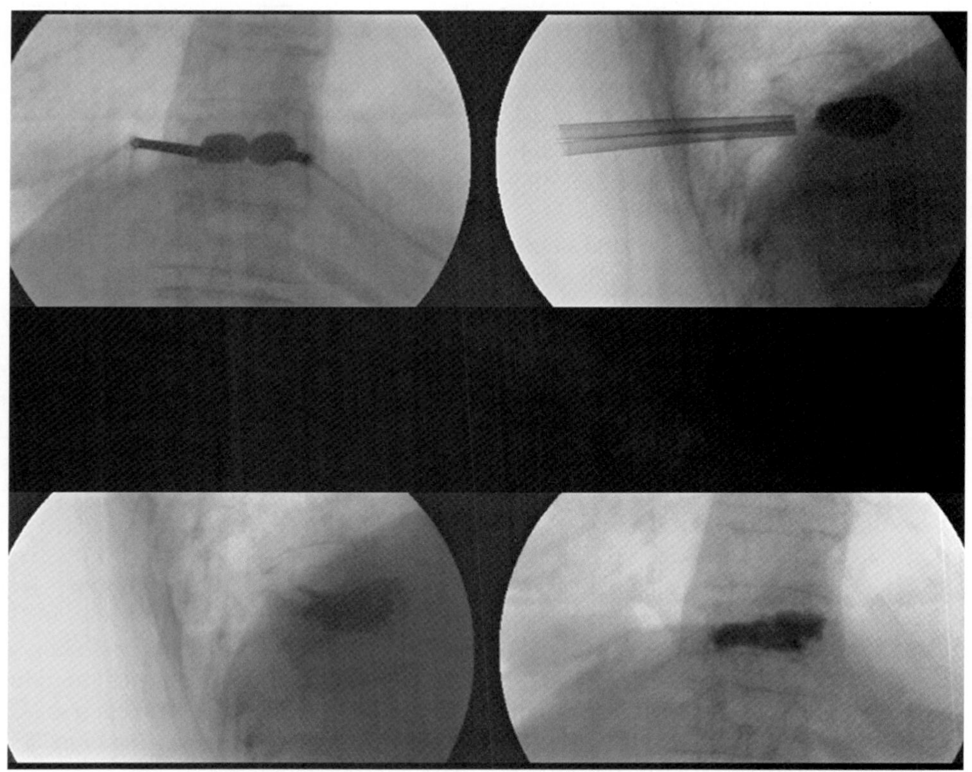

Figure 13.12. With kyphoplasty, a balloon tamp is first inserted into the fractured bone. It is inflated until a bone void is created and/or reduction of the fracture is achieved (top row). The balloon is then deflated and bone cement is inserted to fill the void and maintain reduction and stabilization of the fracture.

or short time inversion recovery (STIR) magnetic resonance images (MRIs), or selective uptake on a bone scan. In the author's experience, patients with fractures as old as 1–2 years can still have dramatic pain relief, provided the image studies are positive. Progressive painless collapse, documented radiographically, is an indication for kyphoplasty because of its unique ability to restore vertebral height. Local spine infection (i.e., active osteomyelitis) and unreversible coagulopathy are relative contra-indications to both procedures.

Outcomes of vertebroplasty and kyphoplasty are among the best for any spine procedure. Rates of pain relief are reportedly between 90–100%. A recent study of patients undergoing kyphoplasty, stabilization of the fractures lead to significant functional improvements *(50)*. In a large multi-center study, kyphoplasty enabled reliable restoration of vertebral body height if performed within 3 months of the injury *(18)*. Other reports have been more modest, reporting only 50–60% height restoration *(50)*. Vertebroplasty, while providing lasting pain relief, has not reliably demonstrated the ability to restore height *(16)*, though the rates of functional improvement, longstanding pain relief, and complications are comparable to the most favorable reports of kyphoplasty.

It is important to note there are no randomized controlled trials of vertebroplasty or kyphoplasty compared to conservative care in the literature. However, there are a number of uncontrolled, prospective cohort studies that have made these comparisons. In a prospective, non-randomized comparison, Diamond et al. *(51)* found significantly better pain relief at 6 weeks with vertebroplasty compared to conservative care; there was no statistical difference at 6-months and 1-year follow-up. In a similar study of kyphoplasty, Kasperk *(52)* found that visual analog pain scores were better in patients who underwent kyphoplasty than conservative treatment for compression fractures that were at least 1 year old. In arguably the best current evidence concerning the efficacy of vertebroplasty, Alvarez et al. *(53)* compared 101 patients who underwent vetebroplasty versus 27 patients who were offered the procedure but refused. There were significantly better improvements in pain, function, and general health scores at 3-months follow-up; however, at 6-months and 1-year follow-up, these differences were no longer statistically significant. From these data, one can conclude that vertebral augmentation provides ealier improvements than conservative care in those with osteoporotic compression fractures.

It has been suggested that augmenting a vertebral body with cement could lead to increased stresses at adjacent osteoporotic vertebrae and thus adjacent level fractures. Though fractures adjacent to an augmented level undeniably occur, it is not clear if these fractures are a sequelae of the procedure or the natural history of the disease. Rates of adjacent level fractures after kyphoplasty/vertebroplasty seem to be comparable to the rate of new fractures documented in so-called conservatively treated patients. In a frequently cited study, Lindsay et al. *(54)* found an 11.5% incidence of a subsequent fracture in 1 year. A comparable number (11.25%) was reported by Harrop et al. *(55)* after kyphoplasty for primary osteoporosis. In the recent series by Alvarez et al. *(53)*, conservatively treated patients had a new fracture rate of 30% compared to an 11% rate after kyphoplasty. In the least, these data suggest that subsequent fracture are not uncommon, but that vertebral augmentation does not appreciably increased their occurrence.

Senile burst fractures can also occur in the osteoporotic spine, though they are much less common than compression fractures. They occur almost exclusively in the T12 or L1 vertebrae (Figure 13.13) *(56)*. In contrast to simple compression fractures, burst fractures by definition have retropulsion of posterior vertebral body fragments into the spinal canal. This results in canal compromise that, if severe enough, can compress the spinal cord or cauda equina and result in neurologic deficit *(57–59)*. Treatment with vertebroplasty or kyphoplasty is contraindicated in this situation.

Open surgical treatment, including anterior decompression by removing the offending bony fragments, is indicated for severe cases. After subtotal vertebrectomy, the missing bone is replaced with a strut composed of autograft or allograft bone, or a cylindrical titanium mesh cage filled with morcelized bone graft. The graft or cage should have as broad a surface as possible to

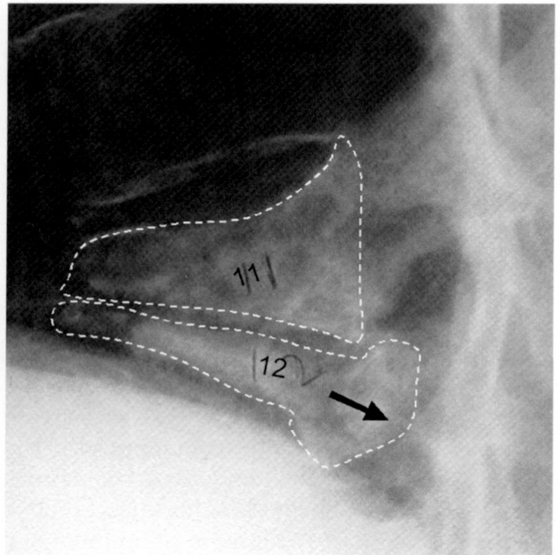

Figure 13.13. A senile burst fracture (bottom, T12) can be distinguished from a simple compression fracture (top, T11) by the presence of posteriorly displaced vertebral body fragments that can impinge upon the spinal cord or cauda equina.

evenly disperse forces to the vertebral endplates. It is generally recommended to stabilize the vertebral bodies with anterior instrumentation, such as plates and screws. Posterior instrumentation and fusion is also performed in a staged manner to provide additional stability and increase the chance for solid bone healing. As the morbidity of such an operation is considerable, it should be reserved for patients with neurological compromise or intractable pain from progressive deformity.

Odontoid (C2) Fractures

Odontoid (or dens) fractures are common in the elderly population. The usual mechanism of injury is a fall forward where the patient's forehead strikes the ground or piece of furniture. This produces an extension moment on the upper cervical spine that places forces at the so-called waist of the odontoid process (Figure 13.14). With this mechanism, fractures are almost always posteriorly displaced; this is in contrast to fractures in younger persons, in which displacement is usually anterior. A bimodal distribution of odontoid fractures in young and older people has long been recognized. Because the ratio of the spinal canal diameter to the spinal cord diameter is approximately three to one in this region, even large amounts of displacement do not cause significant neural compression. Thus, neurologic deficits are infrequent.

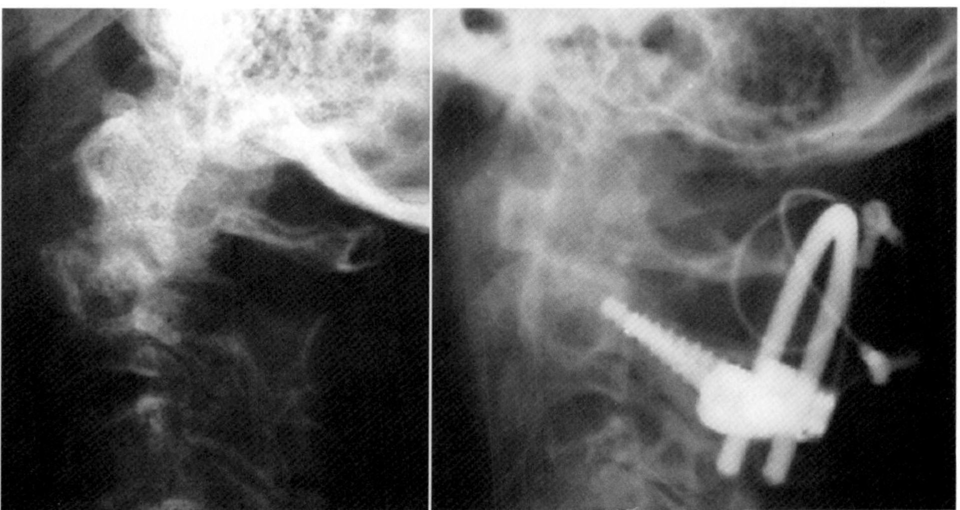

Figure 13.14. Odontoid fractures are common in the elderly (left), often presenting with posterior displacement, as the mechanism is usually falling forward causing a blow to the forehead of face. In some cases, stabilization is recommended, which usually involves a posterior C1-C2 fusion with instrumentation (right).

There are sharp and wide differences in philosophies of the optimal treatment of odontoid fractures in older patients. There are some who support that all fractures should be operatively stabilized, provided the patient can safely tolerate a surgery. There are others who feel that non-operative management is the initial treatment of choice, reserving operative fixation for those with neurological deficits.

Non-operative treatment can include application of a soft collar, hard collar, or halo fixator device. Recent data has indicated a high rate of failure and complications (including death) with the use of halo fixators in older patients. Because of this, most surgeons elect to use a soft or hard collar as a means of non-operative treatment. Although halo fixation can better align fractures, collars act simply to provide immobilization.

Surgical treatment may be best reserved for those patients with active lifestyles, substantial displacement, or associated neural deficit. Operative stabilization can include an anterior odontoid screw or posterior C1-C2 fusion. Both have their own advantages and disadvantages. Because of the rate of odontoid screw pull-out in soft-osteoporotic bone, performance of a posterior fusion with instrumentation may be preferred.

Distal Radius Fractures

Distal radius fractures are another common injury in elderly patients. The most common mechanism of injury is force on an outstretched hand, a maneuver that is frequent when an older person attempts to break a fall after tripping on a loose rug or electrical cord. The soft metaphyseal bone of the distal radius fails under this impact. Along the osteoporosis time line, fractures of the distal radius occur earlier than hip fractures. They should be interpreted as an indicator of significant bone loss and a warning sign that a hip fracture may be imminent. Compared with the general population, patients who have sustained an osteoporotic distal radius fracture are at twice the risk for a subsequent hip fracture *(60)*.

As with most orthopedic injuries, various treatment options exist. Decision-making is influenced by fracture pattern and location and the patient's functional demands. Non-displaced fractures should be treated in a well-molded cast for approximately 6 weeks. Longer periods of immobilization can lead to worsened osteopenia and wrist stiffness.

Fractures of the metaphysis of the distal radius are common. Typically, the distal fragment tilts into extension. Small amounts of angulation may be acceptable. However, greater degrees of tilt are indications for closed reduction. Closed reduction relies on forces placed on the bone through the skin. As the skin in elderly patients can be quite fragile, care must be taken not to deglove the region. Gentle reduction maneuvers also decrease the chance for worsening the comminution at the fracture site. With small amounts of comminution, the fracture can be held in an acceptable position using a cast. With more comminution, a cast may allow re-displacement. In these injuries, it is preferable to maintain the alignment using a fixation device. Traditionally, this is accomplished with either an external fixator or a plate. These devices derive their stability from screw-thread purchase. In osteoporotic bone this can be suboptimal, which may lead to construct failure. Surgery is reserved for patients who have substantially displaced fractures and for active patients in whom wrist function is vital to maintain their independence.

Low profile plates with fixed angle capabilities have been developed for the distal radius specifically to address poor fixation issues in osteoporotic bone *(61)*. Conceptually, the plates act as a mini-blade plate that supports the fracture through the dense bone directly underneath the articular surface. Variations of these devices have been developed for both the dorsal and volar surface of the radius. A common feature is that the screws lock to the plate, which has advantages in osteoporotic bone. Although they can be quite effective, proper use is technically demanding. Use of these devices requires gentle technique to avoid further damage to the bone.

Injectable bone cements such as Norian SRS have been developed to aid in the treatment of osteoporotic distal radius fractures, as they may offer mechanical support to stably reduced fractures. Though not a replacement for surgery, this technique can be used as an adjunct to cast treatment. In one randomized prospective series, better wrist function was noted using Norian SRS bone cement when compared with cast treatment alone *(62)*. Importantly, use of the bone cement reduces the time in the cast to 2 weeks versus 6 weeks. It does not appear to affect maintenance of the initial reduction.

There have been a number of recent studies analyzing the treatment outcomes of distal radius fractures in the elderly. Hegeman et al. *(63)* found external fixation to be adequate in small series of patients. Though the rate of malunion was high, indicating that the fractures healed in an unacceptable position, the functional outcomes were acceptable. In contrast, a randomized controlled study *(64)* showed no malunions with external fixation compared to cast treatment in elderly patients.

Tibial Plateau Fractures

Proximal tibia fractures can occur in the bone supporting the knee. When they involve the articular surface of the knee joint, they are referred to as tibial plateu fractures. In osteoporotic patients, it is common to see an isolated portion of the articular surface pushed down (i.e., depressed) into the soft cancellous metaphysis of the proximal tibia. This produces an incongruent articular surface, which can lead to painful arthritis later on. Minor tibial plateau fractures have recently been recognized as a cause of occult knee pain in elderly persons *(65,66)*.

Fixation of tibial plateau fractures relies on restoration of the joint surface. With large fragments, open reduction and screw fixation is preferred (Figure 13.15). When only a portion of the joint surface is depressed, the reduction can be performed through a less invasive approach. A small window can be made in the cortex along the proximal shaft. A bone tamp can then be inserted underneath the articular fragment to push it back into place. Bone graft can be packed to support the reduction, and screws introduced using a percutaneous approach may be inserted to strengthen the repair.

In the proximal tibia, compression of the osteoporotic cancellous bone can lead to large voids or gaps. Despite anatomic or near anatomic reduction of the main fragments, these gaps can persist. They may be filled with bone graft or bone cement,

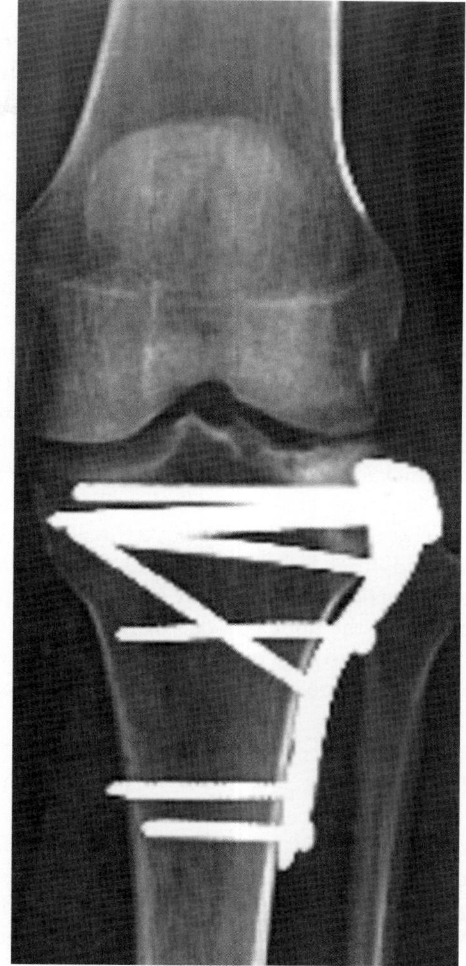

FIGURE 13.15. Anteroposterior radiograph of a tibial plateau fracture treated with a plate and screw construct.

known as PMMA. PMMA can be inserted as a viscous liquid so that it assumes the exact shape of the void or gap. It quickly hardens to provide stable support to the surrounding bone. The disadvantage of PMMA is its non-resorbability, which can result in a rim of tissue reaction or lysis around its borders. This can compromise fixation, and may increase the risk for infection. PMMA can also be used to improve the fixation of screws in osteopenic bone. Similarly, it is injected in a liquid state into the screw hole. The screw is then inserted and the cement is allowed to harden around it, creating a strong bond between the bone and metal. Despite these techniques, fracture fixation in the elderly is still substantially challenged. One study demonstrated that internal fixation of tibial plateau fractures in elderly patients (older than 60 years) is associated with a 79% failure rate compared to a 7% in younger patients *(67)*.

The Less Invasive Stabilization System (LISS) has been recently developed. It enables better fixation in osteoporotic bone using a minimally invasive approach. Plates are inserted through a small slit-like incision along the lateral and distal part of the knee. The plate is then guided along the cortex without actually opening the skin or dissecting the muscle overlaying the bone. Using a special guide, screws are inserted into the plate through stab-wound incisions. In contrast to standard plates in which the screw is able to toggle within its hole, the screws of the LISS plate have threads around their heads that lock them into the plate. Thus, every screw derives its stability not only from purchase within the bone but also from its fixation to the plate. Promising results using this device in osteoporotic bone have been reported *(68)*.

Conclusions

Fractures in elderly patients exhibit a number of unique treatment challenges. Although recent advancements in invasive treatment methods such as vertebroplasty, kyphoplasty, intramedullary devices, and BMPs have promised improved fracture care, future efforts in osteoporosis prevention, treatment, and fracture prevention may prove more impactful in improving the elderly population's quality of life.

References

1. Battacharyya T, Iorio R, Healy WL. Rate of and risk factors for acute inpatient mortality after orthopaedic surgery. J Bone Joint Surg Am 2002;84:562–572.
2. Hamlet WP, Lieberman JR, Freedman EL, et al. Influence of health status and the timing of surgery on mortality in hip fracture. Am J Orthop 1997;26:621–627.
3. Zuckerman JD, Skovron ML, Koval KJ, et al. Postoperative complications and mortality associated with operative delay in older patients who have a fracture of the hip. J Bone Joint Surg Am 1995;77-A:1551–1556.
4. Barr JD, Barr MS, Lemley TJ, et al. Percutaneous vertebroplasty for pain relief and spinal stabilization. Spine 2000;25:923–928.
5. Lorich DG, Geller DS, Nielson JH. Osteoporotic pertrochanteric hip fractures: management and current controversies. Instr Course Lect 2004;53:441–452.
6. Wang JW, Li W, Xu SW, et al. Osteoporosis influences the middle and late periods of fracture healing in a rat osteoporotic model. Chin J Traumatol 2005;8:111–116.
7. Govender S, Csimma C, Genant HK, et al. Recombinant human bone morphogenetic protein-2 for treatment of open tibial fractures. J Bone Joint Surg Am 2002;84-A:2123–2134.
8. Friedlander GE, Perry CR, Cole JD, et al. Osteogenic protein-1 (bone morphogenetic protein-7) in the treatment of tibial nonunions. J Bone Joint Surg Am 2001;83-A:S151–S158.
9. Boden SD, Zdebick TA, Sandhu HS, et al. The use of rhBMP-2 in Interbody fusion cages. Spine 2000;25:376–381.
10. Goh JC, Shah KM, Bose K. Biomechanical study on femoral neck fracture fixation in relation to bone mineral density. Clin Biomech 1995;10:304–308.
11. Spangler L, Cummings P, Tencer AF, et al. Biomechanical factors and failure of transcervical hip fracture repair. Injury 2001;32:223–228.
12. Keating JF, Grant A, Masson M, et al. Randomized comparison of reduction and fixation, bioplar hemiarthroplasty, and total hip arthroplasty. Treatment of displaced intracapsular hip fractures in healthy older patients. J Bone Joint Surg Am 2006;88:249–260.
13. Hoerer D, Volpin G, Stein H. Results of early and delayed surgical fixation of hip fractures in the elderly: a comparative retrospective study. Bull Hosp Jt Dis 1993;53:29–33.
14. Moran CG, Wenn RT, Sikand M, et al. Early mortality after hip fracture: is delay before surgery important? J Bone Joint Surg Am 2005;87:483–489.
15. Koval KJ, Cooley MR. Clinical pathway after hip fracture. Disabil Rehabil 2005;27:1053–1060.
16. Alvarez L, Alcaraz M, Perez-Hiqueras A, et al. Percutaneous vertebroplasty: functional improvement in patients with osteoporotic compression fractures. Spine 2006;31:1113–1118.
17. Deramond H, Depriester C, Galibert P, et al. Percutaneous vertebroplasty with polymethylmethacrylate. Technique, indications, and results. Radiol Clin North Am 1998;36:533–546.
18. Garfin SR, Yuan H, Lieberman IH. Early outcomes in the minimally-invasive reductions and fixation

of compression fractures. Proc North Am Spine Soc 2000:184–185.

18a. Rao RD, Singrakhia MD. Painful osteoporotic vertebral fracture: pathogenesis, evaluation, and roles of vertebroplasty and kyphoplasty in its management. J Bone Joint Surg Am 2003;85: 2010–2022.

19. Spivak JM, Weiss MA, Cotler JM, et al. Cervical spine injuries in patients 65 years and older. Spine 1994;19:2302–2306.

20. Apfelbaum RI, Lonser RR, Veres R, et al. Direct anterior screw fixation for recent and remote odontoid fractures. J Neurosurg 2000;93:227–236.

21. Hanigan WC, Powell FC, Elwood PW, et al. Odontoid fractures in elderly patients. J Neurosurg 1993;78:32–35.

22. Kuntz Ct, Mirza SK, Jarell AD, et al. Type II odontoid fractures in the elderly: early failure of nonsurgical treatment. 2000;8:e7.

23. Namkung-Matthai H, Appleyard R, Jansen J, et al. Osteoporosis influences the early period of fracture healing in a rate osteoporotic model. Bone 2001;28:80–86.

24. Meyer RA, Tsahakis PJ, Martin DE, et al. Age and ovariectomy impair both the normalization of mechanical properties and the accretion of mineral by the fracture callus in rats. J Orthop Res 2001;19: 428–435.

25. Simmons E, Kuhele J, Lee J, et al. Evaluation of metabolic bone disease as a risk factor for lumbar fusion. Spine J 2002;2:99S.

26. Egermann M, Baltzer AW, Adamaszek S, et al. Direct adenoviral transfer of bone morphogenetic protein-2 cDNA enhances fracture healing in osteoporotic sheep. Hum Gene Ther 2006;17:507–517.

27. Kanayama M, Hashimoto T, Shigenobu K, et al. A prospective randomized study of posterolateral lumbar fusion using osteogenic protein-1 (OP-1) versus local autograft with ceramic bone substitute: emphasis of surgical exploration and histologic assessment. Spine 2006;31:1067–1074.

28. Villavicencio AT, Burneikiene S, Nelson EL, et al. Safety of transforaminal lumbar interbody fusion and intervertebral recombinant human bone morphogenetic protein-2. J Neurosurg Spine 2005;3: 436–443.

29. Vaccaro AR, Patel T, Fischgrund J, et al. A 2-year follow-up pilot study evaluating the safety and efficacy of op-1 putty (rhbmp-7) as an adjunct to iliac crest autograft in posterolateral lumbar fusions. Eur Spine J 2005;14:623–629.

30. Vaccaro AR, Anderson DG, Patel T, et al. Comparison of OP-1 Putty (rhBMP-7) to iliac crest autograft for posterolateral lumbar arthrodesis: a minimum 2-year follow-up pilot study. Spine 2005;30:2709–2716.

31. Boden SD, Kang J, Sandhu HS, et al. Use of recombinant human bone morphogenetic protein-2 to achieve posterolateral lumbar spine fusion in humans: a prospective, randomized clinical pilot trial: 2002 Volvo Award in clinical studies. Spine 2002;27:2662–2673.

32. Johnsson R, Stromqvist B, Aspenberg P. Randomized radiostereometric study comparing osteogenic protein-1 (BMP-7) and autograft bone in human noninstrumented posterolateral lumbar fusion: 2002 Volvo Award in clinical studies. Spine 2002;27:2654–2661.

33. Burkus JK, Transfeldt EE, Kitchel SH, et al. Clinical and radiographic outcomes of anterior lumbar interbody fusion using recombinant human bone morphogenetic protein-2. Spine 2002;27:2396–2408.

34. Bono C, Lee C. Critical analysis of trends in fusion for degenerative disc disease over the last twenty-years: influence of technique on fusion rate and clinical outcome. Spine J 2002;2:47S–48S.

35. Nakajima A, Shimoji N, Shiomi K, et al. Mechanisms for the enhancement of fracture healing in rats treated with intermittent low-dose human parathyroid hormone (1–34). J Bone Miner Res 2002;17:2038–2047.

36. Huang RC, Khan SN, Sandhu HS, et al. Alendronate inhibits spine fusion in a rat model. Spine 2005;30:2516–2522.

37. Xue Q, Li H, Zou X, et al. The influence of alendronate treatment and bone graft volume on posterior lateral spine fusion in a porcine model. Spine 2005;30:1116–1121.

38. Cao Y, Mori S, Mashiba T, et al. Raloxifene, estrogen, and alendronate affect the processes of fracture repair differently in ovariectomized rats. J Bone Miner Res 2002;17:2237–2246.

39. Peter CP, Cook WO, Nunamaker DM, et al. Effect of alendronate on fracture healing and bone remodeling in dogs. J Orthop Res 1996;14:74–79.

40. Resnick DK, Choudhri TF, Dailey AT, et al. Guidelines for the performance of fusion procedures for degenerative disease of the lumbar spine. Part 17: bone growth stimulators and lumbar fusion. J Neurosurg Spine 2005;2:737–740.

41. Abeed RI, Naseer M, Abel EW. Capacitively coupled electrical stimulation treatment: results from patients with failed long bone fracture unions. J Orthop Trauma 1998;12:510–513.

42. Phieffer LS, Goulet JA. Delayed unions of the tibia. J Bone Joint Surg Am 2006;88:206–216.

43. Johansson T, Jacobsson SA, Ivarsson I, et al. Internal fixation versus total hip arthroplasty in the

treatment of displaced femoral neck fractures: a prospective randomized study of 100 hips. Acta Orthop Scand 2000;2000:597–602.

44. Ravikumar KJ, Marsh G. Internal fixation versus hemiarthroplasty versus total hip arthroplasty for displaced subcapital fractures of femur-13 year results of a prospective randomised study. Injury 2000;31:793–797.
45. Keating JF, Grant A, Masson M, et al. Randomized comparison of reduction and fixation, bipolar hemiarthroplasty, and total hip arthroplasty. Treatment of displaced intracapsular hip fractures in healthy older patients. J Bone Joint Surg Am 2006;88:249–260.
46. Crawford CH, Malakani AL, Cordray S, et al. The trochanteric nail versus the sliding hip screw for intertrochanteric hip fractures: a review of 93 cases. J Trauma 2006;60:325–328.
47. Utrilla AL, Reig JS, Munoz FM, et al. Trochanteric gamma nail and compression hip screw for trochanteric fractures: a randomized, prospective, comparative study in 210 elderly patients with a new design of the gamma nail. J Orthop Trauma 2005;19:229–233.
48. Schlaich C, Minne HW, Bruckner T, et al. Reduced pulmonary function in patients with spinal osteoporotic fractures. Ostoeoporos Int 1998;8:261–267.
49. Leidig-Bruckner G, Minne HW, Schlaich C, et al. Clinical grading of spinal osteoporosis: quality of life components and spinal deformity in women with chronic low back pain and women with vertebral osteoporosis. J Bone Miner Res 1997; 12:663–675.
50. Lieberman IH, Dudeney S, Reinhardt MK, et al. Initial outcome and efficacy of «kyphoplasty» in the treatment of painful osteoporotic vertebral compression fractures. Spine 2001;26:1631–1638.
51. Diamond TH, Champion B, Clark WA. Management of acute osteoporotic vertebral fractures: a nonrandomized trial comparing percutaneous vertebroplasty with conservative therapy. Am J Med 2003;114(4):326–328.
52. Kasperk C, Hillmeier J, Noldge G, et al. Treatment of painful vertebral fractures by kyphoplasty in patients with primary osteoporosis: a prospective nonrandomized controlled study. J Bone Miner Res 2005;20:604–612.
53. Alvarez L, Alcaraz M, Perez-Higueras A, et al. Percutaneous vertebroplasty: Functional improvement in patients with osteoporotic compression fractures. Spine 2006;31:1113–1118.
54. Lindsay R, Silverman SL, Cooper C, et al. Risk of new vertebral fracture in the year following a fracture. JAMA 2001;285:320–323.
55. Harrop JS, Prpa B, Reinhardt MK, et al. Primary and secondary osteoporosis' incidence of subsequent vertebral compression fractures after kyphoplasty. Spine 2004;29:2120–2125.
56. Chavda DV, Brantigan JW. Burst fractures of the twelfth thoracic vertebra in a middle aged man with osteoporosis. Nebr Med J 1994;79:193–199.
57. Nguyen HV, Ludwig S, Gelb D. Osteoporotic vertebral burst fractures with neurologic compromise. J Spinal Disord Tech 2003;16:10–19.
58. Tanaka T, Kubota M, Fujimoto Y, et al. Conus medullaris syndrome secondary to an L1 burst fracture in osteoporosis. A case report. Spine 1993;18:2131–2134.
59. Korovessis P, Maraziotis T, Piperos G, et al. Spontaneous burst fracture of the thoracolumbar spine in osteoporosis associated with neurological impairment: a report of seven cases and review of the literature. Eur Spine J 1994;3:286–288.
60. Kannus P, Parkkari J, Sievanen H, et al. Epidemiology of hip fractures. Bone 1996;18 (Suppl):57S–63S.
61. Ring D, Jupiter JB. Treatment of osteoporotic distal radius fractures. Osteoporos Int 2005;16 (Suppl):S80–S84.
62. Sanchez-Sotelo J, Munuera L, Madero R. Treatment of fractures of the distal radius with a remodellable bone cement: a prospective, randomised study using Norian SRS. J Bone Joint Surg Br 2000;82-B:856–863.
63. Hegeman JH, Oskam J, Vierhout PA, et al. External fixation for unstable intra-articular distal radial fractures in women older than 55 years. Acceptable functional end results in the majority of the patients despite significant secondary displacement. Injury 2005;36:339–344.
64. Moroni A, Vannini F, Faldini C, et al. Cast vs external fixation: a comparative study in elderly osteoporotic distal radial fracture patients. Scand J Surg 2004;93:64–67.
65. Cabitza P, Tamim H. Occult fractures of tibial plateau detected employing magnetic resonance imaging. Arch Orthop Trauma Surg 2000;120:355–357.
66. Luria S, Liebergall M, Elishoov O, et al. Osteoporotic tibial plateau fractures: an underestimated cause of knee pain in the elderly. Am J Orthop 2005;34:186–188.
67. Ali AM, El-Shafie M, Willett KM. Failure of fixation of tibial plateau fractures. J Orthop Trauma 2002; 16:323–329.
68. Schandelmaier P, Stephan C, Krettek C, et al. Distal fractures of the femur. Unfallchirurg 2000;103: 428–436.

Index

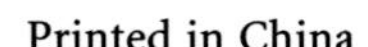
Printed in China